Social Disparities in Health and Health Care

Series Editors:

For other titles published in this series, go to
www.springer.com/series/8142

Linda M. Burton · Susan P. Kemp
ManChui Leung · Stephen A. Matthews
David T. Takeuchi
Editors

Communities, Neighborhoods, and Health

Expanding the Boundaries of Place

Springer

Editors
Linda M. Burton, Ph.D
James B. Duke Professor of Sociology
Duke University
Durham, NC
USA
lburton@soc.duke.edu

Susan P. Kemp, Ph.D
Associate Professor
School of Social Work
University of Washington
Seattle, WA
USA
spk@u.washington.edu

ManChui Leung
Department of Sociology
University of Washington
Seattle, WA
USA
mleung8@u.washington.edu

Stephen A. Matthews, Ph.D
Associate Professor
Department of Sociology and Faculty
Director Geographic Information
Analysis Core
Population Research Institute
The Pennsylvania State University
University Park, PA
USA
sxm27@psu.edu

David T. Takeuchi, Ph.D
Professor
School of Social Work and Department
of Sociology
University of Washington
Seattle, WA
USA
dt5@u.washington.edu

ISBN 978-1-4419-7481-5 e-ISBN 978-1-4419-7482-2
DOI 10.1007/978-1-4419-7482-2
Springer New York Dordrecht Heidelberg London

Printed on acid-free paper

Springer is part of Springer Science+Business Media (www.springer.com)

Foreword

The concept of "place" has growing significance in health research. Where you live contributes to risk and incidence of disease, morbidity, and mortality. Additionally, where you live determines in part the resources available to you, such as education, housing, transportation, and access to health care. Studies have shown the importance of "windows of susceptibility" as the environment "gets under your skin" to affect a person's health. However, conceptualizing and measuring environment and place inconsistently have had incongruent implications for assessment, prevention, and treatment. Clearly, place matters.

Differences in the availability and access to resources affect overall population outcomes for health and disease. The cancer research literature, for example, points to how cancer screening and treatment is affected by where a person lives. Generally, people living in rural areas have poor access to health-care services, including limited access to new technologies and therapies. And, while the "urban health advantage" emphasizes the positive aspects of urban living, metropolitan areas are often characterized by substantial differences in income and health. The de facto segregation of neighborhoods illustrates the strong association of place and opportunity, whether it be educational, economic, or social. Thus, while urban and rural areas pose different sets of challenges, the concept of place provides a useful model to account for these respective rural–urban differences.

Over the last 20 years, scientific evidence has been growing regarding the health effects associated with the unfettered expansion of built environments, conceptualized largely as the physical environment. A high-quality built environment, such as one with access to parks and recreational facilities, and access to grocery stores and markets with fresh fruits and vegetables, can provide residents with the potential to eat well, exercise, and maintain healthier lifestyles. In contrast, the concentration of fast food restaurants, lack of healthful choices for food, crime, and density of liquor and cigarette outlets in disadvantaged neighborhoods may exacerbate the poor health of the residents. However, we also need to consider the environmental stressors, as well as the social and cultural determinants of health, and how they determine health outcomes. As crises increase around the world and people are displaced from their homes and lands, the concept and measurement of place is critical in understanding health outcomes and in developing responsive and effective interventions.

Past and current studies have been important in delineating factors related to place and its relation to health or disease risk. However, much of the research in this area has not been grounded in theory and has not used well-validated constructs. While we are moving toward an era of personalized medicine and tailoring interventions for different populations, we have yet to understand what it is about place, where people live and their geographic realities, that may influence the effective use of interventions for that individual, neighborhood, and community. The development and dissemination of both primary and secondary interventions have been limited by the fact that we have not been able to comprehensively incorporate contextual factors in health. We have yet to address the geographical differences that lie within our own borders while still considering the impacts of global movements and migrations of specific populations. Thus, we need to provide more sophisticated, in-depth, and nuanced conceptualizations of space and the various dimensions of place as we study its effects on health. We need to consider and address the methodological and statistical challenges in how we operationalize place and how we conduct spatial analyses.

The Division of Cancer Control and Population Sciences at the National Cancer Institute, is pleased to have helped support the meeting that led to this book. We believe that the authors have provided important conceptual and empirical contributions to the exploration of why and how place matters in health. Moreover, we believe that these contributions can lead to improved assessment, prevention, and treatment of disease, as the growing body of evidence about the importance of place is incorporated into primary and secondary interventions as well as health policy.

Shobha Srinivasan
Robert T. Croyle

Preface

Introduction
Communities, Neighborhoods, and Health: Expanding the Boundaries of Place

I like geography. I like to know where places are.
Tom Felton, actor (2002)

It's not down on any map; true places never are.
Herman Melville, author (1851, p. 99)

Place, as a context for framing analyses of social inequality and health, has seen a resurgence of interest over the past decade. One reason for this renewed focus on place is the recognition that improving the health of individuals through screening and treatment does little to reduce the prevalence of chronic diseases in communities. Similarly, some of the attention to place is, in some respects, linked to the development of analytic tools that allow for the assessment of multiple hierarchical forms of statistical associations. For the most part, studies supposedly about the effects of place have actually been based on the aggregated characteristics of individuals as measured in the census or other surveys (Gieryn 2000). Typically, the proportion of variance in health behaviors explained by these measures of place have been relatively small, prompting some to suggest that place has only a limited effect on individual behavior. Alternatively, Macintyre et al. (2002) and others suggest that weak place effects are more likely due to inadequate conceptualization, operationalization, and measurement. Based on different reviews of theoretical works and empirical analyses, there is a compelling need to move to multifaceted conceptions of place that encompass geographic location, material form, infrastructure as well as meaning (Cummings et al. 2007; Gieryn 2000; Macintyre et al. 2002).

Place is more than a spatial backdrop for social interaction or a proxy for neighborhood variables. Place is a socio-ecological force with detectable and independent effects on social life and individual well-being (Werlen 1993). Places reflect and reinforce social advantages and disadvantages by extending or denying life-chances to groups located in salutary or detrimental locales (Gieryn 2000). Social processes (e.g., segregation, marginalization, collective action) happen through the intervening mechanism of place (Habraken 1998) with important effects on health and well-being. The effects of place on health and health behaviors are far from uniform across population groups and health outcomes.

If place attachments can facilitate social engagement and a sense of security and well-being, then the loss of place can have devastating implications for psychological well-being (Fullilove 1996). Understanding place – and the related constructs of displacement and emplacement – is critical for understanding societal inequalities. Displacement and detachment occurs when populations are forced to leave places of origin (e.g., immigrants, refugees), constrained by tightening bounds (e.g., prisoners, children in foster care), entrapped in places that become unhealthy over time (e.g., residents of some central cities), or simply, "without place" (e.g., homeless adults and children). Displacement or dislocation is one of the major sources of poor mental health globally (Mollica 2000). Indigenous populations were displaced from their homelands, other groups were brought in as slaves and indentured laborers, and still others migrated to the USA in order to create new lives and/or to escape genocide, wars, and political persecution. Our current understanding of the complex and multidimensional reciprocal dynamics between people and place is limited. We must further explore the mechanisms and processes of how people influence place and by which place "gets under the skin" (Cummins et al. 2007; Taylor et al. 1997).

We began this introduction with two quotes that capture some of the ways place is used in daily life. The quotes also raise some of the tension that exists in scholarship and research on place. Despite the general enthusiasm for the study of place and the potential it has for better understanding the distribution of health and illness in different communities, there is little consensus regarding how the construct should be conceptualized and measured. This book raises some of these issues and provides different disciplinary perspectives about how place can be investigated and used in studying health and illness. The chapters in this book examine the research on place and health, identify innovations in the study of place and health, and provide guidance for developing the future directions of research in this area. Some of the ideas for individual chapters were presented at a conference and specially convened working group held on May 7–8, 2009 in Seattle, Washington. Because discussions of place can be a personal issue, the authors have taken the opportunity to meld some of their personal biography and insights into their scholarship.

The book is organized into three parts. In Part I, *Place Foundations*, five chapters present some conceptual and methodological ideas that help frame the remaining chapters. In Chap. 1, "Place, History, Memory: Thinking Time Within Place," Susan Kemp focuses on time, and particularly on history, drawing on the wealth of knowledge from different disciplines to examine issues of temporality in studies of human and place relationships. Kemp discusses the potential conceptual and methodological opportunities for bringing a historical perspective to bear on scholarship on place and health. She argues for better understanding of the histories sedimented in the places of the present, the economic, social, political, and cultural trajectories of these places, and the particular historical and temporal associations they evoke in people, individually and collectively.

Technology has enabled researchers to link a wide array of data to different units of geographic spaces. This complex, systematic, and formalized technology often is not matched with the conceptual development of the construct of place. Michael F. Goodchild in "Formalizing Place in Geographic Information Systems" confronts this tension in Chap. 2 by focusing on several perspectives which include the current methods of geographic representation in digital form, inherent ambiguities, the case of the gazetteer, the role of volunteered geographic information, and place as an expression of context. Goodchild provides some examples for operationalizing place in research such as deriving definitions from people about geographic spaces, use of mathematical functions and searching the internet for usage patterns.

Stephen A. Matthews, in Chap. 3, expands the discussion of place by introducing the concept of spatial polygamy. In "Spatial Polygamy and the Heterogeneity of Place: Studying People and Place via Egocentric Methods," Matthews argues that we belong to multiple nested and nonnested places and challenges us to think about the appropriateness of conventional measures of space, such as census tracts, that are based on assumptions of bounded, static, and isolated geographic units. The chapter provides two examples using different types of empirical research to better understand the relationships between people and places. First, in an ethnographic study, Matthews shows how people use multiple places to balance individual and families roles and responsibilities, and second, in a secondary analysis of US Census data to investigate the spatial relationships between places.

One of the pressing questions confronting social scientists who study health is: How do social inequities actually influence an individual's health? More specifically, and keeping with the theme of this book, how does place get under the skin? In Chap. 4, "Placing Biology in Breast Cancer Disparities Research," Sarah Gehlert, Charles Mininger and Toni Cipriano-Steffans consider this issue by providing empirical evidence about place effects on breast cancer. The authors use data from research studies conducted under the auspices of the Center for Interdisciplinary Health Disparities Research. Four studies, two on animals and two on humans, provide examples about how place effects are embodied. While the data are aimed at addressing disparities in breast cancer, they provide compelling lessons for other types of health issues.

Race and place are often linked in American society. The historical record documents how some racial groups have been excluded from certain geographic locations, displaced from their homelands, forced to resettle in certain geographic areas, and, in some cases, relocated and interned in geographic areas far from their homes. These events show that racial and socioeconomic stratification are created, reinforced and maintained by place dynamics. Chapter 5, "Race, Place, and Health," considers how place-based social, psychological, geographic, and physical processes are racialized, which reinforce discrimination and social disadvantage. ManChui Leung and David T. Takeuchi show how residential segregation and displacement shape places and people with important effects on health and well-being across and between racial and ethnic groups.

Part II, *Missing Place, Invisible Places* examines settings, populations, and issues often missing, ignored and overlooked in the empirical literature on place and health. One of these areas is research on rural communities since most of the focus on place and health has been on the largest urban centers. Linda Burton, Raymond Garrett-Peters and John Eason address this limitation in Chap. 6, "Morality, Identity, and Mental Health in Rural Ghettos" by investigating mental health issues in rural ghettos. Rural ghettos are residentially segregated places that have high concentrations of disadvantage and contextual stigma and exist within small, geographically isolated towns and their adjacent pastoral communities. This chapter investigates the power of place on mental health by examining the role of rural ghettos in shaping the well-being of their residents and those who live in close proximity. Two dimensions of place are examined – location as morality and as identity. The challenges in these emerging ghettoized sections of rural communities present challenges to residents' perceptions, beliefs, and practices regarding their "rural moral codes" and their "rural place identities."

Thousands of visitors come to Aspen, Colorado, many of whom are wealthy. They come to see the beauty of Aspen and enjoy the luxury of a resort area. But how do service workers, composed mainly of immigrants, view the same place? Lisa Sun-Hee Park and David Naguib Pellow consider this intriguing question in Chap. 7, "The Case of the Missing Mountain: Migration and the Power of Place." They provide a window into the strategies immigrants use to become emplaced within Aspen, an area where their contributions to the local economy and culture are ignored. With rich quotes from their interviews with immigrants, they find that emplacement strategies tend to fall into three categories: public emplacement, everyday emplacement, and questioning environmental privilege. Their chapter provides insights about how people in a common place create and recreate boundaries that define and redefine their position in that space.

In Chap. 8, Karen Albright, Grace Chung, Allison De Marco, and Joan Yoo add the dimension of time to their discussion of immigration and health in "Moving Beyond Geography: Health Practices and Outcomes Across Time and Place." They examine three distinct immigrant communities and show how the culture, identities, and experiences affect health behaviors and outcomes. In the first example, they consider Chinese immigrants in England and the importance of Chinese identity and its effects on health. A small town Roseto, Pennsylvania provides the second example, where Italian immigrants and subsequent generations who settled in the town have low mortality rates compared to other geographic areas in Pennsylvania. The authors consider the epidemiological paradox in their final example and the facts that may contribute to this phenomenon.

Religion and spirituality are often seen as potentially important factors in health and illness. Frequently studied as individual variables that may help people cope, enhance stability and meaning to lives, and provide social networks resources that lend support, guidance, and information during difficult times. Jennifer Abe, in Chap. 9, "Sacred Place: An Interdisciplinary Approach for the Social Sciences" argues that current views of religiosity and spirituality are almost exclusively decontextualized individual behaviors and attitudes. She directs our attention to an examination of sacred places and how they contribute to an understanding of the ways in which places, when experienced as sacred, may mediate well-being. She also examines the role of specific "place-making" activities in these places, activities that sustain their sacred meaning to persons and communities over time but may also contribute to health and well-being.

In Chap. 10, "Dis-placement and Dis-ease: Land, Place, and Health among American Indians and Alaskan Natives," Karina Walters, Ramona Beltran, David Huh, and Teresa Evans-Campbell stimulate the scholarship on place by highlighting how historical trauma losses and disruptions tied to place or land effect the health of American Indians and Alaska Natives. They share empirical findings related to land loss and place on the physical and mental health among a national sample of gay, lesbian, bisexual, and transgender American Indians and Alaska Natives.

Part III, *Justice in Places,* is comprised of two chapters how place can be used for meaningful social change. In Chap. 11, Devon Peña combines passion and scholarship to address how places and people in these places are denied access to opportunities and how they take action against inequities in their communities. In "Structural Violence, Historical Trauma and Public Health: The Environmental Justice Critique of Contemporary Risk Science and Practice," Peña focuses on the issues of environmental justice and provides a critique of efforts to include communities in the decision making process. He highlights how environmental racism affects people of color and low-income communities who suffer disproportionate exposure to health risks from pollution in residential areas and workplace hazards. Peña argues that to resolve problems created by environmental racism requires more than individuals acting by themselves, but communities and collectives uniting behind a common cause.

Michael S. Spencer, Amanda Garratt, Elaine Hockman and Bunyan Bryant in Chap. 12, also address environmental justice issues but with a unique twist. They focuses on communities that have Head Start programs in Detroit, Michigan. "Environmental Justice and the Well-Being of Poor Children of Color" highlights a study which uses a community-based participatory research approach to increase awareness of environmental hazards confronting these communities. Spencer and colleagues describe how features of places can be used to enact meaningful social change in a community. By using Photovoice, a participatory action methodology, they are able to blend photography and social action, and use it as a tool to provide empirical data and allow communities to address environmental problems in their communities.

We end this edited volume with a special epilogue "Attachment and Dislocation: African-American Journeys in the USA." Carol Stack, in her ground-breaking works, *All Our Kin* and *Call to Home*, used ethnography as a method of critical inquiry to call attention to people living in poverty in urban America. She deftly describes how the social conditions of the times, especially those driven by public policies, affect the daily lives of women and their children. In Chap. 13, Stack reflects on her studies and provides additional insights about people and their places. She describes four methodological uncertainties that resulted from her ethnographic studies: The Historian's question; the Demographer's question; the Superintendent's dilemma; and Clyde's dilemma. Disentangling these uncertainties allowed her to decipher the complexities of the return migration movement and place ethnographic and demographic data across generations of families. Stack concludes her chapter with some lessons for researchers.

Linda M. Burton
Susan P. Kemp
ManChui Leung
Stephen A. Matthews
David T. Takeuchi

References

Cummins, S., S. Curtis, A.V. Diez-Roux, S. Macintyre. 2007. "Understanding and representing 'place' in health research: a relational approach". *Social Science and Medicine* 65:1825–1838.
Fullilove, M.T. 1996. "Psychiatric implications of displacement: Contributions from the psychology of place". *The American Journal of Psychiatry* 153:1516–1523.
Gieryn, T.F. 2000. "A space for place in sociology." *Annual Review of Sociology* 26:463–493.
Habraken, N.J. 1998. *The Structure of the Ordinary, Form and Control in the Built Environment.* Edited by Jonathan Teicher. Cambridge, MA: MIT Press.
Macintyre, S., A. Ellaway, S. Cummins. 2002. "Place effects on health; how can we conceptualize and measure them?" *Social Science and Medicine* 55:125–139.
Melville, H. 1851. *Moby-Dick.* 2004 edition. London: CRW Publishing Limited.
Mollica, R.F. 2000. "Waging a new kind of war. Invisible wounds". *Scientific American* 282(6): 54–57.
Morreale, M. and L. Guastafeste. "Tom Felton Talks About Reading, Collecting, and Being Draco" *Scholastic News.* (2020 words). Retrieved on April 17, 2010. (http://teacher.scholastic.com/scholasticnews/indepth/harry_potter_movie/interviews/index.asp?article=tom_felton&topic=1).
Taylor, S.E., R.L. Repetti, and T. Seeman. 1997. "Health Psychology: What Is an Unhealthy Environment and How Does It Get Under the Skin?" *Annual Review of Psychology* 48:411–447.
Werlen, B. 1993. *Society, Action and Space: An Alternative Human Geography.* London: Routledge.

Acknowledgments

We could not have organized the *Place, Health and Equity* conference and completed the *Communities, Neighborhoods and Health: Expanding the Boundaries of Place* book project without the support and assistance provided by our funders, sponsors, and several key individuals. The primary funders for this book project include the National Cancer Institute and the National Institute on Drug Abuse. Their funding helped support the costs to convene invited speakers and discussants for the May 2009 conference. The University of Washington could not have been a better host institution. The support from across the University of Washington community reflected broad interdisciplinary interest around the issue of place, social inequality, and health. Our co-sponsors at the University of Washington were, in alphabetical order, the Center for Studies in Demography and Ecology, the College of Built Environment, the College of the Environment, the Department of Anthropology, the Department of American Ethnic Studies, the Department of Geography, the Department of Political Science, the Department of Sociology, the Diversity Research Institute, the Division of Social Sciences – College of Arts and Sciences, the School of Nursing, the School of Public Health, the School of Social Work, and the West Coast Poverty Center. Finally, Edwina Uehara, Dean and Professor, School of Social Work, University of Washington has provided support throughout the project – she not only opened the conference, she opened her home.

Consistent with the complexity and multidimensionality of place, this book has dynamic ties to many places. The editors and participants in this project came together for 48 hours at one locale, the University of Washington in Seattle. While Seattle was the physical meeting place and central node for over 2 years, the spatial network of voice and digital conversations extended across the USA and beyond via fixed desktops and landlines, and mobile laptops and cell phones. This book was not the product of one place, one time, or one person. It is a product of multiple places, multiple times, and multiple people.

Linda M. Burton
Susan P. Kemp
ManChui Leung
Stephen A. Matthews
David T. Takeuchi

Acknowledgments

Contents

Contributors

Jennifer Abe, Ph.D
Associate Professor, Department of Psychology and Associate Dean for the Bellarmine College of Liberal Arts, Loyola Marymount University, Los Angeles, CA, USA

Karen Albright, Ph.D
Assistant Professor, Department of Community and Behavioral Health, Colorado School of Public Health, University of Colorado Denver, Anschutz Medical Campus, Denver, CO, USA

Ramona Beltran, MSW, Ph.D
Post-Doctoral Fellow, Department of Psychology Addictive Behaviors Research Center and School of Social Work Indigenous Wellness Research Institute, University of Washington, Seattle, USA

Bunyan Bryant, Ph.D
Professor, School of Natural Resources and the Environment, University of Michigan, Ann Arbor, MI, USA

Linda M. Burton, Ph.D
Professor of Sociology and Director of Undergraduate Studies Duke University, Durham NC, USA

Grace Chung, Ph.D
Assistant Professor, Department of Child Development & Family Studies, College of Human Ecology, Seoul National University, Seoul, South Korea

Toni M. Cipriano-Steffens, MA
Senior Research Professional, Center for Interdisciplinary Health Disparities Research, The University of Chicago, Chicago, IL, USA

Allison De Marco, MSW, Ph.D
Investigator Frank Porter Graham Child Development Institute, University of North Carolina at Chapel Hill, Chapel Hill, NC, USA

John Major Eason, Ph.D
Assistant Professor, School Criminology and Criminal Justice,
Arizona State University, Phoenix, AZ, USA

Teresa Evans-Campbell, Ph.D
Associate Professor, School of Social Work, University of Washington,
Seattle, WA, USA

Amanda Garratt, MS, MSW
School of Natural Resources and the Environment and School of Social Work,
University of Michigan, Ann Arbor, MI, USA

Raymond Garrett-Peters, MS
Department of Sociology, North Carolina State University, Raleigh, NC, USA

Sarah Gehlert, Ph.D
Director and Principal Investigator, Center for Interdisciplinary
Health Disparities Research, The University of Chicago, Chicago, IL, USA

Michael F. Goodchild, Ph.D
Professor Department of Geography, University of California,
Santa Barbara, CA, USA

Elaine Hockman, Ph.D
Adjunct Assistant Professor, School of Natural Resources and the Environment,
University of Michigan, Ann Arbor, MI, USA

David Huh, MS
Department of Psychology, University of Washington, Seattle, WA, USA

Susan P. Kemp, Ph.D
Associate Professor, School of Social Work,
University of Washington, Seattle, WA, USA

Laura Kohn-Wood, Ph.D
Associate Chair and Associate Professor, University of Miami,
School Education, Department of Educational and Psychological Studies,
Merrick Building 3190B, Coral Gables, FL 33146, USA

ManChui Leung
Department of Sociology, University of Washington, Seattle, WA, USA

Stephen A. Matthews, Ph.D
Associate Professor, Department of Sociology and Faculty Director,
Geographic Information Analysis Core, Population Research Institute,
The Pennsylvania State University, University Park, PA, USA

Charles Mininger, AM
Research Assistant, Center for Interdisciplinary Health Disparities Research,
The University of Chicago, Chicago, IL, USA

Lisa Sun-Hee Park, Ph.D
Associate Professor, Department of Sociology, University of Minnesota, Minneapolis, MN, USA

David Naguib Pellow, Ph.D
Professor of Sociology, University of Minnesota, Minneapolis MN, USA

Devon G. Peña, Ph.D
Professor of Anthropology and American Ethnic Studies
University of Washington, Seattle, WA, USA

Michael S. Spencer, Ph.D, LMSW
Associate Dean of Educational Programs, School of Social Work, University of Michigan, Ann Arbor, MI, USA

Carol B. Stack, Ph.D
Professor Emeritus, Department of Women's Studies and Graduate School of Education, University of California, Berkeley, CA, USA

David T. Takeuchi, Ph.D
Professor, School of Social Work and Department of Sociology, University of Washington, Seattle, WA, USA

Karina L. Walters, Ph.D
Associate Professor of Social Work, School of Social Work, University of Washington, Seattle, WA, USA

Joan Yoo, Ph.D
Assistant Professor, Department of Social Welfare, College of Social Sciences, Seoul National University, Seoul, South Korea

Part I
Place Foundations

Chapter 1
Place, History, Memory: Thinking Time Within Place

Susan P. Kemp

> *Any reconceptualisation of place in health research must also pay more attention to the significance of time – both historical and biographical*
>
> Popay et al. (2003:398)

Flourishing interest in place as a critical mediator of human well-being has brought with it calls for researchers to move beyond understandings of place as simply "here" – local, fixed, bounded, and, frequently, ahistorical – to more fully engage the dynamics of place, over time and across spatial scales. A "relational" view of place (Cummins et al. 2007) conceptualizes it as process rather than entity – a fluid, dynamic field of constantly interacting elements, within and beyond itself. Inherent in this shift away from conventional, static notions of place is renewed interest in the role of time as a salient factor in place/health relationships. Cummins et al. (2007), for example, propose the development of research approaches that focus on not only "the life course of individuals, but also the social and economic trajectories of the places which they inhabit" (p. 1,832). Popay et al. (2003) have likewise argued for a more thorough-going focus on time, and specifically history, in research on place and health, particularly in relation to health disparities. This chapter, written from the vantage point of a scholar of place with historical training, rather than a health disparities researcher, attempts to add further dimensionality to these proposals.

From an "upstream perspective" (Williams et al. 2008), inequalities in health are by definition "an historical phenomenon" (Popay et al. 2003:382). Over time, sociospatial processes such as racial segregation, suburbanization, urban disinvestment, and gentrification manifest in apparently intransigent place-based disparities (Anderson 1987; Pulido et al. 1996). In turn, these inequitable patterns of environmental and social risk differentially impact individual and collective health and well-being (Massey 2004). Efforts to understand contemporary health experiences in the context of larger sociospatial processes, unfolding over time,

S.P. Kemp (✉)
Associate Professor, School of Social Work, University of Washington, Seattle, WA, USA
e-mail: spk@u.washington.edu

L.M. Burton et al. (eds.), *Communities, Neighborhoods, and Health*,
Social Disparities in Health and Health Care 1, DOI 10.1007/978-1-4419-7482-2_1,

can thus provide "a more dynamic framework for understanding the relationship between individual human agency, social structure and health inequalities" (Popay et al. 2003:399).

Nested within and linked to these larger historical patterns are the more intimate, but equally consequential, place histories and memories of individuals and groups. Although place experiences are universally influential in human development (Casey 2001), genealogical ties to place and land are particularly important to the identity and well-being of many communities of color. Around the world, indigenous peoples define themselves through ties to ancestral places (see, e.g., Basso 1996). Historically and in the present, African Americans have found respite and collective renewal in "homeplaces" set apart from the places and spaces of a racist society (Burton et al. 2004; hooks 1990a). Given these cultural and spiritual connections, the loss or degradation of place that frequently accompanies oppression and marginality can be particularly devastating for racial and ethnic minority populations. Studies of collective memory (Johnson 1998), historical trauma (Evans-Campbell 2008), and urban renewal (Fullilove 2004), for example, point to the reverberating influence of histories of place-based oppression and displacement on the contemporary functioning and well-being of marginalized individuals and groups.

Despite evidence pointing to the relevance of history, broadly constructed, in health outcomes, and scattered calls for greater attention to history and temporality in research on health and place (e.g., Popay et al. 2003), the vast majority of studies in this area are cross-sectional and present-focused (see, e.g., Frumpkin 2006). Although longitudinal studies of place and health are becoming more common [for example in the application of life course perspectives to research on health inequalities (see, e.g., Wadsworth 1997)], many focus linearly on the implications of earlier place experiences for health outcomes (e.g., Curtis et al. 2004), rather than on their interrelations over time. Qualitative studies, whether cross-sectional or longitudinal, reach more deeply into the dynamics of person/place experiences, but even here a thorough-going focus on the implications of time, history, and memory for differential health outcomes is lacking. Sustained attention to the place histories of those marginalized and oppressed groups most at risk of differential health experiences and outcomes is likewise comparatively rare. Without further conceptual and methodological specification, therefore, it seems likely that the historical dimensions of place and place experience will remain on the peripheries of health disparities research.

In response, this chapter draws on an array of interdisciplinary scholarship to expand arguments for the relevance of an historical lens in research on place and health. Its central working assumption is that the economic, social, political, and cultural histories of places interact with human experience, individually and collectively, in ways that have implications for health outcomes in general, and health disparities in particular. To elaborate these core ideas, the chapter explores three dimensions pertinent to a more dynamic, historicized approach to place: the histories of places; collective place histories and memories; and personal, or biographical place histories, memories, and attachments.

This multilevel approach is consistent with the suggestion by Popay et al. (2003) that adding an historical dimension to conceptualizations of place within health research entails two interlocking tasks: first, exploration of "the conceptualisation and measurement of place within a historical location as the location in which macro social structures impact on individual lives" and second, consideration of how "places, conceptualised in this way, are understood within lay experience of the everyday life world" (p. 399). In a similar vein, Mallinson et al. (2003) argue that "research seeking to understand the contribution of particular places to health inequalities must both conceptualize places as social phenomena with histories, and consider the ways in which the meanings people give to places and the social relationships that develop within them have emerged over time" (p. 773).

Following a brief framing discussion of conceptual approaches to questions of time and place, the body of the chapter attempts to add specificity to these proposals. The concluding section draws implications for methodological directions. Before moving forward, I should however note that although several bodies of literature point to the relevance of an historical perspective for research and scholarship on place disparities and health, the material presented here is by no means definitive. Rather, my aim is to provoke interest in the historical and temporal dimensions of place and person/place relationships, suggest promising avenues for conceptual and methodological exploration, and encourage further work in this area.

Thinking Time Within Place

In *Space and Place*, his landmark exploration of place experience, Tuan (1977) pointed out that "How time and place are related is an intricate problem" (p. 179). He went on to propose three potential approaches to untangling their mutual implication. The first, typical of research on health and place (Cummins et al. 2007), conceptualizes "time as motion or flow and place as a pause in the temporal current" (p. 179). A second approach views place meanings and attachments "as a function of time" (p. 179). From this perspective, length of time in place becomes a proxy for the strength (or weakness) of place attachments and the salience of places in people's lives. Tuan's third approach conceptualizes place as "time made visible, or place as a memorial to times past" (p. 179).

Each of these approaches has generated important bodies of work, the insights from which continue to be influential. All rely, however, on two, often linked assumptions. First, that place is "here" – bounded, static, "paused" (indeed, Tuan argues that stasis is essential to the development of a sense of place). Second, that the implications of place/time relationships in human life are linearly causal; whether prospectively (place experiences in the past influence current outcomes), or retrospectively (past histories, now gone but embedded in present places, shape current outcomes) Time's arrow is directional. On both counts Tuan's typology, conceptually at least, separates place and time.

Relational views of place, on the other hand, aim not to untangle time and place but to bring them together, recognizing their essential "stickiness" (Dodghson 2008) and conceptualizing place as inherently fluid, changing, and "on the move" (Cummins et al. 2007). Reflecting cultural theorist Raymond Williams' observation that "places comprise an ensemble of forces that somehow much be examined together," geographer Alan Pred (1984) defined place as "a historically contingent process" (p. 280) – a state of "becoming" that is constantly being made and remade by individual, collective, and institutional practices, and by structural forces. Doreen Massey (1995) likewise argued for the inseparability of place and time, noting that across multiple dimensions, "places stretch through time" (p. 188). She noted that "[t]he past is present in places in a variety of ways" (p. 186), including the materiality of buildings and monuments, the resonance of the past in place names and words, and the living archives of people's individual and collective memories.

For Massey, as for other relational theorists (see, e.g., Cresswell 2002), place and time are inseparable: people and places interact over time in complex, mutually influential, nonlinear, and inherently recursive relationships. Furthermore, while the past influences the present, the present also reaches out to and engages with the past, since people's current relationships to places, in their diversity and heterogeneity, necessarily evoke "multivocal" understandings of the past. "What has come together, in this place, now," Massey asserted, "is a conjunction of many histories and many places" (Massey 1995:191; see also Pred 1990). People in places have different life trajectories, varied racial, ethnic, cultural, class, and gender experiences, and a range of prior geographies. Given this diversity, the histories of places evoke multiple responses with, potentially, differential implications for health, development, and well-being (Popay et al. 2003).

Three key points can be distilled from these ideas. First, a relational approach to place necessarily involves attention to place trajectories, examined on multiple, interlocking dimensions from the structural to the personal. Second, adequate understanding of "place" must grapple not only with the fundamental relationality of people and place but with the implications of these interactions over time, collectively and within individual lives. Third, place histories are not experienced uniformly; rather, multiple histories (and historical trajectories) coexist in any place. In the following sections, the implications of these admittedly complex ideas for scholarship on health disparities are explored on multiple levels, beginning with place histories and moving from there to the intersections of history and memory, including social memories, collective memories, and personal place memories.

Histories of Places, Places of History

In an evocative phrase, Kevin Lynch (1972) asked "what time is this place?" At the sociostructural level, the relevance of this question to health inequalities is illustrated by studies illuminating the historical processes at the heart of differentials in contemporary place-based patterns of health risks. Geographer Kay Anderson's (1987) powerful historical study, for example, examined the role of a potent, mutually reinforcing combination of media representations, public health interventions, and urban policy strategies in constructing Vancouver's Chinatown as a segregated site of difference. Over time, this elite discourse marginalized and racialized both Chinatown and the Chinese. Susan Craddock's (2000) deeply spatial public health history, *City of Plagues*, likewise explored the role of discourses of disease, contagion, and deviance as central mechanisms in the construction of San Francisco's Chinatown as a segregated enclave at the turn of the twentieth century. Fine-grained historical studies such as these unveil historical "map[s] of health discrimination…the product of selective placement, entrapment and displacement" (Smith and Easterlow 2005:174), and provide an important starting point for deeper understanding of the roots of health disparities. Exploration of the unfolding implications of these histories for contemporary health disparities requires, however, longitudinal studies such as the one described below.

Selecting two of Los Angeles' most polluted communities, Pulido et al. (1996) used historical methods (including historical census data, archival sources, secondary sources, and site observations) to explore the sociospatial pathways by which the disparate levels of health risks in these two neighborhoods were created. Their findings show the importance of an historical perspective in illuminating contemporary conditions of environmental injustice. Importantly, they also show how different sets of historical processes give rise to apparently similar contemporary place environments. The history of one community is marked by racialized urban planning policies focused on the community itself, beginning with the development early in the twentieth century of segregated housing for Latino workers located close to heavy industry but at a distance from housing also being developed for white workers (which, in turn, was more distant from the factories and their pollutants). In the second community, high levels of pollution result from the placing of heavy industry not in the community but proximal to it and the homes of its minority residents, who serve as an available labor force for the plants. Although, over time, both communities have become "negatively racialized landscapes (p. 431) burdened with unacceptable levels of environmental toxins, their different historical trajectories have implications for understanding them as places in the present. By approaching race and class as "historically and geographically specific social relations that are spatially constituted" (p. 420), this study illuminates both the differential mechanisms by which these communities become disproportionally vulnerable to health risks and their shared reality that decades of racialized policies (not race and class per se) have contributed to contemporary environmental risks.

Studies such as those presented here make visible the sociostructural mechanisms underlying contemporary health inequalities. Absent this perspective, negative health outcomes in poor communities of color may be interpreted primarily in cultural or behavioral terms, rather than as the downstream effect of historical processes of racialization and segregation (see, e.g., Kwate 2008).

History/Memory/Place

Place histories (in the sense described above) exist in recursive, dynamic relationship with social, collective, and personal memories of place. In his brilliant exploration of the entwining of history and memory, *Remembering Ahanagran*, historian Richard White (1998) cautioned that "only careless historians confuse history and memory" (p. 4). Nonetheless, his book is centrally interested in "those places where histories and memories meet" (p. 6). As pointed out, "Memory and identity are too powerful to go unquestioned and too important to be discarded as simply inventions" (p. 6). For scholars of place, attention to the intersection of place histories and place meanings – the ways in which places are "interpreted, narrated, felt, understood, and imagined" (Gieryn 2000:467) – is, I propose, essential to fully understanding people/place interactions. Three dimensions of this meaningful interface are elaborated below: social memories, collective memories, and personal place memories.

Social Memories in Place

Through "places of memory" such as statues, memorials, museums, and buildings, societies represent and maintain the past. Frequently, these representations are determined and defined by dominant groups, resulting in contemporary place topographies in which some histories are sustained and others are lost, ignored, or obliterated (Dwyer 2000; Lowenthal 1975; Till 2003). Everyday places are thus complex historical tapestries, filled with visible markers of some histories, identities, and cultural preferences, and the erasure, or forgetting, of other histories, identities, and priorities. Examples abound of the complex patterns of social memory and forgetting embodied in place geographies, including landscapes of violence and trauma (Foote 2003), civil rights memorials (Dwyer 2000), and powerful exemplars of spatial erasure, such as the Place de la Concorde in Paris, formerly the Place de la Révolution, where all signs of its revolutionary past as the site of the guillotine have been erased (Allen 2009), and Natchez, Mississippi, where a site that African American residents revere as hallowed ground because it was once the city's slave market is now an "inconspicuous intersection" (Hoelscher 2006:57) where all traces of this early history have long been destroyed.

Many sites of memory are immediately recognizable, but more subtle forms of historical inscription also send powerful messages about identity and belonging (Legg 2007). Sociospatial processes such as gentrification, restoration, historic preservation, urban renewal, and the redevelopment of public housing reconstruct places (and place aesthetics) in ways that may or may not coincide with lived experiences and histories, particularly those of marginalized groups. In a study of processes of urban change and gentrification in Stoke Newington, for example, Patrick Wright (1985) explored the different responses of incoming residents to this blue collar community. Invoking historical preservation, upwardly mobile new residents focused on "restoring" and renovating their homes, in the process erasing, reimagining, and/or contesting the aesthetic and cultural preferences of both longstanding working class residents and new waves of immigrant residents. As a neighborhood changes, Wright concluded, its changing social structure is represented in place, setting "the worlds inhabited by some groups...against the needs and interests of others...The sense of history plays a part in all of this" (p. 111).

Given the inherent heterogeneity within most communities, particularly in urban settings, contestations over place and its sociohistorical meaning take many forms. Using the example of petitions to rename the area around Ninth Street in Washington DC (an historically African American neighborhood) as "Little Ethiopia," for example, Nieves (2008) showed how debates over place can arise between established minority communities, for whom settings have historic significance, and newer waves of immigrants seeking recognition and validation in a new country. Nieves' study illustrates Massey's (1995) argument that places are always "multivocal," and highlights the importance of careful attention to the diverse and shifting ways that history and identity are "inscribed in the landscapes of marginalized groups" (p. 24).

By no means all of this inscription is top-down. In richly creative ways, marginalized groups resist the social erasure of their place histories, creating oppositional memorials and landscapes to affirm invisible histories, mark sites of violence and oppression, and acknowledge struggles for civil rights (Dwyer 2000). These "struggle[s] of memory against forgetting" (hooks 1990b:147), take many different forms. In Natchez, Mississippi, African American residents have begun to assert "counter-narratives" to the "landscapes of memory and race" (Hoelscher 2006:55) embodied in the city's careful preservation of its plantation history, – including gospel performances, public readings of personal stories, and efforts to preserve and mark places with historical associations to slavery. In Oakland, CA, landscape architect Walter Hood collaborates with local residents to construct sites of memory affirming the history of Oakland's African American community. In New York City, the colorful, flag-draped casitas of Puerto Rican immigrants (Hayden 1995) and the urban gardens of the homeless (Balmori and Morton 1993), testify to the power and importance of vernacular places as sites of renewal and resistance.

For our purposes, three important points emerge from these discussions. First, the visible and invisible traces of history in everyday places have meaning in contemporary lives, and thus, potentially, important implications for place and health. As Jacobs (1996) has observed, "It is precisely in the local that it is possible to see how the past ... inheres in place. This is not an archaic residue, but an active and influential occupation" (p. 35). Places convey powerful messages about identity, inclusion or exclusion, safety, and recognition, which in turn link to health and well-being (Manzo 2008).

Second, efforts to understand this meaningful landscape, both explicit and implicit, are essential. Because "places conceal their histories" (Cresswell 2004), seeing the "shapes of time" in place, particularly the place histories of marginalized groups, is more difficult than assessing its surface features. Nonetheless, as Hoelscher (2006) noted, "just because a landscape has been obliterated does not mean that its memories have been erased. They just might take a little more effort to see" (p. 59). Evocatively, Bell (1997) writes of the "ghosts of place," a phenomenological but frequently invisible landscape in which historical place experiences link to and become part of the "places where we feel we belong and do not belong" (p. 813). Efforts to "see" these ghosts of place typically involve close ethnographic observation of daily place activities, along with efforts to elicit lay perspectives on place and its meaning in people's lives (Popay et al. 2003).

Third, looking toward intervention, the growing literature on oppositional landscapes and sites of memory underscores both the resistance and agency of marginalized communities and the importance of history to these efforts to resist domination. Urban cultural landscapes are "the people's history" (Hayden (1995) p. 227); excavating and affirming these vernacular histories, so often muted, distorted, or erased, is thus essential to the collective well-being of oppressed communities.

Collective Place Memories

Till (2003) points out that "[t]he dense experiential and social qualities of place and landscape…not only frame social memory, they also situate and spatially constitute group remembrances" (p. 291). The work of Maurice Halbwachs (1980 [1950]) on collective memory is fundamental to scholarship in this area. Halbwachs conceptualized memory as inherently social, collective, and communicative: in his view, what we think of as "personal" memories are in reality co-constructed among people through shared narratives, stretching over time, that link with and shape personal remembrances. Elaborating on these ideas, Legg (2007) noted that "[t]he specific nature of personal memories in a particular period and place will depend upon the social conditioning of individual memory: what we are encouraged to remember; what we are told to forget; what is hidden from us; and what is invented to submerge us in a particular tradition" (p. 458).

Spatiality and place are central to both the scaffolding and the persistence of collective memories. "Every collective memory," Halbwachs (1980 [1950]) suggested, "unfolds within a spatial framework" (p. 140). Hayden (1995) concurs, noting that "[u]rban landscapes are storehouses for these social memories" (p. 9). Place, in other words, is the reference point and ground for memory, in both its personal and collective sense (Crang and Travlou 2001).

Collective spatial memories are inherently dynamic and productive, a vital component of individual and communal place attachment, identity, meaning, and well-being in the present and over time. In the latter sense, they represent the "living bond of generations" (Halbwachs 1980 [1950]:63), a sturdy thread connecting past, present, and future. Relevant across groups and cultures, collective place memories have particular salience in oppressed communities (White 1998), which frequently have experienced segregation, displacement, and removal. For indigenous peoples, generational ties to place are the bedrock of cultural identity, a "geopsyche" that involves a deep connection to the earth and the life-world (Cajete 2000) and is vital to individual and collective well-being. Brutal histories of colonization and spatial oppression have thus been particularly devastating for Native Americans. The trauma resulting from these experiences reverberates from one generation to the next, transmitted through collective memories and stories (Sotero 2006). Experiences of war, genocide, and slavery have had similar generational impacts in other communities of color.

Drawing conceptually on Halbwachs' work on collective memory along with work on historical trauma and Holocaust survivors, for example, Johnson (1998) proposed that traumatic place memories associated with slavery and racism (e.g., lynching, sharecropping), transmitted across generations through collective stories and memories of the land, may in part account for African Americans' relative lack of interest in outdoor recreation and wilderness places (in contrast to cultivated gardens or developed places). By opening up the potential relationships between an historically produced "black land aesthetic" and contemporary responses to place, Johnson's study has implications for scholarship on place and the health experiences of African American communities, for example in relation to obesity.

Personal Place Histories

> In everyday life, people keep track of places. They talk about how the neighborhood has changed; when that building went up; what it was like in the old days; how it feels to live here now. These comments are spontaneous. They belong to the vital obscurities of a life in common – to the love of places, composed from statements that are always heeded but seldom recorded. The reports continue from one generation to the next, proceeding by observation and reflection, by question and answer, by memory and anecdote.
>
> Walter (1988:1)

Humanistic geographers have long asserted the central importance of place histories in people's life experiences and developmental trajectories. Relph (1976) describes places, actual, imagined, and remembered, as "centres of special personal significance" (p. 11). Phenomenologists such as Edward Casey (2001) and Jeff Malpas (1999) likewise center place at the heart of embodied experience: for Casey (2001), place is "the immediate ambience of my lived body and its history, including the whole sedimented history of social and cultural influences and personal experiences that compose my life-history" (p. 404).

Place experiences resonate across the life course, shaping sense of self in the world along with attitudes to the world in general. These ideas are powerfully demonstrated in the work of Glen Elder (1974), whose landmark longitudinal study, *Children of the Depression*, elegantly demonstrated the reverberating impact of major social and contextual experiences over the individual life course, and beyond. Elder concluded that individual lives are embedded in and powerfully shaped by conditions and events occurring during the historical periods during which the person lives: "lives are lived in specific historical times and places…if historical times and places change, they change the way people live their lives" (Elder 2001, cited in Sotero 2006:1). These personal place histories have implications not only within but across lives, for example when adults who experienced the Depression as children carry frugal habits and a strong work ethic forward into their own families as adults. Elder's evocative notion of "linked lives" provides additional support for the importance of careful attention to the longterm implications of formative place experiences.

Early experiences in formative places result in lifelong preferences for, or aversions to, particular places and place experiences. Downing (2003), an interior design scholar, calls these "place scripts," noting that "[e]veryone retains in memory sites of significance: places that surround us with a sense of well-being or from which we recoil in distress or fear; places of vulnerability or power; of dependence or independence" (pp. 215–216). Whether good or bad, for "better or worse" (Manzo 2005), these place memories are triggered by and reawakened in present environments.

The historical and temporal dimensions of place experience have implications for efforts to better understand the mechanisms by which everyday places "get under the skin," particularly in relation to aspects of place experience that may not be fully captured in present studies. Popay et al. (2003) argue that "[a]ttention to the meanings people attach to their experiences of places and how this shapes social action could provide a missing link in our understanding of the causes of inequalities in health" (p. 401). An historical lens seems very relevant, for example, to studies of the microdynamics of place use by different groups, such as Burton and Graham's (1998) ethnography of the daily lives of young urban mothers of color. Through close-grained, long-term observation of the comings and goings of young adults in the neighborhood across the day – the ebb and flow of "neighborhood time" (p. 8), as they called it – Burton and Graham's study brought into view the daily and weekly rhythms of the neighborhood's "contextual clock" (p. 8), particularly the "different temporal use of public spaces by ethnically diverse families" (p. 8). Stretching the frame of the analysis to include history potentially opens up other questions about these spatiotemporal dynamics. How, for example, do individual and collective place histories, memories, and "scripts" shape the mundane patterns of everyday lives and geographies?

Displacement

Given the salience of place histories and attachments to identity and well-being (Manzo 2008), what are the implications of spatial dislocation – an experience routinely experienced by the poor and communities of color – for individual and collective health and well-being?

In his classic study of urban renewal in West Boston, Fried (1963) found that nearly half of the 250 women in his study experienced pervasive, long-lasting grief following relocation. Noting that more powerful grief reactions correlated with strong attachments to place and community, Fried posited that displacement resulted in a fragmenting of "spatial identity" – a "sense of belonging some-place, in a particular place which is quite familiar and easily delineated, in a wide area in which one feels 'at home'" (p. 154). Importantly, he also placed these impacts in a temporal context, noting that loss of place disrupts "one's relationship to the past, to the present, and to the future" (p. 153). Fried concluded that "grieving for a lost home is evidently a widespread and serious social phenomenon following in the wake of urban dislocation" (p. 167), that this grief response has significant mental health implications, and that efforts to help people maintain a "sense of continuity" (p. 169) despite spatial change are therefore vitally important.

More recent work affirms Fried's findings. In his Australian study of the loss of beloved places to highway development, urban renewal, hydro dams, and natural disasters, Peter Read (1996) likewise found pervasive and frequently unresolved grief, a condition which he termed "place bereavement." Tellingly, he also noted that "no a single person in any of the accounts we have followed received any kind of counselling for the grief and trauma associated with their lost place. Many received, instead, the unsolicited advice to get on with their lives" (p. 197). Reflecting across the case studies in the book, Read argued that in general there is a lack of attention to the "psychological effects of place deprivation" (p. 197).

Fullilove's (2004) detailed ethnographic study, *Root Shock*, documented the cultural, social, and psychological impacts of urban renewal projects in several African American communities in the Northeast. Between 1949 and 1973, by Fullilove's estimation, 1,600 black neighborhoods were demolished by urban renewal, with devastating implications not only for many residents but for the fragile ecologies of the communities themselves. For African Americans who migrated to northern industrial cities during the First and Second Great Migrations, "newcomer neighborhoods were the beginning and end of their options for housing" (p. 24). Although these neighborhoods were racialized, segregated, and increasingly, pathologized by the larger society, they became, Fullilove argued, "a group of islands of black life" and culture (p. 27). For African American residents, these neighborhoods thus had a double reality: although they were marked by degradation and stigma, they were also important sources of refuge and cultural renewal in a deeply racist society.

The loss of their homes and communities was thus deeply traumatic for many residents, with impacts that "increased the vulnerability of the uprooted not simply for a few years, but for many decades to come" (Fullilove 2004:99). Fullilove characterized these displacement effects as "root shock," defined as a "traumatic stress reaction to the destruction of all or part of one's emotional ecosystem" (p. 11). Fundamental to root shock, she suggested, was "the disrupted context, exterior to the individual and the group" (p. 12). Integral to this loss of context, furthermore, was the loss of historically and culturally meaningful connections to place. As one resident said, "While no one regrets the vanishing of the old slums, we also remember we once had neighborhoods" (p. 172). Observing the reverberating consequences of this upheaval for the residents of these communities and their extended family networks (including her own), Fullilove (2004), like Fried, concluded that separation from place "is an operation best done with care" (p. 11).

Clearly, the quality, safety, or toxicity of a particular place are not determining factors in the strength of people's place attachments; studies such as those described above show that people are attached to places "for better or worse" (Manzo 2005). Regardless of their valence, place attachments typically go deep. As Carol Stack (1996) observed in her study of the "call to home" animating the return migration of African Americans from the urban Northeast to the rural South, "the road from home leads out into the world and back" (p. 16). Despite the pain and trauma associated with the duress of living with overt racism, Stack noted, the subjects of her study "never really departed" (p. 16) from Southern homeplaces; in later life, for all their ambivalence about the South, the pull to home became stronger than the will to stay in the northern cities.

Key to how well people navigate experiences of spatial change, it appears, are (1) the nature of people's place attachments, (2) their past histories of displacement or removal, and (3) the degree of involvement or control they have over what is happening to them (Brown and Perkins 1992). For many marginalized communities, however, these factors represent a double jeopardy. On one hand, ties to place, land, and home have particular resonance, both cultural and social. On the other hand, spatial dislocation and lack of spatial control frequently are perduring experiences, over generations and in the present. Careful attention to the ramifications of histories of displacement for marginalized groups thus seems central to scholarship on the role of place in health disparities.

In so doing we should also ask what factors support individual and collective resilience in the face of historical and contemporary experiences of place-based risk. Not all experiences of place disruption have negative outcomes. Indeed, the studies cited above, along with others that explore the implications for health and well-being of dislocations such as migration, immigration, and natural disasters (see, e.g., Aguilar-San Juan 2005; Mazumdar et al. 2000), also make clear people's capacities to resiliently make themselves and their communities into place in new settings.

Place, History, Memory: Methodological Implications

The methodological implications of a deepened emphasis on history and time in scholarship on health and place tilt toward more expansive and varied use of qualitative approaches. Nonetheless, adequate exploration of people/place trajectories also requires attention to quantitative indicators of differentials. Indeed, a relational approach, which brings together the contextual, compositional, and collective elements of place (Cummins et al. 2007), by definition points to the value of multiple methods in health disparities research.

Longitudinal studies, both qualitative and quantitative, are essential to uncovering the sociospatial processes at the core of health disparities and their implications in individual and collective experience. Studies of macrostructural processes such as the one by Pulido et al. (1996) described earlier, make essential contributions to efforts to tease out the larger sociostructural mechanisms influencing collective health and well-being. Historical GIS (global information systems technologies) (Knowles 2002) also seem a very promising tool for mapping sites of social memory and tracing their implications over time.

As Singer and Ryff (1997) point out, longitudinal approaches can range from studies of individual lives (including case studies, biographies, autobiographies, and narratives) to prospective surveys of collective experiences unfolding over time, providing they focus centrally on both accumulating risks to health, and the mechanisms, operating in multiple domains over time, by which inequalities influence health outcomes. Singer and Ryff's ecumenical approach to longitudinal methods is both refreshingly expansive and consistent with other writing in this area. Smith and Easterlow (2005), for example, argue for longitudinal studies which explore not only contextual effects, but the ways in which "health conditions may be "mapped onto" places by people as they negotiate a path through the markets and institutions that shape and encase their lives" (p. 178).

Moving downstream to lived experience and the place experiences embodied in collective and personal histories and memories, qualitative methods come to the fore. As Hoelscher (2006) pointed out, "A landscape's meaning does not come neatly packaged, inherently ready to be deciphered or to be simply 'read' as a transparent and unproblematic text. Stories need to be told and linked to the landscape…" (p. 53). Not surprisingly, narrative methods – ranging from in-depth interviews to visual narratives such as writing, drawing, art, and photography – are central to surfacing place histories and stories (Eyles 2008). Popay et al. (2003) encourage more expansive use of lay narratives in health disparities research. Historical methods such as oral histories and life histories are likewise ideally suited to the exploration of place histories, particularly in relation to tracing the "ghosts of place" resident in personal memories and recollections (Wallace 2006; Mallinson et al. 2003).

Expanding conventional narrative approaches, geographer Mei-Po Kwan is breaking new ground in her use of geo-narratives, which link narrative methods (oral histories, life histories, and personal stories) and global information systems technologies to "illuminat[e] the social, cultural, and institutional contexts in which experiences were constituted, shaped, and enacted" (Kwan and Ding 2008:448). Importantly for our purposes, Kwan and Ding note that geo-narratives, which illuminate the time-geographies of daily lives, are particularly useful for "studying hidden histories and geographies, the place-based lives and memories of disadvantaged people, minority groups, and others whose views have been ignored" (George and Stratford 2005, cited in Kwan and Ding 2008:448).

Places come into being through the everyday practices of individuals and groups. Ethnographic methods such as participant observation, which seek fine-grained understanding of what people *do* in place, as well as how they make meaning within it, thus make an essential contribution to fully dimensional explorations of place histories and experiences. Walter (1988) described the process of getting out into place and learning its history and embedded meanings literally from the ground up as "studying with his legs" (p. 11). Beyond participant observation, promising strategies for exploring the historical dimensions of place experience include "walking interviews" (Carpiano 2009), visual methods such as photovoice, video, and mapping (Dennis et al. 2008), and geo-ethnography, which brings the spatial mapping capacities of GIS together with ethnographic approaches to simultaneously explore multiple dimensions of lived experience in place (Matthews et al. 2005).

Concluding Thoughts

Reflecting on the neglect of human experience in research on place, Walter (1988) identified the Aristotelian separation of person and place typical of Western scholarship as the field's fundamental "epistemological stumbling block" (p. 211). Although this bifurcation of people and place remains an obstinate divide, my aim in this chapter has been to prod health scholars to revisit their equally problematic tendency to separate time and place. As Lucy Lippard (1997) has so eloquently observed, "place is latitudinal and longitudinal within the map of a person's life. A layered location replete with human histories and memories, place has width as well as depth" (p. 7). Adequately engaging this plenitude necessarily involves careful attention to all its dimensions, including its inherent dynamism. Doing so is not easy, conceptually or methodologically. Yet setting place outside of history flattens human experience, reducing it to the single plane of the present, and obscuring the deep-rooted social, political, and economic mechanisms at the core of health disparities, and thus of the work this field aims to do. On both counts, therefore, I encourage efforts to reconnect place and history within health disparities research.

References

Aguilar-San Juan, K. 2005. "Staying Vietnamese: Community and place in Orange County and Boston." *City & Community* 4(1):37–65.

Allen, D. A. 2009. "Memory and place: Two case studies." *Places* 21(1):56–61.

Anderson, K. J. 1987. "The idea of Chinatown: The power of place and institutional practice in the making of a racial category." *Annals of the Association of American Geographers* 77(4):580–598.

Balmori, D. and M. Morton. 1993. *Transitory gardens, uprooted lives*. New Haven, CT: Yale University Press.

Basso, K. H. 1996. *Wisdom sits in places: Landscape and language among the Western Apache*. Albuquerque, NM: University of New Mexico Press.

Bell, M. M. 1997. "The ghosts of place." *Theory and Society* 26(6):813–836.

Brown, B. B. and D. D. Perkins. 1992. "Disruptions in place attachment." pp. 279–304 in *Place attachment*. Edited by I. Altman and S. Low. New York: Plenum Press.

Burton, L. M. and J. E. Graham. 1998. Neighborhood rhythms and the social activities of adolescent mothers. *New Directions in Adolescent Development* 82:7–22.
Burton, L. M., D. M. Winn, H. Stevenson and S. L. Clark. 2004. "Working with African American clients: Considering the homeplace in counseling and therapy practices." *Journal of Marital and Family Therapy* 30(4):397–410.
Carpiano, R. M. 2009. "Come take a walk with me: The 'Go-Along' interview as a novel method for studying the implications of place for health and well-being." *Health & Place* 15:263–272.
Cajete, G. 2000. *Native science: Natural laws of interdependence*. Santa Fe, NM: Clearlight Publishers.
Casey, E. S. 2001. "Body, self, and landscape: A geophilosophical inquiry into the place-world." pp. 403–425 in *Textures of place: Exploring humanistic geographies*. Edited by P. Adams, S. Hoelscher, and K. E. Till. Minneapolis, MN: University of Minnesota.
Craddock, S. 2000. *City of plagues: Disease, poverty, and deviance in San Francisco*. Minneapolis, MN: University of Minnesota Press.
Crang, M. and P. S. Travlou. 2001. "The city and topologies of memory." *Environment and Planning D: Society and Space* 19:161–177.
Cresswell, T. 2002. "Introduction: Theorizing place." pp. 11–32 in *Mobilizing place, placing mobility: The politics of representation in a globalized world*. Edited by G. Verstraete and T. Cresswell. New York: Rodopi.
Cresswell, T. 2004. *Place: A short introduction*. New York: Blackwell Publishing.
Cummins, S., S. Curtis, A. V. Diez-Roux and S. Macintyre. 2007. "Understanding and representing 'place' in health research: A relational approach." *Social Science & Medicine* 65:1825–1838.
Curtis, S., H. Southall, P. Congdon and B. Dodgeon. 2004. "Area effects on health variation over the life-course: Analysis of the longitudinal study sample in England using new data on area of residence." *Social Science & Medicine* 58(1):57–74.
Dennis, S. F. Jr., S. Gaulocher, R. M. Carpiano and D. Brown. 2008. "Participatory photomapping (PPM): Exploring an integrated method for health and place research with young people." *Health & Place* 15:466–473.
Dodghson, R. A. 2008. "Geography's place in time." *Geografiska Annaler B* 90(1):1–15.
Downing, F. 2003. "Transcending memory: Remembrance and the design of place." *Design Studies* 24:213–235.
Dwyer, O. J. 2000. "Interpreting the Civil Rights movement: Place, memory, and conflict." *Political Geography* 52(4):660–671.
Elder, G. H. Jr. 1974. *Children of the great depression: Social change in life experience*. Chicago, IL: University of Chicago Press.
Evans-Campbell, T. 2008. "Historical trauma in American Indian/Native Alaska communities." *Journal of Interpersonal Violence* 23(3):316–338.
Eyles, J. 2008. "Qualitative approaches in the investigation of sense of place and health relations." pp. 59–69 in *Sense of place, health, and quality of life*. Edited by J. Eyles and A. Williams. Burlington, VT: Ashgate.
Foote, K. E. 2003. *Shadowed ground: America's landscapes of violence and tragedy* (Revised edn.). Austin, TX: University of Texas Press.
Fried, M. 1963. "Grieving for a lost home." pp. 151–171 in *The urban condition: People and policy in the metropolis*. Edited by L. J. Duhl. New York: Basic Books.
Frumpkin, H. 2006. "The measure of place." *American Journal of Preventive Medicine* 31(6):530–532.
Fullilove, M. T. 2004. *Root shock: How tearing up city neighborhoods hurts America, and what we can do about it*. New York: Ballantine Books.
Gieryn, T. F. 2000. "A space for place in sociology." *Annual Review of Sociology* 26:463–496.
Halbwachs, M. 1980 [1950]. *The collective memory*. New York: Harper & Row.
Hayden, D. 1995. *The power of place: Urban landscapes as public history*. Cambridge, MA: MIT Press.
Hoelscher, S. 2006. "The white-pillared past: Landscapes of memory and race in the American South." pp. 39–72 in *Landscape and race in the United States*. Edited by R. H. Schein. New York: Routledge.

hooks, b. 1990a. "Homeplace: A site of resistance." pp. 41–49 in *Yearning: Race, gender, and cultural politics*. Boston, MA: South End Press.
hooks, b. 1990b. "Choosing the margin as a space of radical openness." pp. 145–154 in *Yearning: Race, gender, and cultural politics*. Boston, MA: South End Press.
Jacobs, J. M. 1996. *Edge of empire: Postcolonialism and the city*. New York: Routledge.
Johnson, C. Y. 1998. "A consideration of collective memory in African American attachment to wildland recreation places." *Human Ecology Review* 5(1):5–15.
Knowles, A. K. 2002. *Past time, past place: GIS for history*. Redlands, CA: ESRI.
Kwan, M.-P. and G. Ding. 2008. "Geo-narrative: Extending geographic information systems for narrative analysis in qualitative and mixed-methods research." *The Professional Geographer* 60(4):443–465.
Kwate, N. A. O. 2008. "Fried children and fresh apples: Racial segregation as a fundamental cause of fast food density in black neighborhoods." *Health & Place* 14:2–44.
Legg, S. 2007. "Reviewing geographies of memory/forgetting." *Environment and Planning A* 39:456–466.
Lippard, L. R. 1997. *Lure of the local: Senses of place in a multicentered society*. New York: The New Press.
Lowenthal, D. 1975. "Past time, present place: Landscape and memory." *Geographical Review* 65(1):1–36.
Lynch, K. 1972. *What time is this place?* Cambridge, MA: MIT Press.
Mallinson, S., J. Popay, E. Elliott, S. Bennet, L. Bostock, A. Gatrell, C. Thomas and G. Williams. 2003. "Historical data for health inequalities research: A research note." *Sociology* 37(4):771–780.
Malpas, J. 1999. *Place and experience: A philosophical topography*. New York: Cambridge University Press.
Manzo, L. C. 2005. "For better or worse: Exploring multiple dimensions of place meaning." *Journal of Environmental Psychology* 25(1):67–86.
Manzo, L. C. 2008. "The experience of displacement on sense of place and well-being." pp. 87–104 in *Sense of place, health, and quality of life*. Edited by J. Eyles and A. Williams. Burlington, VT: Ashgate.
Massey, D. 1995. "Places and their pasts." *History Workshop Journal* 39(Spring):182–192.
Massey, D. S. 2004. "Segregation and stratification: A biosocial perspective." *Du Bois Review* 1(1):7–25.
Matthews, S. A., J. E. Detwiler and L. M. Burton. 2005. "Geo-ethnography: Coupling geographic information analysis techniques with ethnographic methods in urban research." *Cartographica* 40(2):75–90.
Mazumdar, S., S. Mazumdar, F. Docuyanan and C. M. McLaughlin. 2000. "Creating a sense of place: The Vietnamese Americans and Little Saigon." *Journal of Environmental Psychology* 20:319–333.
Nieves, A. D. 2008. "Revaluing places: Hidden histories from the margins." *Places* 20(1):21–25.
Popay, J., G. Williams, C. Thomas and A. Gatrell. 2003. "Theorizing inequalities in health: The place of lay knowledge." pp. 385–409 in *Health and social justice: Politics, ideology, and inequity in the distribution of disease*. Edited by R. Hofrichter. New York: Jossey-Bass.
Pred, A. 1984. "Place as historically contingent process: Structuration and the time-geography of becoming places." *Annals of the Association of American Geographers* 74(2):279–297.
Pred, A. 1990. *Making histories and constructing human geographies: The local transformation of practice, power relations, and consciousness*. Boulder, CO: Westview Press.
Pulido, L., S. Sidawi and R. O. Vos. 1996. "An archeology of environmental racism in Los Angeles." *Urban Geography* 17(5):419–439.
Read, P. 1996. *Returning to nothing: The meaning of lost places*. New York: Cambridge University Press.
Relph, E. C. 1976. *Place and placelessness*. London: Pion.
Singer, B. and C. Ryff. 1997. "Racial and ethnic inequalities in health: Environmental, psychosocial, and physiological pathways." pp. 89–122 in *Intelligence, genes, and success: Scientists*

respond to "The Bell Curve." Edited by B. Devlin, S. Fienberg, D. Resnick, and K. Roeder. New York: Springer-Verlag.

Smith, S. J. and D. Easterlow. 2005. "The strange geography of health inequalities." *Transactions of the Institute of British Geographers* NS30:173–190.

Sotero, M. M. 2006. "A conceptual model of historical trauma." *Journal of Health Disparities Research and Practice* 1(1):93–108.

Stack, C. 1996. *Call to home: African Americans reclaim the rural South.* New York: Basic Books.

Till, K. E. 2003. "Places of memory." pp. 289–301 in *A companion to political geography.* Edited by J. Agnew, K. Mitchell, and G. Toal. Malden, MA: Blackwell.

Tuan, Y.-F. 1977. *Space and place: The perspective of experience.* Minneapolis, MN: University of Minnesota Press.

Wadsworth, M. E. 1997. "Health inequalities in the life course perspective." *Social Science & Medicine* 44: 859–869.

Wallace, G. 2006. "Recreating the ghosts of place: Community struggle through loss and healing." *Illness, Crisis & Loss* 14(1):23–42.

Walter, E. V. 1988. *Placeways: A theory of the human environment.* Chapel Hill, NC: The University of North Carolina Press.

White, R. 1998. *Remembering Ahanagran: Storytelling in a family's past.* New York: Hill and Wang.

Williams, D. R., M. V. Costa, A. O. Odunlami and S. A. Mohammed. 2008. "Moving upstream: How interventions that address the social determinants of health can improve health and reduce disparities." *Journal of Public Health Management Practice* 14(6):S8–S17.

Wright, P. 1985. *On living in an old country: The national past in contemporary Britain.* London: Verso.

[illegible] The Hill Gard[illegible] by [illegible]

[illegible] (ed.) [illegible] Press.

[illegible] and [illegible] (19[illegible]) [illegible] of health [illegible]

[illegible] model of [illegible]

[illegible] pp. [illegible]

[illegible] Sports of Landscape [illegible]

[illegible] Landscape, L. Mitchell, and D. Revill. Middlesex: [illegible]

[illegible] Space and place: The perspective of experience. [illegible] of Minnesota Press.

[illegible] (19[illegible]) The [illegible] in the [illegible]

[illegible] the [illegible] of place [illegible]

[illegible]

Chapter 2
Formalizing Place in Geographic Information Systems

Michael F. Goodchild

Introduction

The concept of place has a long history in geography and related disciplines, but has been plagued by a fundamental vagueness of definition: what, exactly, does the term mean? Within any one area of application, such as the study of migration, it may be possible to approach precision, but definition has remained elusive across the wide spectrum of domains in which the term is used.

In the mid-1960s, it became possible to reduce the contents of maps to digital form for the first time (Foresman 1998), allowing them to be processed by the new digital computers that were then becoming available. The first driving motivation was simple measurement, given the historic frustration with obtaining even the most basic measures of mapped features, such as length and area, from paper copies (Maling 1989). In time, it became possible to see and exploit the advantages of computer-based handling of map data in many areas besides measurement – in the editing processes of map compilation, in managing complex geographically distributed operations, and in scientific research. By 1980, the concept of a geographic information system (GIS) had taken hold, as a system that would support a vast array of operations on geographic information, and a first commercial software products began to appear. Today GIS is a major computer application, used in and indispensable to many forms of human activity. The average citizen is likely to encounter a simple form of GIS in seeking driving directions from Web services, zooming to his or her local neighborhood using Google Earth, or tracking jogging routes with a global positioning system (GPS).

It is easy to underestimate the profound effect that the development of GIS has had on all aspects of geographic data production, analysis, and use. Instead of the tedium and inherent errors of map measurement, it offers precision. Instead of

M.F. Goodchild (✉)
Professor Department of Geography, University of California, Santa Barbara, CA, USA
e-mail: good@geog.ucsb.edu

L.M. Burton et al. (eds.), *Communities, Neighborhoods, and Health*,
Social Disparities in Health and Health Care 1, DOI 10.1007/978-1-4419-7482-2_2,

vaguely defined locations, it captures and manages coordinates to as many decimal places as the data can justify (and frequently many more). And more importantly, it formalizes many of the previous vague terms of geographic research. In order to represent geographic information in the precise environment of a digital computer, with its binary alphabet of 0s and 1s, it is necessary to reduce everything being represented to a simple code, using agreed and explicit rules. Because of this, GIS has often been accused of taking an excessively simplistic view of the complexity of many geographic ideas (Pickles 1995); but when those ideas are rigorously defined and readily formalized, as they hopefully are in scientific applications, then the benefits are obvious in the ease with which data can be analyzed, visualized, modeled, and shared.

The purpose of this chapter is to explore the formalization of one such concept, place. In essence, the chapter addresses the relationship between the informal world of human discourse on one hand, and the formal world of digitally represented geography on the other. Much effort over the past four decades has gone into ensuring the accuracy of digital geographic data, into ensuring that terms used by one community are understood by another, and into ensuring that the GIS enterprise meets the norms of scientific research (Goodchild et al. 1999). Special attention has been devoted to concepts that are inherently vague, such as the definition and limits of many geographic features (Burrough and Frank 1996). The chapter addresses the formalization of place, and returns at the end to the question of whether place is simply too vague to be formalized, except in very narrowly defined circumstances.

The next section discusses alternative definitions and examples. This is followed by sections on inherent ambiguities, on placenames and the formal gazetteer, on the role of volunteered geographic information or user-generated geographic content, and on defining place as context. The final substantive section reviews the role of place as one of a number of fundamental spatial concepts.

Definitions and Examples

A *GIS* can be defined as a computer application designed to perform virtually any conceivable operation on geographic information. It is a means of acquiring, storing, communicating (Sui and Goodchild 2001), and analyzing what is known about the geographic world. In turn, *geographic information* can be defined as knowledge about the geographic world; as information linking properties to locations on or near the Earth's surface. Every item of information in a GIS must be associated with some location, expressed in the coordinates of latitude/longitude or some equally universal system. Finally, a map is a compilation of one or more types of geographic information, or *layers*, for a defined area. Maps are typically printed on flat paper, which requires that the true curved surface of the Earth be distorted through the use of a *projection*. Much geographic information is now dynamic, including a vast number of real-time information sources fed through the Internet, so the concept of an inherently static map as a repository of geographic information is today somewhat limiting.

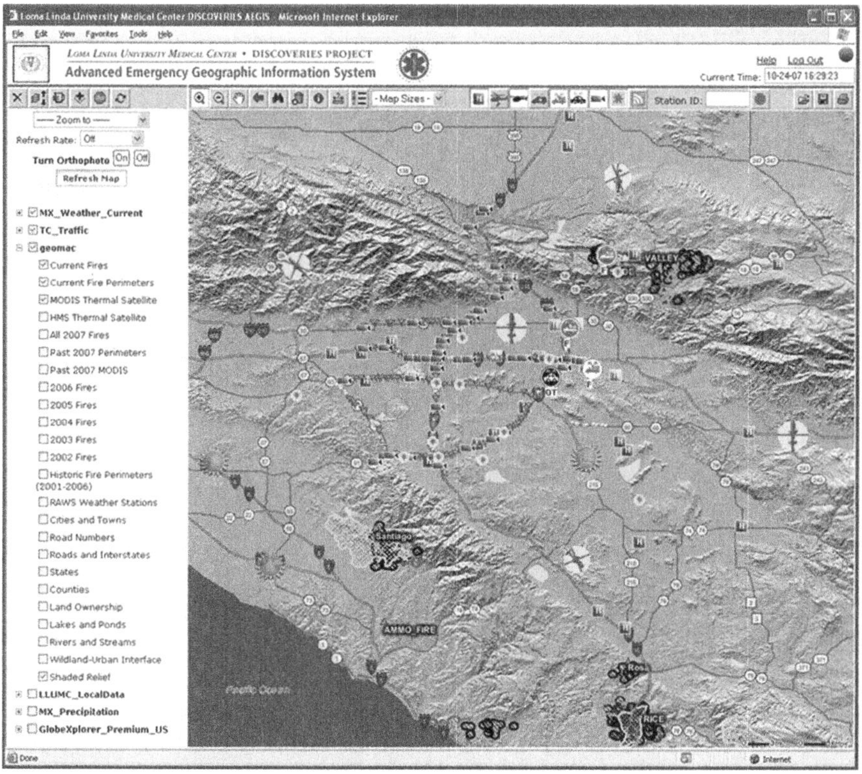

Fig. 2.1 Screen shot of the Advanced Emergency GIS, showing the situation during an outbreak of wildfires in Southern California in 2007. Each clickable icon denotes the availability of real-time information about a feature or asset relevant to the emergency, such as a rescuer vehicle, hospital, or freeway camera

Figure 2.1 shows an example of this modern concept of a map: a display of real-time information in the Advanced Emergency GIS, developed through a collaboration between ESRI, the leading vendor of GIS software, and the Loma Linda University Medical Center. It shows the situation during a fire emergency in Southern California, with icons depicting real-time sources of information, such as the locations of rescue vehicles and helicopters, the perimeters of the fires, and the locations of hospitals and freeway surveillance cameras. The actual display from which this screen shot was obtained is dynamic, allowing the user to zoom, pan, click on icons to obtain more information, and plan actions.

Figure 2.2 illustrates the power of GIS as an engine for visualization and analysis. The list on the left represents a typical table of data – a list of states in alphabetical order, with one variable, median value of housing in the state, exemplifying the vast amount of information that is available from official sources through programs such as the decennial Census. On the right is a map showing the same variable, along with major freeways. Seeing the data in spatial perspective

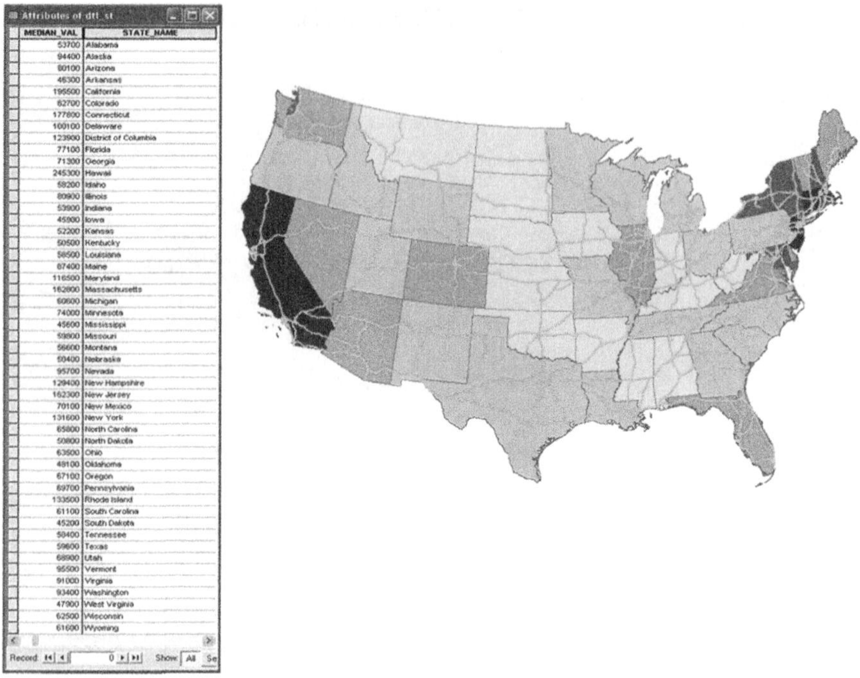

MEDIAN_VAL	STATE_NAME
53700	Alabama
94400	Alaska
80100	Arizona
46300	Arkansas
195500	California
82700	Colorado
177800	Connecticut
100100	Delaware
123900	District of Columbia
77100	Florida
71300	Georgia
245300	Hawaii
58200	Idaho
80900	Illinois
53900	Indiana
45900	Iowa
52200	Kansas
50500	Kentucky
58500	Louisiana
87400	Maine
116500	Maryland
162800	Massachusetts
60600	Michigan
74000	Minnesota
45600	Mississippi
59800	Missouri
56600	Montana
50400	Nebraska
95700	Nevada
129400	New Hampshire
162300	New Jersey
70100	New Mexico
131600	New York
65800	North Carolina
50800	North Dakota
63500	Ohio
48100	Oklahoma
67100	Oregon
69700	Pennsylvania
133500	Rhode Island
61100	South Carolina
45200	South Dakota
58400	Tennessee
59600	Texas
68900	Utah
95500	Vermont
91000	Virginia
93400	Washington
47900	West Virginia
62500	Wisconsin
61600	Wyoming

Fig. 2.2 Contrasting the insights available from a table (*left*) and a map (*right*). The same information (median value of housing by state) is displayed in both, but the map places that information in context, allowing a range of inferences to be drawn from the spatial pattern

immediately suggests a number of questions that would not be as readily suggested by the table: why is high housing value a phenomenon of the Northeast and California? Why are houses in Delaware cheaper than those in neighboring Maryland? Why is housing in New Hampshire more expensive than in its neighbor Vermont? Making an alphabetical list of states removes from view any of the insights that can be gained from spatial context, with the exception of Indiana/Illinois and Florida/Georgia, which are adjacent both in space and in the alphabetically ordered table.

Ambiguities

One of the complications of GIS stems from the vast number of ways in which simple items of geographic information can be coded. Information may be available about points, lines, or areas, and may include a vast array of attributes that are often quantitative (e.g., population) but also qualitative (text descriptions, images, and sound). To be useful as a means of communicating geographic knowledge, however, the coding scheme must be both replicable, in the sense that two people would independently arrive at the same code, and understood by both sender and receiver of information. Unfortunately, lack of standards and rigorous definitions has meant that all too often geographic information is not *interoperable*, in other words intelligible and informative across divides of distance, discipline, or application (Goodchild et al. 1999).

Consider, for example, the message "It's cool today in Seattle for the time of year." This is by definition geographic information, since it relates a property (cool) to a place (Seattle). But its efficacy relies on the receiver sharing the same understanding of "cool for the time of year" and "Seattle." To transmit the message in GIS, Seattle would have to be represented precisely, perhaps as a point centered downtown, or perhaps as a polygon delimiting the city boundary. The attribute "cool for the time of year" could be sent as text despite its inherent ambiguity, or replaced by a Celsius measurement along with the 30-year normals.

Vagueness is endemic in geographic information (Duckham 2009), despite efforts to remove it through the use of such scientific scales as Celsius. Figure 2.3 reproduces a postcard sent in the 1980s by geographer Peter Gould from Cape Hatteras, NC to my colleague Waldo Tobler at his home in Santa Barbara. The use of latitude/longitude instead of a conventional street address suggests that this coordinate system is sufficiently interoperable to guarantee understanding. But although the address is given to the nearest second of arc (roughly 30 m), the point turns out to be approximately 400 m from Tobler's house, 90 m of which can be accounted for by a 1983 change in the reference ellipsoid that is used to define North American latitudes and longitudes. The other 310 m is presumably due to the difficulty of

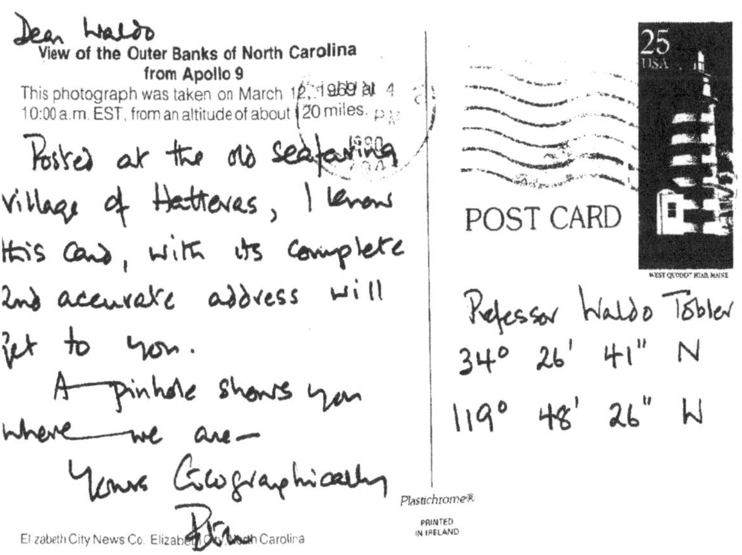

Fig. 2.3 Reproduction of a postcard sent in 1980 from Cape Hatteras, NC, by Prof. Peter Gould. Despite the use of latitude/longitude to code and formalize street address, the card was successfully delivered to Prof. Waldo Tobler in Santa Barbara, CA by the US Postal Service

determining latitude and longitude accurately from a highway map, or whatever source the sender used. More generally, it is true to say that all geographic information is subject to uncertainty, because of limitations of measuring instruments, vagueness of definitions, lack of essential documentation, and a multitude of other sources. Thus, addressing uncertainty, and visualizing its magnitude, has become a major research issue in the field (Zhang and Goodchild 2002). On the other hand, the apparent precision of the products of a GIS, whether in the form of maps or numbers, is clearly one of its attractive features, and it has been difficult at times to persuade the users of GIS to address uncertainty explicitly.

Digital Gazetteers

The vagueness of place, and the interface between the informal world of human discourse and the formal world of GIS, is nowhere as apparent as with the gazetteer. A gazetteer is defined as a table of records about named features, each record containing three elements: a location defined in a suitable coordinate system, a type of the feature using a controlled vocabulary, and a name (Goodchild and Hill 2008). Gazetteers reflect the modernist view that every feature should have a single, officially recognized name. Digital gazetteers are an essential though hidden part of many Web sites, since they allow placenames provided by users to be converted into coordinates, and used to provide associated services such as driving directions.

There has been much interest recently in automating the use of placenames, especially when they occur in text. The term *geoparsing* is often used to describe the process of detecting placename references in text and automating their formalization, a process that has found abundant applications in gathering of intelligence from email and phone conversations. Many entries in Wikipedia are now *geotagged* by the addition of hidden codes (*microformats*) that represent location in a formal coordinate system. The geoparsing task is enormously difficult, however, because of the role of context in defining the meaning of placenames. For example, the placename *Shanghai* can appear in English as a verb (to kidnap), and the placename *Los Angeles* may have different meanings when spoken in New York or in San Bernardino, CA. A simple example is provided by the clustering of geotags that has appeared recently around the small town of Boston, NY, because of confusion in geoparsing texts that contain lists of major US cities.

Formalization of placenames, in other words removal of ambiguity, poses very substantial research challenges. The identification of places is a subjective, cognitive act (e.g., the Italian term *poggio* for a rounded hill has no single-word English equivalent), is culturally situated (e.g., bordering countries can give different names to features), and is often time-variant (e.g., Lake Bonneville is now dry). In the case of Lake Tahoe, all three elements of its gazetteer entry are ambiguous: it has had at least six names through history; it is alternatively classified either as a lake or a reservoir; and its location varies depending on the scale of the source mapping. Hastings (2008) has argued that the three elements should be strictly prioritized in addressing ambiguity. Location should be treated first, since all locations assigned to a feature will be similar; type should be second, because conflicting types will be semantically related even in a controlled vocabulary; and name should be last, because alternative names need have no resemblance to each other.

While gazetteers normally limit themselves to officially recognized features, Montello et al. (2003) have addressed the problem of formalizing informal or vernacular features. Using the example of Downtown Santa Barbara, they have shown how experiments with human subjects can be used to elicit a feature's geographic limits, and how such limits can be represented in a GIS, despite a lack of complete consensus. Jones (e.g., Jones et al. 2008) has conducted a number of experiments aimed at automatically eliciting similar geographic limits from vernacular placenames used in Web text.

Volunteered Geographic Information

The production of gazetteers has traditionally been the responsibility of authorities, such as the US Geological Survey, and its equivalent national mapping agencies in other countries. These agencies have ensured that naming is standardized, so that users can communicate without ambiguity. It is important to realize, however, that this modernist approach is confined to the past century or two. If we go back to 1507, for example, we find an instance of naming that involved no authority, but nevertheless came in time to be accepted as standard by much of humanity (Fernández-Armesto 2007). I refer to the naming of America, which occurred in that year in St-Dié-des-Vosges, a small town in Eastern France. Martin Waldseemüller and Vautrin Lud needed a name to identify the large land mass that explorers had found to the west of the Atlantic. They were excited to receive letters from Florence that appeared to give credit to Amerigo Vespucci for being first to recognize the land as a New World, a new continent. They feminized his first name, and placed the word "America" on the map of what we would now call South America. Although it seems that they later regretted their decision (Fernández-Armesto 2007), the map had by then been widely distributed and the name stuck. No government agency was involved, and Waldseemüller had no recognizable form of authority.

In today's postmodern world such practices are becoming common once again, supported by the participatory information technology that we today know as the Web and that permit ordinary citizens with no authority, training, or financial reward to publish names for features that reflect their own interests, cultural, or linguistic affiliations, or whatever suits their fancy. This form of *user-generated content* is part of a larger movement often termed Web 2.0, to distinguish it from earlier visions of the Web as a top-down mechanism for information dissemination.

An excellent example of a postmodern, Web 2.0 equivalent of the gazetteer is Wikimapia, a site that uses procedures somewhat similar to the better-known Wikipedia to placenames on maps, or as the site itself proclaims, to "describe the whole world." Wikimapia allows users to find features in a familiar map interface, to outline their limits as polygons, and to provide descriptions that may be as short as a single name, or as long as an extensive text – together with hyperlinks to other Web-based information. The number of entries in Wikimapia is currently approaching 11 million, which is roughly twice as many as in the world's most extensive gazetteer. Wikimapia entries may be formally recognized or vernacular, and the descriptions are in many cases far richer than those of a gazetteer, which are limited to a simple type.

Many hundreds of examples of such citizen-created VGI can be found on the Web, ranging from entertaining efforts to map the use of language to serious citizen science. In the latter category are such programs as the Christmas Bird Count of the Audubon Society and Project Budburst, a large-scale effort to provide phenological data. Hundreds of millions of volunteered, geo-registered photographs are now available at the Flickr site, and Open Street Map is an international effort to create a detailed global map using volunteer effort.

Effort such as these have powerful practical implications for studies of place, since information elicited from the average citizen can potentially help us to define and thus formalize associated concepts. Zook and Graham (2009) have made extensive analyses of VGI, searching for culturally significant terms that can be used to delimit community. By searching for instances of "Jesus" and "Allah," for example, they are able to make detailed maps of the distributions of Christianity and Islam within Europe. By searching for instances of "Polish" they have produced detailed delimitations of the Polish community in Chicago.

Place as Context

Like many terms, *place* performs a variety of functions in different settings. Social scientists are most likely to be interested in its role in defining context, or the geographic area within which humans live their lives. As such it is likely to be of value in linking individual behavior to context, in studies of links between humans and their environment. For example, it may be helpful in studies of the effects of air pollution, or in links between obesity and urban design (Lopez 2007). Place often is used in the sense of *action space*, or the space within which humans carry out habitual aspects of their lives, such as shopping, work, recreation, and sleeping. Such spaces are largely unique to the individual, and likely also to vary through time as habits change, as spaces are learnt, or as people migrate. Place is often used in the sense of *community* or *neighborhood*, implying an informal relationship to an area surrounding the individual's place of residence. In this case also, the boundaries of place are likely to be specific to the individual and time dependent, and perhaps inherently vague.

Set against this perspective of individual, time-dependent definitions are the various administrative *tesselations*. A tesselation can be defined as a partitioning of space into irregularly shaped areas, such that every location lies in exactly one area. Counties, states, local municipalities, and census tracts all satisfy this definition. All are administrative in origin and fixed (though most are annoyingly subject to revision from time to time). As formalizations of place, they are highly unsatisfactory, allowing none of the individual variations or time dependence discussed above. However, their role as *reporting zones* for social statistics makes them particularly attractive for research, to the degree that many researchers are willing to overlook their inherently unsatisfactory aspects and to adopt an individual's containing reporting zone as a convenient surrogate for that individual's neighborhood.

One of the most egregious examples is the US county, an administrative unit that is often used for research, since an abundance of data are available for these units. Far from reflecting a single scale or level of geographic detail, the counties of the conterminous US vary by a factor of 10^4 in area (from Manassas City County, VA to San Bernardino County, CA) and 10^5 in population (from Yellowstone National Park County, MT to Los Angeles County, CA).

Techniques have been developed for estimating statistics for specialized areas, and in principle these might be used to provide better definitions of context. Statistical agencies such as the US Bureau of the Census may be willing to provide custom tabulations for specialized areas, and more generally methods of *areal interpolation* provide a stop-gap solution. In areal interpolation, we define areas for which statistics are available as *source zones*, and areas for which statistics need to be estimated as *target zones*. The simplest of these methods (Goodchild and Lam 1980) apportions counts for source zones according to the areas of overlap between them and target zones, based on the assumption that populations are uniformly distributed within source zones. A variety of more elaborate techniques have been investigated, based on different assumptions about spatial distributions (e.g., Goodchild et al. 1993; Tobler 1979).

Figure 2.4 shows an example application of the simplest technique. The population of Los Angeles County, which is concentrated near the coast, is clearly better represented in the interpolated estimates for three-digit ZIP boundaries, since these are generally smaller than counties in areas of high density.

Spatial convolution describes a different set of techniques that are perhaps more useful in approaching individual definitions of place. Instead of equating context with the contents of some administratively defined unit that happens to contain the individual's location, these methods define context geometrically and centered on the individual. One might, for example, define context as a circle of radius x centered on the individual. The value of x would have to be set, of course, but could be rationalized based on some program of empirical research. Using GIS, this circle could then be overlaid on reporting-zone boundaries, areas of overlap computed, and estimates made using these areas as weights. A rather more sophisticated and theoretically more acceptable version would weight according to distance, using a suitable mathematical function to provide the weights.

Figure 2.5 shows a simple illustration of this approach. The shaded polygons represent three reporting zones, which have been overlaid with a raster of cells. Each zone's population (or whatever variable is most relevant to the context) is distributed among the cells that overlap it based on area. The cells are then summed using weights computed from a decreasing function of distance known as a *kernel* function. The method bears a strong resemblance to *density estimation* (Silverman 1986).

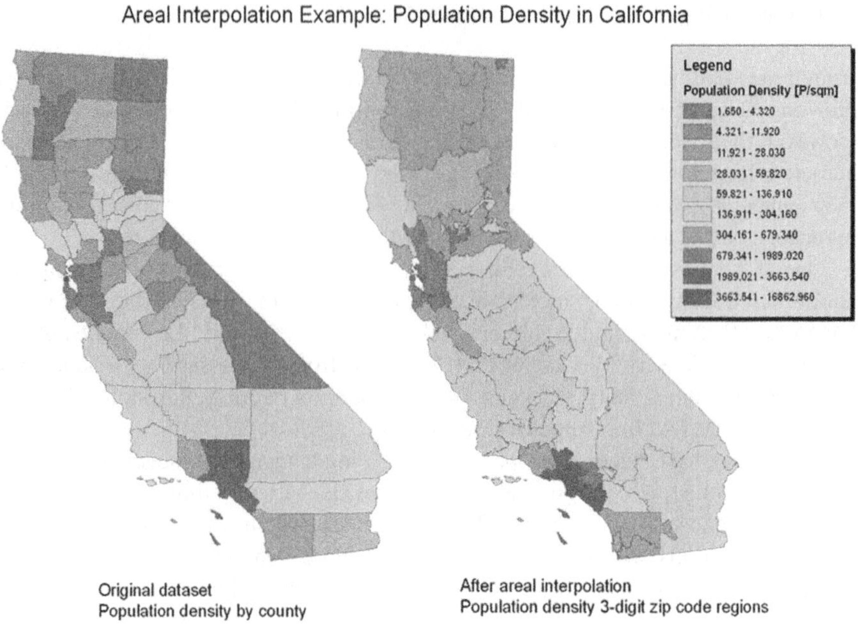

Fig. 2.4 Areal interpolation of population density from the source zones (the counties of California) to target zones defined by the first three digits of ZIP codes

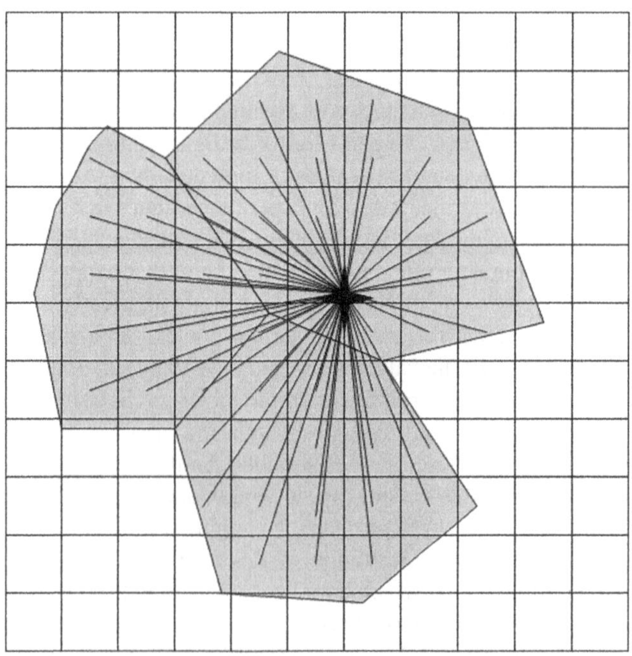

Fig. 2.5 A simple example of convolution to obtain an estimate of the context of a person located at the point shown. Statistics associated with three polygonal reporting zones are assigned to an overlay of cells, weighted according to distance from the point, and summed

Place as a Spatial Concept

We have seen in this chapter how the concept of place underlies many investigations of the nature of geographic reality, and the processes that play themselves out on the geographic landscape. As such it ranks with many other spatial concepts, from the simplest (location and distance) to the most advanced (spatial dependence and spatial heterogeneity) that provide many of the primitive elements of disciplines that deal with phenomena distributed in space and time. There have been many attempts over the past few decades to enumerate these concepts and to study how an understanding of them is acquired during the cognitive development of humans. Gardner (1999), for example, has argued that these concepts are the foundation of a distinct form of intelligence, one of a number of such discrete intelligences that underlie human learning and reasoning (Eliot 1987).

The concepts of spatial intelligence have recently been the subject of a major report by the National Research Council on *spatial thinking*, which the report describes as "pervasive" and "vital across a wide range of domains of practical and scientific knowledge; yet it is underrecognized, undervalued, underappreciated, and therefore underinstructed" (NRC 2006). At the Center for Spatial Studies at the University of California, Santa Barbara, we have constructed a comprehensive directory to this literature (http://www.teachspatial.org), and identified almost 200 fundamental concepts from the literatures of many disciplines.

Concluding Comments

The digital world that has come to dominate information in the twenty-first century is harsh and unforgiving, requiring as it does that all knowledge be expressed in a code of just two symbols, 0 and 1. Rigid rules are required to translate information into this alphabet, rules that are in many cases alien to the much less formal world of the humanities and social sciences. The advantages, however, are obvious: digital information can be shared, analyzed, and verified in ways that are impossible with less rigorously structured forms.

This chapter has examined the concept of *place* from this perspective. Comparisons are often drawn between place and *space*, arguing that the latter is rigidly scientific but substantively uninteresting. What role, for example, have latitude and longitude ever played in explaining society? Place is a rich concept, yet its inherent vagueness appears to make it irrelevant to the brave new world of digital scholarship.

Like other words such as system and object, place as a term is overloaded with alternative meanings. Separating those meanings may allow some of them to be defined with sufficient rigor to be formalized. This chapter has presented several examples of this nature, and shown how GIS techniques can be used to operationalize place in specific areas of research, whether it be by eliciting definitions of place from human subjects, by the use of mathematical functions in convolution, or by searching the Web for patterns of usage.

Several conferences over the past few years have drawn attention to the growing interest in spatially detailed analyses of human dynamics. Yet at this time, there is no single, comprehensive text on the topic, and courses in universities are few and far between. Given time, perhaps a new field will emerge at this intersection between digital technology, social science, and digital data. If it does, the concept of *place* will clearly occupy a central position.

Acknowledgments I thank Donald Janelle and Karl Grossner for their work in building the teachspatial.org site with its ontology of spatial concepts.

References

Burrough, P.A. and A.U. Frank, editors, 1996. *Geographic Objects with Indeterminate Boundaries.* London: Taylor and Francis.

Duckham, M., 2009. Keynote paper: representation of the natural environment. In N. Mount, G. Harvey, P. Aplin, and G. Priestnall, editors, *Representing, Modeling, and Visualizing the Natural Environment*, pp. 11–20. Boca Raton: CRC Press.

Eliot, J., 1987. *Models of Psychological Space: Psychometric, Developmental and Experimental Approaches.* New York: Springer-Verlag.

Foresman, T.W., editor, 1998. *The History of Geographic Information Systems: Perspectives from the Pioneers.* Upper Saddle River, NJ: Prentice Hall.

Fernández-Armesto, F., 2007. *Amerigo: The Man Who Gave His Name to America.* New York: Random House.

Gardner, H., 1999. *Intelligence Reframed: Multiple Intelligences for the 21st Century.* New York: Basic Books.

Goodchild, M.F., L. Anselin, and U. Deichmann, 1993. A framework for the areal interpolation of socioeconomic data. *Environment and Planning A* 25: 383–397.

Goodchild, M.F., M.J. Egenhofer, R. Fegeas, and C.A. Kottman, editors, 1999. *Interoperating Geographic Information Systems.* Boston: Kluwer Academic Publishers.

Goodchild, M.F. and L.L. Hill, 2008. Introduction to digital gazetteer research. *International Journal of Geographical Information Science* 22(10): 1039–1044.

Goodchild, M.F. and N. Lam, 1980. Areal interpolation: a variant of the traditional spatial problem. *Geoprocessing* 1: 297–312.

Hastings, J.T., 2008. Automated conflation of digital gazetteer data. *International Journal of Geographical Information Science* 22(10): 1109–1127.

Jones, C.B., R.S. Purves, P.D. Clough, and H. Joho, 2008. Modelling vague places with knowledge from the Web. *International Journal of Geographical Information Science* 22(10): 1045–1065.

Lopez, R.P., 2007. Neighborhood risk factors for obesity. *Obesity* 15: 2111–2119.

Maling, D.H., 1989. *Measurement from Maps: Principles and Methods of Cartometry.* New York: Pergamon.

Montello, D.R., M.F. Goodchild, J. Gottsegen, and P. Fohl, 2003. Where's downtown? Behavioral methods for determining referents of vague spatial queries. *Spatial Cognition and Computation* 3(2,3): 185–204.

National Research Council (NRC), 2006. *Learning to Think Spatially: GIS as a Support System in the K-12 Curriculum.* Washington, DC: National Academies Press.

Pickles, J., editor, 1995. *Ground Truth: The Social Implications of Geographic Information Systems.* New York: Guilford.

Silverman, B.W., 1986. *Density Estimation for Statistics and Data Analysis.* London: Chapman and Hall.

Sui, D.Z. and M.F. Goodchild, 2001. Guest editorial: GIS as media? *International Journal of Geographical Information Science* 15(5): 387–389.

Tobler, W.R., 1979. Smooth pycnophylactic interpolation for geographical regions. *Journal of the American Statistical Association* 74(367): 519–536.

Zhang, J.-X. and M.F. Goodchild, 2002. *Uncertainty in Geographical Information*. New York: Taylor and Francis.

Zook, M. and M. Graham, 2009. Mapping the GeoWeb: The spatial contours of Web 2.0 cyberspace. Paper presented at the Annual Meetings of the Association of American Geographers, Las Vegas.

Chapter 3
Spatial Polygamy and the Heterogeneity of Place: Studying People and Place via Egocentric Methods

Stephen A. Matthews

This map possibly isn't the way things are. But it is one of the ways they could be.

Pratchett (1995) – The Discworld Mapp

Introduction

For most of the past 20 years, I have lived in a Metropolitan Statistical Area (MSA). My commute to the university is 4 miles, a comfortable 25–40 min between my front door and the office door, via a drop-off at a childcare center. The commute from my place of residence to place of work passes through eight census tracts or along streets that provide invisible dividing lines between adjacent census tracts. Along the way, I also cross or travel along numerous other invisible boundaries passing through census blocks, census block groups, elementary school catchment areas, middle school catchment areas, county subdivisions, planning zones, voting precincts, state congressional districts, and ZIP codes (see Fig. 3.1). If I deviate off my routine commute, I will cross over many other additional boundaries, some more fuzzy than others, that include T-communities (see Grannis 1998, 2008), Catholic parishes, store catchment areas, and pizza delivery areas to name just a few. None of these boundary lines are visible on the ground. While some of these multiple boundaries are formally acknowledged by local government, various agencies, and the US Post Office, many are probably not known by the local residents. Even if these boundary lines were known to residents, they would probably not match up with the residents' subjective definition of their neighborhood or other neighborhoods in the MSA. More importantly, I would argue that the bounded

S.A. Matthews (✉)
Department of Sociology, Population Research Institute,
The Pennsylvania State University, University Park, PA, USA
e-mail: sxm27@psu.edu

L.M. Burton et al. (eds.), *Communities, Neighborhoods, and Health*,
Social Disparities in Health and Health Care 1, DOI 10.1007/978-1-4419-7482-2_3,

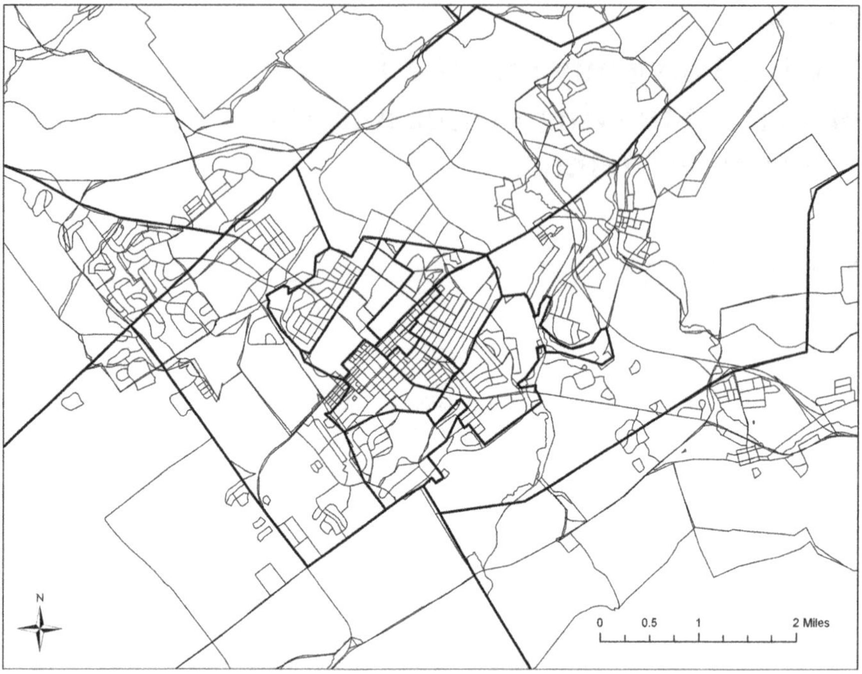

Fig. 3.1 Part of the State College, Pennsylvania MSA. The *faint lines* represent the overlay of several different statistical boundary areas (including census blocks, block groups, state legislative areas, and ZIP codes). The census tract statistical areas are shown in the *thicker line*

statistical areas do not capture the spatial behavior or movement of most residents during the course of their typical day.

I emphasize my place of residence (my statistical neighborhood), my commute, and the nested and nonnested nature of "place(s)" – variously defined – in this way because in the academic world of social and health science research, the residential census tract has become the "statistical unit" of choice for linking individuals to a place. It is still rare that we think about linking individuals to multiple or hierarchically nested or hybridized places. Therefore, if I were the subject of a sociological or health study, the measured attributes of my place (i.e., my residential census tract) would be linked to any individual level measures about me utilizing a geocoded street address or geographic code for my area of residence. This approach not only privileges area-based definitions of the residential neighborhood, but it also assumes that the factors that mediate determinants of health can be found and more importantly measured (I assume without error) at this level or unit of analysis, and often *only* at this level. This is "the local trap" (Cummins 2007). If all census tracts were the same size – they are not – this would suggest that the mechanisms and processes by which place "gets under the skin" (Taylor et al. 1997) are also scale invariant. We ignore what we know about how the multivariate relationships between ecological variables can change as units of analysis change (for a demonstration of the modifiable areal unit problem, see Fotheringham and Wong 1991). We are also assuming that the relationships between variables and outcomes are stationary across places. And, as the place of analysis is treated as an isolated island, we also ignore any possible mediating role of attributes found in adjacent or nearby extra-local places. And, we typically do not collect information on respondent mobility to extra-local places. There are other problematic assumptions made too. The conventional approach is usually static in that links between the individual and the place, and the attributes of place, occur only at one point in time. Finally, unless data are collected on residential histories of the respondent, the research privileges current residential location. In summary, there would appear to be a lot of omitted data on the respondent and how they use space as well on embedded, adjacent and other types of hybrid places. Terry Pratchett, a leading British science fantasy author, made a very insightful observation that relates to how researchers make choices regarding an appropriate scale of analysis in ecological and/or multilevel modeling, about map design, spatial autocorrelation, and spatial nonstationarity (where the relationship between variables varies across places). To paraphrase Pratchett (1995), the results we see based on conventional methods that embed an individual in a bounded, static, single-level, and isolated place may not be the way things are but it is one of the ways it could be. We need to explore the other ways things could be too.

My goal in this chapter is to raise awareness about the assumptions many of us make in our research, me included, and to move toward new ways of thinking about people and place, and place attachment. I will introduce and define spatial polygamy and briefly critique the measure of place based on residential units such as the census tracts. It is important to note that the critique of the assumption of bounded, static, and isolated units in studies of place is not new.

To illustrate this, I will review some literature from sociology and geography and some from almost a century ago. The empirical sections of the paper introduce two different types of research that seek to explore and better understand relationships between people and place. Using data gathered in ethnographic studies, I will show the complexity of lived lives and how the use of multiple place(s) varies in juggling different individual and family responsibilities among low-income and minority families. I believe that local places do matter for low-income and minority families but I will demonstrate that while their spatial range may be more constrained than those with access to resources they too are users of nonresidential places. That is, the material I present should not be used to suggest that the residential place is unimportant for individuals with less autonomy and control over their own lives, less freedom of movement or who spend time at a limited set of locations such as children, the disabled, and the elderly. We just need to know about the ties to nonresidential places too. An approach based on secondary data from the US Census demonstrates a different way in which research on places can be more explicit about issues of scale and the spatial relationships between places. These two very different examples will be followed by a brief discussion of the research potential afforded by developments in new tracking technologies, innovative data collection methods, and methodological tools.

Spatial Polygamy

We know from personal experience that key anchor points or nodes (e.g., the places we work, worship, shop, play, and receive health) and journeys between anchor points are important to us in terms of how we perceive and define as well as use and interact with places (see Lynch 1960; Lee 1968; Gould and White 1974; Tuan 1974, 1977; Michelson 1976; Golledge and Stimson 1997). The relative importance of these anchor points varies across space and time. Structured daily routines differentiate home place and workplace. Other less frequent activities take us to potentially new sets of places where we shop or find entertainment. The temporal rhythm of these activities may vary and the journeys to and between them may include coupled activities and/or be tasks undertaken alone or with others; this is true of daily commuting, weekly shopping, monthly visits to friends/relatives, and annual vacations. Our lives are complex. But so far we are only scratching the surface. If we extend the temporal horizon, many of us will likely have attachments to places of birth, childhood, family vacations, college, marriage, and all the places lived in accumulated over our lifetime thus far. Some individuals have attachment to places and times through ancestors too (see Walters et al., Chap. 10). And, while some places may be distant temporally and spatially, the continual development of communication technologies and the Internet provide ways of visiting the people in a social network and the places of attachment.

The spatial polygamy, I speak of in the title of this paper, is a characterization of how most of us think about, use, and relate to specific places. The essence of the spatial polygamy argument is that people, for the most part, are not loyal to a single place. Many of us enjoy intimate relations with multiple places, and we do so simultaneously. The simultaneity of attachment to multiple places can reside *within* a person and may do so throughout long periods of their lives. That is, as most international migrants will tell you the phrase "you can take the person out of the country but you cannot take the country out of the person" seems to hold true. For example, I have no doubts about who I will be supporting in the World Cup soccer match between England (my place of birth) and the USA in June 2010. I have no doubts because even though I have spent roughly equal amounts of time in both countries, the first memories and experiences are formative in terms of developing language, social skills, behaviors, traits, and identity, including place-based identity. You cannot tell, or perhaps you can, but I write in an English accent.

The simultaneity of place attachments can also occur *within* a short-time frame (e.g., a day). Within a typical day, many of us will spend some time at home, some at work, and perhaps at some places in between the two. Our spatial range or activity space may be bounded, but we are mobile and will visit different type of places for different reasons. A pure simultaneity exists when we visit or are tied to two or more places at once; a task facilitated via use of communication technologies and the Internet. This may be an extreme example, but as I write this chapter I am sitting at home in the USA wondering whether England will be victorious against South Africa in a cricket match being played in Cape Town and if a tennis player in

Melbourne, Australia will be the first male Brit to win a "major" in 70+ years. I should note that Andy Murray is a Scot, but the English have the bad habit of referring to anyone from Scotland, Wales, or Northern Ireland as British when it brings credit to them through a higher place-based labeling. I can also use more traditional ways of transporting myself to another time and place via reading fiction and nonfiction. I can even visit imagined places such as the science fantasy novels of Terry Pratchett in his Discworld series.

Some may claim that there are people who are loyal to one place and that only one place matters. This may be so but unless we are talking about ties based on nationality and relatively large geographic areas, I suspect that places as defined by statistical boundaries, boundaries that most of us could not identify, that mark off our residential census tract or our residential ZIP code are not the *one* place we think of. Let me try to defend my claim. We will start with some observations about the census tract. Although I focus my critique and attention on census tracts, it is important to note that some researchers have used other geographically defined "statistical" units such as the ZIP code (which on a personal level I have trouble defending) or school district (which I do not).

The Residential Census Tract as Place?

Today researchers, of many different stripes, are comfortable using data on, and aggregating data to, census tracts, and these statistical units are synonymous with definitions of neighborhood and by extension place. The advantage of census tracts is based on the perception that they are "standardized, quasi-neighborhood units" (Lee et al. 2008).

The census tract is officially defined as a compact, recognizable, and homogeneous territorial unit with relatively permanent boundaries; they usually have between 2,500 and 8,000 residents and an optimum population of about 4,000 people (U.S. Census Bureau 1997). But while there is quite considerable heterogeneity in the population size of census tracts, the phrase most commonly stated by researchers about them is that their average population size is approximately 4,000 people. Does anyone check this? In 2000, in the lower 48 states, the mean population size was approximately 4,300 and a quarter of all census tracts had either fewer than 2,500 or greater than 8,000 residents. An equally important issue is that census tracts (and other units) have very different daytime and night time populations in terms of both total numbers and composition. The area around downtown and the university campus where I work easily accommodates upwards of 40,000 temporary residents during the middle of the day but the resident population is one-tenth that number. This diurnal variation is dwarfed by the 110,000 people who call the hallowed ground in the football stadium "home"; a stadium that on 8 days per year is in population terms the third largest MSAs in the state of Pennsylvania after Philadelphia and Pittsburgh. I realize that these are extreme examples but I mention these as a reminder that the census variables most of us utilize are based on the characteristics of the population of residence on a single census enumeration night (at least until the American Community Survey is available). I also want to suggest that more use should be made of noncensus data on the built, social, and physical landscape of places, including census tracts. Noncensus data might reveal very different characteristics and functional uses of the places of interest to us.

Now let us consider the compactness of census tracts. Briefly, the heterogeneity in the size of the geographic footprint of the census tract is enormous but this is rarely, if ever, mentioned (though I acknowledge that some researchers do use area to create a measure of population density). The impression one gets from many papers, however, is that a census tract is a census tract is a census tract. They might as well be equal in size and shape. Descriptive statistics in a published article might provide the mean and standard deviation of a variable (e.g., the poverty rate) at the census tract level but how many times are the mean and standard deviation of the area of the census tracts in the study area presented. Perhaps it does not matter how big or small census tracts are. Well, my residential census tract, falling within the city limits, just 4 miles from downtown and containing approximately 4,300 residents is a census tract with a land area of 31.8 square miles. Admittedly, 31.8 square miles put my residential MSA census tract in the top 10% of all metro census tracts based on area but that would be missing the point.

In 2000, in the MSA counties in the lower 48 states, the mean size of a census tract was 13.7 square miles. I wonder how many readers would have guessed that number and/or can visualize what an average census tract looks like on the ground? Of course, the distribution of census tract sizes is highly skewed. In MSA counties in the lower 48 states, the median size of a census tract is approximately 1.25 square miles and three-quarters of all MSA census tracts are less than 4.5 square miles. Is this skew all because of the large census tracts found in Riverside-San Bernardino-Ontario, CA MSA? If only it were that simple. The median tract size in 2000 was less than 1 square mile in 22 of the top 100 MSAs but over 3 square miles in 13 others. Three square miles are equivalent to the area of a circle with a radius of approximately 1 mile. Among the top 100 MSAs, the interquartile range for census tract size among the low-density MSAs was 1 square mile in size at the 25th percentile to over 10 square miles at the 75th percentile. In 23 of the top 100 MSAs, there are census tracts that are less than a square mile in size and other census tracts that are over 500 square miles.

What does this all mean? Well perhaps, it suggest that when we start to measure factors that might mediate the role of the built and social environment on health and other outcomes, it would be wise to avoid binary measures such as presence/absence of these resources (e.g., food stores, alcohol outlets, clinics, parks, and schools) without appropriate consideration for the heterogeneity of both population and geographical size and shape of census tracts across a study area. We also might want to look at the resources in, and the relationship between, adjacent or nearby census tracts. We live in a continuous world not one bounded by arbitrary boundaries. For example, despite the large size of my residential tract when based on assets, or lack thereof, my residential census does not contain a large grocery store, a high school, a hospital, or a mall, and my daughter's elementary school – usually seen as an anchor institution within a local neighborhood – is in an adjacent census tract. My census tract does have parks, alcohol outlets, a post office as well as both fast food and full-service restaurants. Do I really live in a food desert area lacking a grocery store but containing fast food restaurants? Well yes, if a food desert is defined using either a count or a binary indicator (i.e., presence/absence) of grocery stores and fast food outlets based on census tracts. What about my family's spatial behavior? We must buy our groceries somewhere. Indeed, in looking at the resources, we use as a family the majority of them are outside my residential tract. I also do not live at the center of my census tract, so when I say my daughter's school is in an adjacent census tract, it is important to note that it is within a mile of home if you flew or about a mile-and-a-half if you drove. These census tract boundaries do mess things up. Is this type of observation new? No.

Spatial Polygamy and Everyday Ties to Nonresidential Places

Galster (2001, p. 2111) noted that urban sociologists "have treated 'neighborhood' in much the same way as the courts have treated pornography: a term that is hard to define precisely but everyone knows it when they see it." Similarly, researchers such as Coulton et al. (2001), Furstenberg et al. (1999), and Lee and Campbell (1997) have all noted that individuals and families, even those living in close proximity to one another, do not share a common definition of neighborhood and moreover when interviewing the *same* respondent over time the definition of neighborhood can change.

While it would be easy to believe that criticisms of boundaries and definitions of neighborhood emerged recently, McKenzie in 1921 (reprinted 1923) wrote that "probably no other term is used so loosely or with such changing content as the term neighborhood, and very few concepts are more difficult to define" (pp. 344–345). He further went on to note – in 1921 no less – that "the concept of neighborhood has come down to us from a distant past and therefore has connotations which scarcely fit the facts when applied to a patch of life in a modern large city" (p. 346). McClenahan (1929, 1946) was among the first to recognize the significance of nonlocal community ties, defining this as "communality." In 1946, McClenahan wrote:

> Any city dweller can test for himself the meaning of his place of local residence.
>
> If he will list his major activities and then spot their focal centers on a map he will quickly discover that his associations and his associates are rarely to be found in the immediate vicinity of his home. Nor will he ordinarily find the home of his best friend in his neighborhood. (pp. 272–273).

During the 1950s, several sociological studies identified the functional rather than spatial organization of society, the rise in mobility across urban space, the rise in anonymity, and the growing lack of identification with residential areas (see, e.g., Foley 1950; Smith et al. 1954; Axelrod 1956; Greer 1956; Bell and Boat 1957).

By the 1960s, urban sociology had been introduced to the "community of limited liability" where local participation depended on attachment to community (Greer 1962) and the "community without propinquity" or spatially dispersed, nonplace communities (Webber 1963). Later still sociologist discussed "community liberation" (Wellman 1979; Wellman and Leighton 1979). At the turn of the century, researchers began to look at new and more complex forms of extended social networks, long-distance travel, and communications; for example "networks in the global village" (Wellman 1999) and the "new mobilities research" (Larsen et al. 2006).

In addition to the lineage within sociology of attachment to place and the complexity of everyday life in and across diverse social contexts, there has been a focus on the *emplacement* of human behavior (Gieryn 2000). We can find evidence of the emplacement of people within nested hierarchies of place in the work of Suttles' (1972), in Jacobs' (1961) levels of neighborhood (the block, the community/district, and the city), and even more generally within Bronfenbrenner's (1979) ecological perspective and typology of multiple, overlapping, individual, and environmental contexts. Given this literature – and an extensive one outside sociology in disciplines such as geography, planning, and environmental psychology – it is surprising that single-level, bounded, static, and isolated census tracts have been the analytical unit of choice when linking people to place.

In my own work, I have explored people's use of places via geo-ethnography (Matthews et al. 2005; Skinner et al. 2005). Geo-ethnography is not a theory but an approach and a descriptive model that can shed light on the interrelatedness of human behavior, time, space, and place(s). The limitations on human behavior caused by temporal and geographic constraints are inescapable but are rarely incorporated into social science frameworks. The convention in time-geography approaches is to look at societal constraints and *potential* activity spaces. In geo-ethnography, however, the focus is on the actual or *realized* activity patterns and the functional ties existing between people and place(s). In this sense, geo-ethnography is similar to the recent studies of commuting data and travel diaries within a geographic information system (GIS) (see Kwan 1999, 2000, 2002) though how data are collected, integrated, and analyzed are quite different; though see Kwan's recent work on geo-narratives (Kwan and Ding 2008).

Geo-ethnography involves the extraction of references to place(s) and journeys from field notes and data generated in ethnographic studies. As noted above in other papers, I and others have discussed the significance of and meaning of place(s) and social networks in the lives of low-income families (see also Roy et al. 2004; Matthews unpublished manuscript). Here I am glossing over a complex process and downplaying what we learn from the voices of the families about *their* places and *their* journeys, specifically the choices they make over modes of transportation, the stores they buy food and clothes, their places of work, and the sites of encounter with the medical and social services. That is from the family narratives we do know more about the "how" and "why" questions. For my immediate purposes, the emphasis is on the "where" question, summarizing aggregate patterns and visualizing function ties. I will present data on ten families residing in one "ethnographic" neighborhood in Boston (in the larger ethnographic study data were collected on 43 families living in different areas of the city – see Winston et al. 1999 for an overview of the study design). From the field notes on these ten families, reference to the utilization of 222 unique places (excluding their home place) was identified. All of these places were geocoded and classified into one of nine domains of everyday life: child care, education, food shopping, nonfood shopping, health services, social services, social networks, work, and recreation. The spatial patterning of these 222 places, the distribution of their aggregate functional ties is shown in Fig. 3.2. This pattern might not look surprising or remarkable. To me, that is a good thing as it supports my main argument.

Let us consider the distribution of places in relation to census tract boundaries (see Table 3.1). Of the 222 locations, just 14 (6%) were found in the residential census tract of the participants and only another 47 (or 21% of the total) were located in immediately adjacent (i.e., neighboring) census tracts. Seventy-three percent of all locations used by the families were scattered across the city – these were the places where members of the families work, access childcare, shop for food and nonfood products, access health and social services, interact with social network members, and play (see Table 3.1). This pattern holds up across families in other neighborhoods in the larger study where overall the percent of functional ties to places in the home census tract was just 6% of the total, in adjacent tracts 20%, and thus in non-adjacent tracts 74%. Again, this type of observation is not new.

Research in geography, psychology, sociology, and urban planning finds considerable heterogeneity in spatial behavior and place attachment among people living in the same "neighborhood" (Golledge and Stimson 1997; Sastry et al. 2002). Moreover, given the volume of social science research undertaken on topics such as social support networks, migration and residential relocation, facility accessibility and utilization, participation in local organizations, race/ethnic segregation, marriage markets, commuting, and the spatial mismatch between home and workplace none of the observations about the places we spend time should be of any surprise. McClenahan (1946), Foley (1950), and others all predicted that many lines of functional interdependency extend out from a designated residential district.

In a second ethnography study, based in rural and small town communities, we have incorporated the collection of a 7-day activity log coupled with neighborhood and social network protocols to help generate more complete data on the frequency, duration and the sequencing of trips, the use of local and nonlocal resources, and role of social networks. While residential census tracts in rural areas and small towns are on average larger than within cities, so too are the distances that families traverse – and in many cases the time taken – to go to work, shop, visit family and friends, or receive health care. Figure 3.3 includes a visual representation of the frequency, duration, and sequencing of trips made over 7 days by one respondent. Note the scale bar and the areal size and shape of census tract and ZIP code boundaries, and the number of trips to places outside these boundaries. This is what the real world of invisible boundaries looks like if you map it.

We know much about time and time use (for example, Hochschild 1997; Presser 2003; Jacobs and Gerson 2004) and specifically about changes in household time budgets, the relative time spent at work or at leisure and the effects of such changes

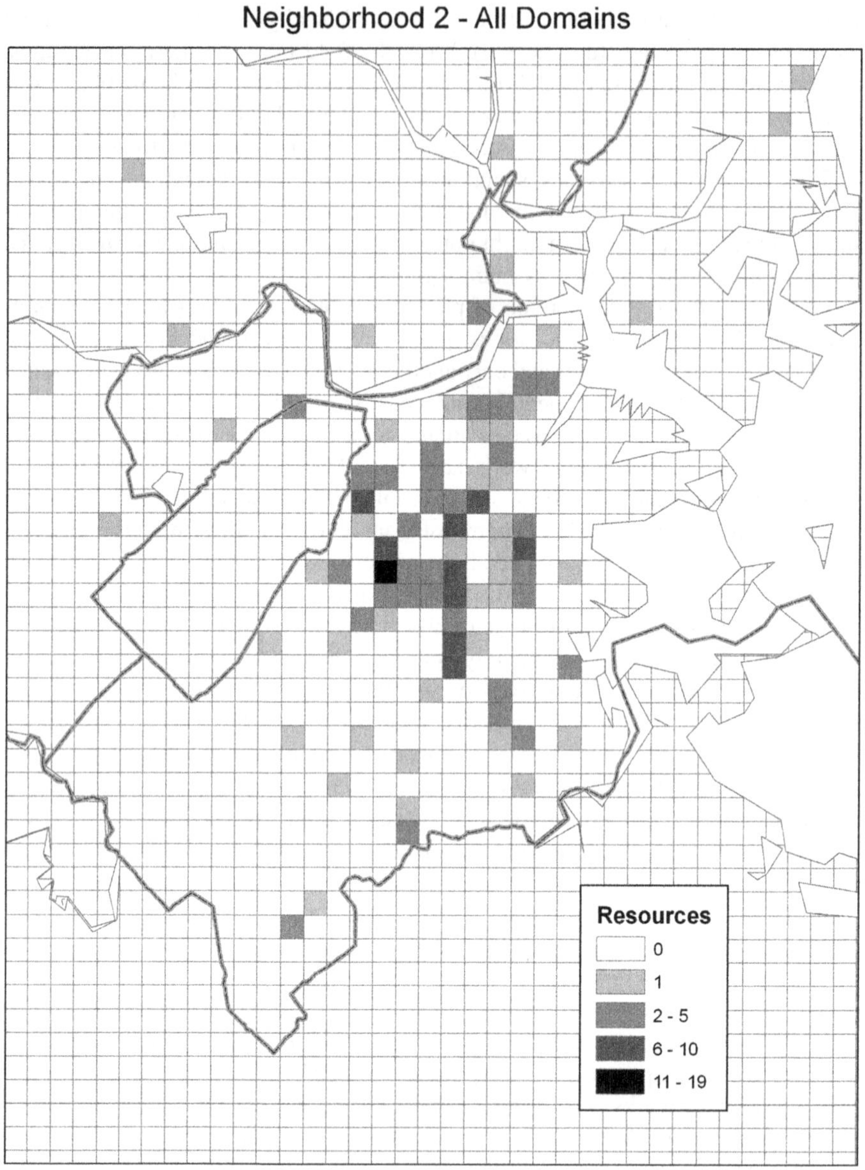

Fig. 3.2 A gridded surface of total family activities or resource sites ($n = 222$) based on ten families residing in one neighborhood. Each grid cell is 500 m by 500 m

in time spent in selected activities on family and child outcomes. However, surprisingly, few social scientists link time to movement across the urban environment and the functional ties to and use of specific places. Figure 3.4 illustrates two ways of viewing the activities of a focal mother over the course of 1 week. The activity

Table 3.1 Residential, adjacent and nonadjacent activity domains (rank-ordered by percent of activities in nonadjacent tracts; highest-to-lowest)

Domain	*N*	Residential tract	Adjacent tract	Nonadjacent tract
Social services	22	4.55	9.09	86.36
Work	11	9.09	9.09	81.82
Nonfood shopping	22	4.55	18.18	77.27
Childcare	15	0.00	26.67	73.33
Health services	45	6.67	20.00	73.33
Education	26	7.69	19.23	73.08
Social network	18	22.22	5.56	72.22
Other services	12	0.00	33.33	66.67
Food shopping	37	5.41	29.73	64.86
Recreation	14	0.00	42.86	57.14
Total	222	6.31	21.17	72.52

Ten families, 222 unique nonhome places

temporal component has been summarized in Fig. 3.4a, in which each shaded box indicate time spent outside the home on a 7-day/24-h grid. While there are many different types of activities, including coupled activities (data not shown), the dominant pattern for this focal mother is one of structure. On 5 of the 7 days, the mother leaves the home in the early hours of the morning and returns home during the evening. Scattered throughout the week are six shorter journeys. This family includes a focal mother, her young child, and her husband.

Now let us look at the spatial patterning of this focal mother's activity log (Fig. 3.4b); the circles represent the residential census tract. What does a focus on the spatial pattern reveal? In the example below try to focus on the *where* of both the mother and the child. On day 1, the mother wakes up early, leaves home with her infant and drives to work via her sister-in-law's house. The sister-in-law provides day care while she is at work for approximately 12-h. Later in the evening, the mother and infant collect the husband from his place of work. On day 2 (a Saturday), the mother goes to work, leaving home slightly later than on day 1 but still putting in long hours. The child stays at home with the husband. On day 3, the mother drives to work this time dropping off the infant with her sister. On day 4, the mother stays at home with her infant and during the course of the day makes one trip out of the house; a walk with her infant to a park and a nearby restaurant. Day 5 includes three short trips, dropping off her husband at work, a visit to a local grocery store, and then collecting her husband at the end of the day. Day 6 follows the same schedule as Day 3. On day 7, the mother travels to work via the sister-in-law's house but on the return journey stops at WalMart, in part because some items she wanted to buy were not available in the local grocery store. At the end of the day, the mother and infant drive to collect her husband from his place of work. Overall then, what looks like five long work days and a great deal of structure masks complex but coordinated childcare arrangements, arrangements that are scattered across people and places. Rather than use a single formal childcare provider, the parents use services from people they know and trust. During the week, the child spends upwards of

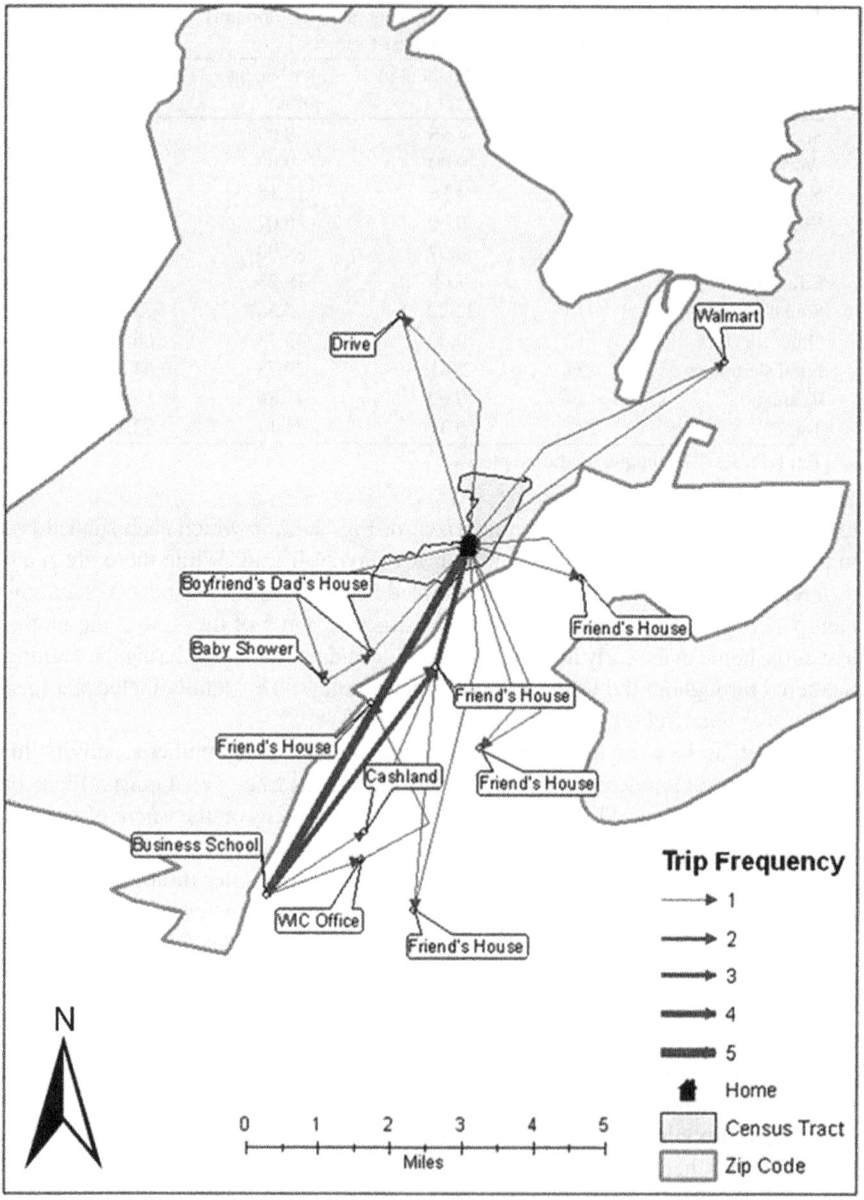

Fig. 3.3 A rural resident's actvity pattern over 1 week. Places visited are overlaid on top of the geographic footprint of the residential census tract and ZIP code

12-h on 4 of the 7 days at two different relatives' homes as well as spending full days at home with either the husband (1 day) or the focal mother (2 days).

This focus on the temporal and spatial together provides new insight on the extent of functional ties and their timing, duration, and sequencing of activities in places.

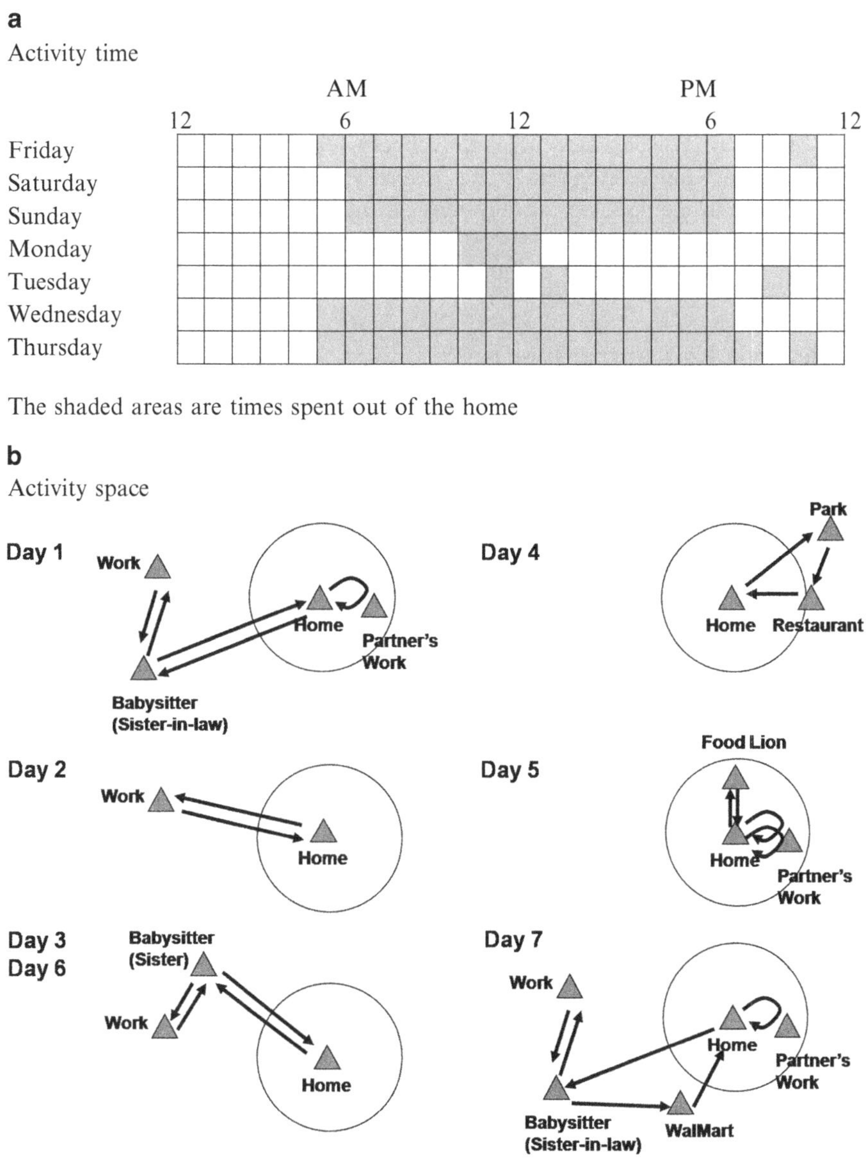

Fig. 3.4 Respondent 7-day activity log by (**a**) time and (**b**) space

The examples from Boston and from the rural, small town ethnography both show that we need to collect and measure functional ties and movement across place as well as better understand the choices and constraints behind each of these functional ties. As noted earlier, we also need to collect detailed data on life course trajectories across places not just focus on a single week of activity. We have only begun to scratch the surface but geo-ethnography can be used to provide insights in to perceptions of place and places and the meanings they hold for an individual. In some preliminary work with Linda Burton, we have conducted neighborhood walkthroughs with participants, tracking movements via global positioning systems (GPS), and recording personal narratives about the places where they grew up and have lived. I will discuss new tracking technologies in my final comments. What the examples in this section reinforce is a need for a reexamination of conceptual, theoretical, and methodological questions on the relationship and functional ties between people and place.

Scale-Free Egocentric Places

To date, I have focused on the measure of people and their activities in places. Now I want to turn briefly to the measure of place. As someone who has worked in the field of GIS for many years, I can confirm that the easiest way to represent place, indeed the easiest one to operationalize, is to use administrative boundaries; though there is little guidance on which one boundary to use. How one operationalizes place, however, changes if the starting point is the individual. In a methodological study looking at residential racial and income segregation, my colleagues and I have been doing just that (see Reardon et al. 2008; Lee et al. 2008). Conventional segregation studies rely heavily on the use of race/ethnic data aggregated to units such as the census tract. Moreover, rarely are analyses presented simultaneously for two or more levels (e.g., the census block group and the census tract) and almost all analysis focuses on isolated units of analysis; that is, they are nonspatial (for an exception, see Wong 2004).

In our work, we move "beyond the census tract" and focus on egocentric local environments (Lee et al. 2008). The approach (described in detail by Reardon et al. 2008) calculates race/ethnic and income segregation measures for circular egocentric local environments of varying size. While this approach draws on small area census data and privileges residential location and the night time population distribution we are not tied to administrative units. We calculate neighborhood measures of race/ethnic and income segregation for nested local environments of 500, 1,000, 2,000, and 4,000 m radii. We argue that these radii reflect a continuum of neighborhoods from pedestrian neighborhoods through elementary catchments and other local institutional jurisdictions on up to areas capturing activities such as shopping, high school attendance, and worship. In this way, we can simultaneously embed an individual within different definitions of place. For any given point (a 50 m × 50 m cell), we can generate the measure of percent black for the census tract in which the cell is found as well as the percent black for any range of specified radii.

Figure 3.5 shows proportion black for each point (i.e., a grid cell on the map of 50 m × 50 m) for part of the Atlanta–Sandy Springs–Marietta, Georgia metropolitan area using a 4,000 m radius. A biweight kernel, an approach that approximates a Gaussian (normal curve) shape, weights nearby locations more heavily

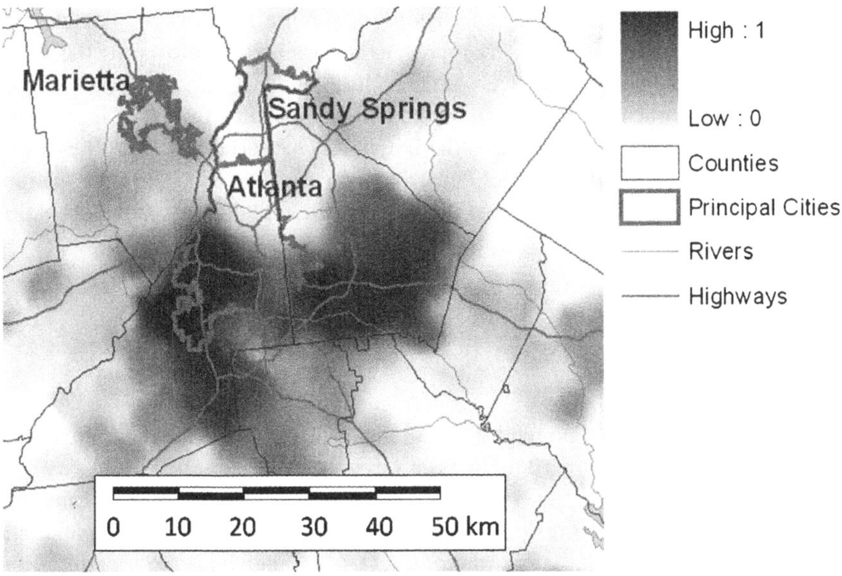

Fig. 3.5 Spatially weighted surface of percent black in part of the Atlanta – Sandy Springs – Marietta metropolitan area, 2000 (using a 4,000 m, biweight kernel). Based on the NSF project Measuring Spatial Segregation (grants SES-0520400 to Reardon and SES-0520405 to Matthews). For more information on the method see Reardon et al. (2008) and http://www.pop.psu.edu/mss

than more distant locations up to the radial distance. That is, when a census tract in central and south Atlanta might be 90% black, we can measure percent black at different scales (e.g., at 4,000 m radii). In parts of Atlanta, black –white segregation occurs at a macroscale, with densely populated black areas being as much as 20 km across. An African-American living in a low-income, high-percent black census tract in the middle of this area in south Atlanta is living in a very different type of place than an African-American living in a low-income, high-percent black census tract on the edge of this area. The difference is based on relative exposure to people of other races/ethnicities. While our approach has its conceptual weaknesses, the replacement of tracts with egocentric local environments will allow investigators to think in a more spatially sophisticated manner about linkages between exposure to risk (e.g., environmental hazards, crime) and access to resources and opportunities (schools, clinics, and grocery stores). The approach we use can easily be extended to other nominal or ordinal census variables.

This segregation work looks at easily constructed geometric local environments as a flexible definition of embedded places. Of course, the real world is not like this. We do not live in an isotropic world or possess perfect knowledge of all people and all places in all directions around us. Rather the inherently asymmetric world constrains movement, knowledge, and interaction. That is, we live in anisotropic world in which movement is easier in some directions than others. For example, compare the aggregate geographic footprint or area of all the locations you can reach within a 15-min walk from where you are standing assuming no barriers or friction of movement to the area you can reach, if you are constrained to follow only the street/sidewalk network (see Chaix et al. 2009). Our spatial segregation surfaces and place-specific profiles that can be generated are refinements over the single-level, nonspatial approaches that dominates the literature. Our surfaces and profiles represent another way the world could be. For us, the next steps should include modifications to account for the real world of street networks, terrain, hydrology, and distribution of the population by day.

Where Next?

The findings from geo-ethnography and the measuring spatial segregation studies are consistent with emerging directions in research on health and place. The geo-ethnography-related examples reinforce the existence of spatial polygamy and suggest that a focus on the residential neighborhood ignores important spatial and temporal dimensions of daily life (and of lives). More data on activity patterns and extra-local ties would enable researchers to better quantify residential and nonresidential exposure (Inagami et al. 2007) to both risks and resources and to better understand the decisions, constraints, and trade-offs faced every day. If we are to get a better handle on the importance of place(s) future studies will likely need to think about collecting space–time information on everyday functional connections at the conceptualization of new projects. This might best be incorporated using GPS, PDAs, and cell phones, and next generation wireless technologies that facilitate intensive longitudinal data collection 24/7 as well as ecological momentary assessments and activity logs that can capture information on the frequency, sequence, and duration of activities as well as data on other characteristics of journeys or movements across the urban environment (e.g., how?, why?, and who with?; see, e.g., Nusser et al. 2006). Recent studies of physical activity (Rodriguez et al. 2005), children and adolescent mobility (Elgethun et al. 2007; Wiehe et al. 2008), and accessibility research have used new tracking and wireless technologies such as GPS, and new forms of data (at least new to social scientists) are already being analyzed. An exciting research area is emerging around the integration of detailed social and spatial networks (see Faust et al. 1999; Entwistle et al. 2007; McCarty et al. 2007).

As the measuring spatial segregation component suggests, the definition of place and the spatial and temporal embeddedness of residential census tracts also need to be acknowledged. While there are challenges, an area of considerable promise for exploring extra-local effects lies at the intersection of multilevel analyses and spatial analysis (Subramanian et al. 2003; Chaix et al. 2005a, b). In an innovative approach, Chaix and colleagues specifically incorporate a continuous notion of space rather than relying on administrative boundary demarcations. Their spatial mixed models provide information not only on the magnitude but also on the scale of spatial variations and provide more accurate standard errors for risk factor effects in studies of both mental disorders in Malmo, Sweden and healthcare utilization in France. Their work suggests that in neighborhood studies, "a deeper understanding of the spatial variations in health outcomes may be gained by building notions of space into statistical models and measuring contextual factors across continuous space" (Chaix et al. 2005b p. 179). Nonnested multilevel models that permit assigning individuals to multiple nonnested contexts could also push the field forward.

While innovation in social and health research on place has been driven by new data, tools, and methods, it is fair to say that theoretical and conceptual development has lagged behind. One of the weakest areas of current practice is the conventional conceptions of place and our tenuous assumptions regarding place (Cummins et al. 2007; Matthews et al. 2009). Place is usually defined as administratively bounded, static, and as a series of isolated islands unconnected to other bounded units, divorced from the myriad of other contextual influences and power relationships that operate at different scales and can shape human behavior (Cummins et al. 2007). The time is ripe for updating our conceptual models of place and to take advantage of emerging technologies, methods, and data. More specifically, the research community should expect to be able to utilize new forms of data on human spatial behavior as well as new data on new measures of the attributes of place. These data should facilitate new ways of thinking about relative and absolute utilization and/or exposure to place, spatial embeddedness, and scales of analysis. Emerging statistical methods and new types of data coupled with reciprocal enhancements in conceptual models will help to push research on place and health forward.

Several commentaries on people and places and on neighborhoods and health have appeared in the sociological, epidemiological, and public health literature in recent years (for a selection, see Pickett and Pearl 2001; Ellen et al. 2001; Mitchell 2001; Sampson et al. 2002; Diez-Roux 2003; O'Campo 2003; Roosa et al. 2003; Frumkin 2006; Bernard et al. 2007; Matthews 2008). Some efficient starting points would include Macintyre et al. (2002), Cummins et al. (2007), and Chaix et al. (2009). And, if you want to experience how others think about interesting places, the warping of the space–time continuum, and affinity to place the science fantasy novels of Terry Pratchett should keep you entertained.

Acknowledgments The work presented in this chapter draws on ideas that have emerged from many years of thinking about people and places and from several projects that draw on geospatial data on both individuals and neighborhoods. Several people pushed and prodded me to pursue this track and/or have collaborated with me; these include, but are not limited to, Sandy Azar, Alan Benjamin, Nyesha Black, Yosef Bodovski, Linda Burton, Steven Cummins, Mark Daniel, Jim Detwiler, Glenn Firebaugh, John Iceland, Donald Janelle, Susan Kemp, Barrett Lee, Susan McHale, Brian McManus, Anne Vernez Moudon, Claudia Nau, David O'Sullivan, Sean Reardon, Luis Sanchez, Carla Shoff, Debra Skinner, David Takeuchi, and Tse-Chuan Yang. Brian McManus, Yosef Bodovski, and Carla Shoff (all of the Geographic Information Analysis Core, Population Research Institute at Penn State) helped prepare the figures. Any errors or misrepresentations that remain are mine. The term "spatial polygamy" I attribute to John Odland (the late Professor of Geography at Indiana University) made during an invited seminar to the Department of Geography at UCLA in the early 1990s. John died in 2009.

References

Axelrod, M. 1956. "Urban Structure and Social Participation." *American Sociological Review* 21 (1):13–18.

Bell, W. and M.D. Boat. 1957. "Urban Neighborhoods and Informal Social Relations." *American Journal of Sociology* 62:391–398.

Bernard, P., R. Charafeddine, K.L. Frohlich, M. Daniel, Y. Kestens, and L. Potvin. 2007. "Health Inequalities and Place: A Theoretical Conception of Neighborhood." *Social Science and Medicine* 65 (9):1839–1852.

Bronfrebrenner, U. 1979. *The Ecology of Human Development: Experiments by Nature and Design.* Cambridge, MA: Harvard University Press.

Chaix, B., J. Merlo, and P. Chauvin. 2005a. "Comparison of a Spatial Approach With the Multilevel Approach for Investigating Place Effects on Health: The Example of Healthcare Utilization in France." *Journal of Epidemiology and Community Health* 59:517–526.

Chaix, B., J. Merlo, S.V. Subramanian, J. Lynch, and P. Chauvin. 2005b. "Comparison of a Spatial Perspective with a Multilevel Analytical Approach in Neighborhood Studies: The Case of Mental and Behavioral Disorders Due to Psychoactive Substance Use in Malmö, Sweden, 2001." *American Journal of Epidemiology* 162 (2):171–182.

Chaix, B., J. Merlo, D. Evans, C. Leal, and S. Havard. 2009. "Neighborhoods in Eco-Epidemiologic Research: Delimiting Personal Exposure Areas: A Response to Riva, Gauvin, Apparicio and Brodeur." *Social Science & Medicine* 69 (9):1306–1310.

Coulton CJ, Korbin J, Chan T, Su M. 2001. Mapping residents' perceptions of neighborhood boundaries: a methodological note. *American Journal of Community Psychology* 29:371–383.

Cummins, S. 2007. "Commentary: Investigating Neighbourhood Effects on Health – Avoiding the 'Local Trap.'" *International Journal of Epidemiology* 36 (920):355–357.

Cummins, S., S. Curtis, A.V. Diez-Roux, and S. Macintrye. 2007. "Understanding and Representing 'Place' in Health Research: A Relational Approach." *Social Science & Medicine* 65 (9):1825–1838.

Diez-Roux, A.V. 2003. "The Examination of Neighborhood Effects on Health: Conceptual and Methodological Issues Related to the Presence of Multiple Levels of Organization." pp. 45–64 in *Neighborhoods and Health*, edited by Kawachi I. and L.F. Berkman. New York, NY: Oxford University Press.

Elgethun, K., M.G. Yost, C.T.E. Fitzpatrick, T.L. Nyerges, and R.A. Fenske. 2007. "Comparison of Global Positioning System (GPS) Tracking and Parent-Report Diaries to Characterize Children's Time-Location Patterns." *Journal of Exposure Science and Environmental Epidemiology* 17:196–206.

Ellen, I.G., T. Mijanovich, and K.-N. Dillman. 2001. "Neighborhood Effects on Health: Exploring the Links and Assessing the Evidence." *Journal of Urban Affairs* 23 (3–4):391–408.

Entwistle, B., K. Faust, R.R. Rindfuss, and T. Kenada. 2007. "Networks and Contexts: Variation in the Structure of Social Ties." *American Journal of Sociology* 112 (5):1495–1533.

Faust, K., B. Entwisle, R.R. Rindfuss, S.J. Walsh, and Y. Sawangdee. 1999. "Spatial Arrangement of Social and Economic Networks Among Villages in Nang Rong District, Thailand." *Social Networks* 21:311–337.

Foley, D.L. 1950. "The Use of Local Facilities in a Metropolis." *American Journal of Sociology* 56 (3):238–246.

Fotheringham, A.S. and D.W.S. Wong. 1991. "The Modifiable Areal Unit Problem in Multivariate Statistical Analysis." *Environment and Planning A* 23:1025–1044.

Frumkin, H. 2006. "The Measure of Place." *American Journal of Preventive Medicine* 31 (6):530–532.

Furstenberg, F.F. Jr., T.D. Cook, J. Eccles, G.H. Jr. Elder, and A. Sameroff. 1999. *Managing to Make It: Urban Families and Adolescent Success.* Chicago, IL: University of Chicago Press.

Galster, G. 2001. "On the Nature of Neighborhood." *Urban Studies* 38 (12):2111–2124.

Gieryn, T.F. 2000. "A Space for Place in Sociology." *Annual Review of Sociology* 26:463–495.
Golledge, R.G. and R.J. Stimson. 1997. *Spatial Behavior: A Geographical Perspective.* New York, NY: Guilford Press.
Gould, P. and R. White. 1974. *Mental Maps.* Harmondsworth, UK: Penguin Books.
Grannis, R.1998. "The Importance of Trivial Streets: Residential Streets and Residential Segregation." *American Journal of Sociology* 103:1530–1564.
Grannis, R. 2008. *From the Ground Up: Translating Geography into Community Through Neighbor Networks.* Princeton, NJ: Princeton University Press.
Greer, S. 1956. "Urbanism Reconsidered: A Comparative Study of Local Areas in a Metropolis." *American Sociological Review* 21:19–25.
Greer, S. 1962. *The Emerging City; Myth and Reality.* New York, NY: Free Press.
Hochschild AR. 1997. *The Time Bind: When Work Becomes Home and Home Becomes Work.* New York, NY: Metropolitan/Holt.
Inagami, S., D.A. Cohen, and B.K. Finch. 2007. Non-Residential Neighborhood Exposures Suppress Neighborhood Effects on Self-Rated Health. *Social Science & Medicine* 65 (8):1779–1791.
Jacobs, J. 1961. *The Death and Life of Great American Cities.* New York, NY: Random House.
Jacobs, J.A., Gerson, K. 2004. *The Time Divide: Work, Family and Gender Inequality.* Cambridge, MA: Harvard University Press.
Kwan, M.-P. 1999. "Gender and Individual Access to Urban Opportunities: A Study Using Space-Time Measures." *The Professional Geographer* 51:210–227.
Kwan, M.-P. 2000. "Interactive Geovisualization of Activity Travel Patterns Using 3-D GIS." *Transportation Research Part C* 8:185–203.
Kwan, M.-P. 2002. "Time, Information Technologies, and the Geographies of Everyday Life." *Urban Geography* 23 (5):471–482.
Kwan, M.-P. and G. Ding. 2008. "Geo-Narrative: Extending Geographic Information Systems for Narrative Analysis in Qualitative and Mixed-Method Research." *The Professional Geographer* 60 (4):443–465.
Larsen, J., J. Urry, and K. Axhausen. 2006. *Mobilities, Networks, Geographies* Aldershot, UK: Ashgate Publishing Limited.
Lee, T.R. 1968. "Urban Neighborhood as a Socio-Spatial Schema." *Human Relations* 21:241–267.
Lee, B.A. and K. Campbell. 1997. "Common Ground? Urban Neighborhoods as Survey Respondents See Them." *Social Science Quarterly* 78:922–936.
Lee, B.A., S.F. Reardon, G. Firebaugh, C.R. Farrell, S.A. Matthews, and D. O'Sullivan. 2008. "Beyond the Census Tract: Patterns and Determinants of Racial Segregation at Multiple Geographic Scales." *American Sociological Review* 73:766–791.
Lynch, K. 1960. *The Image of the City.* Cambridge: MIT Press.
Macintyre, S., A. Ellaway, and S. Cummins. 2002. "Place Effects on Health: How Can We Conceptualise, Operationalise and Measure Them?" *Social Science & Medicine* 55 (1):125–139.
Matthews, S.A. 2008. "The Salience of Neighborhood: Some Lessons from Sociology." *American Journal of Preventive Medicine* 34 (3):257–259.
Matthews, S.A. Unpublished Manuscript. "The Salience of Neighborhood: Some Observations and Lessons from Geo-Ethnography." Department of Sociology, Penn State. Manuscript available from the author.
Matthews, S.A., J. Detwiler, and L.M. Burton. 2005. "Geoethnography: Coupling Geographic Information Analysis Techniques with Ethnographic Methods in Urban Research." *Cartographica* 40 (4):75–90.
Matthews, S.A., A.V. Moudon, and M. Daniel. 2009. "Using Geographic Information Systems (GIS) for Enhancing Research Relevant to Policy on Diet, Physical Activity, and Weight." *American Journal of Preventive Medicine* 36 (4S):171–176.
McCarty, C., J.L. Molina, C. Aguilar, and L. Rota. 2007. "A Comparison of Social Network Mapping and Personal Network Visualization." *Field Methods* 19 (2):145–162.
McClenahan, B. 1929. *The Changing Urban Neighborhood.* Los Angeles, CA: University of Southern California.

McClenahan, B. 1946. "The Communality: The Urban Substitute for the Traditional Community." *Sociology and Social Research* 30:264–274.
McKenzie, R.D. 1923. *The Neighborhood: A Study of Local Life in the City of Columbus, Ohio*. Chicago, IL: University of Chicago Press.
Michelson, W.H. 1976. *Man and His Urban Environment*. Reading, MA: Addison-Wesley.
Mitchell, R. 2001. "Multi-level Modeling Might Not Be the Answer." *Environment and Planning A* 33:1357–1360.
Nusser, S.M., S.S. Intille, and R. Maitra. 2006. "Emerging Technologies and Next-Generation Intensive Longitudinal Data Collection." pp. 254–277 in *Models for Intensive Longitudinal Data*, edited by Walls T.A. and J.L. Schafer. Oxford, UK: Oxford University Press.
O'Campo, P. 2003. "Invited Commentary: Advancing Theory and Methods for Multilevel Models of Residential Neighborhoods and Health." *American Journal of Epidemiology* 157:9–13.
Pickett, K.E. and M. Pearl. 2001. "Multilevel Analysis of Neighborhood Socioeconomic Context and Health Outcomes: A Critical Review." *Journal of Epidemiology and Community Health* 55 (2):111–122.
Pratchett, T. 1995. "I Needed a Map." in *The Discworld Mapp: Being the Onlie True and Mostly Accurate Mappe of the Fantastyk and Magical Dyscworlde*, edited by Pratchett T. and S. Briggs. London, UK: Corgi Books.
Presser HB. 2003. *Working in a 24/7 Economy: Challenges for American Families*. New York, NY: Russell Sage Foundation.
Reardon, S.F., S.A. Matthews, D. O'Sullivan, B.A. Lee, G. Firebaugh, C.R. Farrell, and K. Bischoff. 2008. "The Geographic Scale of Metropolitan Racial Segregation." *Demography* 45 (3):489–514.
Rodriguez, D.A., A.L. Brown, and P.J. Troped. 2005. "Portable Global Positioning Units to Complement Accelerometry-Based Physical Activity Monitors." *Medicine and Science in Sports and Exercise* 37 (11):S572–S581.
Roosa, M.W., S. Jones, J.-Y. Tein, and W. Cree. 2003. "Prevention Science and Neighborhood Influences on Low-Income Children's Development: Theoretical and Methodological Issues." *American Journal of Community Psychology* 31 (1/2):55–72.
Roy, K., C. Tubbs, and L.M. Burton. 2004. "Don't Have No Time: Daily Rhythms and the Organization of Time for Low-Income Families." *Family Relations* 53:168–178.
Sampson, R.J., J.D. Morenoff, and T. Gannon-Rowley. 2002. "Assessing Neighborhood Effects: Social Processes and New Directions in Research." *Annual Review of Sociology* 28:443–478.
Sastry, N., A. Pebley, and M. Zonta. 2002. "Neighborhood Definitions and the Spatial Dimension of Daily Life in Los Angeles." *CCPR Working Paper* 033-04. Los Angeles, CA: California Center for Population Research, UCLA.
Skinner, D., S.A. Matthews, and L.M. Burton. 2005. "Combining Ethnography and GIS Technology to Examine Constructions of Developmental Opportunities in Contexts of Poverty and Disability." pp. 223–239 in *Discovering Successful Pathways in Children's Development: Mixed Methods in the Study of Childhood and Family Life*, edited by Weisner, T. Chicago, IL: MacArthur Foundation, University of Chicago Press.
Smith, J., W.H. Form, and G.P. Stone. 1954. "Local Intimacy in a Middle-Sized City." *American Journal of Sociology* 60 (3):276–284.
Subramanian, S.V., K. Jones, and C. Duncan. 2003. "Multilevel Methods for Public Health Research." pp. 65–111 in *Neighborhoods and Health*, edited by Kawachi I. and L.F. Berkman. New York, NY: Oxford University Press.
Suttles, G. 1972. *The Social Construction of Communities*. Chicago, IL: University of Chicago Press.
Taylor, S.E., R.L. Repetti, and T. Seeman. 1997. "Health Psychology: What Is an Unhealthy Environment and How Does It Get Under the Skin?" *Annual Review of Psychology* 48:411–447.
Tuan, Y. 1974. *Topophilia: A Study of Environmental Perception, Attitudes, and Values*. Englewood Cliffs, NJ: Prentice Hall.
Tuan, Y. 1977. *Space and Place: The Perspective of Experience*. Englewood Cliffs, NJ: Prentice Hall.

U.S. Census Bureau. 1997. *United States Census 2000: Participant Statistical Areas Program Guidelines*. Washington, DC: U.S. Census Bureau.

Webber, M.M. 1963. "Order in Diversity, Community Without Propinquity." Pp. 23–54 in *Cities and Space: The Future Use of Urban Land*, edited by Wingo, L. Baltimore, MD: Johns Hopkins University Press.

Wellman, B. 1979. "The Community Question: The Intimate Networks of East Yonkers." *American Journal of Sociology* 84 (5):1201–1231.

Wellman, B. 1999. *Networks in the Global Village: Life in Contemporary Communities*. Boulder, CO: Westview Press.

Wellman, B. and B. Leighton. 1979. "Networks, Neighborhoods and Communities." *Urban Affairs Quarterly* 14:363–390.

Wiehe, S.E., A.E. Carroll, G.C. Lui, K.L. Haberkorn, S.C. Hoch, J.S. Wilson, and J.D. Fortenberry. 2008. "Using GPS-Enabled Cell Phones to Track the Travel Patterns of Adolescents." *International Journal of Health Geographics* 7:22.

Winston P., R.J. Angel, L.M. Burton, P.L. Chase-Lansdale, A.J. Cherlin, R.A. Moffitt, and W.J. Wilson. 1999. *Welfare, Children and Families Three City Study: Overview and Design Report*. Baltimore, MD: Johns Hopkins University, Welfare, Children and Families Project.

Wong, D.W.S. 2004. "Comparing Traditional and Spatial Segregation Measures: A Spatial Scale Perspective." *Urban Geography* 25:66–82.

[illegible]

Chapter 4
Placing Biology in Breast Cancer Disparities Research

Sarah Gehlert, Charles Mininger, and Toni M. Cipriano-Steffens

The idea that place affects health has been accepted for some time, but the exact nature of the relationship remains unclear. Only a small handful of scholars from a variety of disciplines have posited pathways through which place might affect health, from affecting encounters between providers and patients to shaping identity and protecting psychological equilibrium. None is well-proven. Lacking, too, is consideration of a biological route between place and health. After a brief review of the existing literature on place and health, we present work done at the University of Chicago's Center for Interdisciplinary Health Disparities Research in which we have identified causal links between various levels of determinants of breast cancer, from the neighborhood and community to within the cell, among women newly diagnosed with the breast cancer living on the South Side of Chicago.

The Built Environment and Health

The built environment is one aspect of place that has been related to health. It encompasses all of the artifacts that are placed in the physical space, such as the physical structures, economic concerns, populations, and the type and quality of public throughways, roads, and transit services. These identifiable characteristics in turn provide the context in which interactions between individuals and all other actors, structures, networks, and organizations that inhabit or interact with the neighborhood take place. In this conceptualization, the built environment provides two fundamental functions. First, it generates opportunities for people to interact with one other to create social and economic possibilities. Second, based on the resources, organization, and aesthetic indicators that it provides, the built environment helps to establish the bounds of what is considered acceptable behavior and, thus, can be thought of as an informal means of monitoring behavior. In this regard,

S. Gehlert (✉)
The Brown School, Washington University, One Brookings Dr., St. Louis, MO 63130, USA
e-mail: SGehlert@wustl.edu

L.M. Burton et al. (eds.), *Communities, Neighborhoods, and Health*, Social Disparities in Health and Health Care 1, DOI 10.1007/978-1-4419-7482-2_4,

the built environment is akin to Foucault's conceptualization of the panopticon, with the "unequal gaze" that Foucault describes imbuing residents with the constant possibility of observation. At its maximum utility, the built environment acts to decrease the likelihood of deviation from accepted norms, because of the belief that individuals are being observed, even when they are not (Foucault 1977).

Empirical investigations of the effects of the built environment on health, while never directly testing pathways from one to the other, have suggested factors that might intervene between the two. These factors fall into two categories, namely perceptions of neighborhood characteristics and quality and affect on psychological functioning. The built environment, for instance, has been positively associated with residents' perceptions of their own safety (Taylor et al. 1985) as well as with their perceptions of community collective efficacy (Birtchnell et al. 1988; Sampson et al. 1997; Perkins et al. 1993; Cohen et al. 2000). The built environment also has been posited to alter health through its affect on mental health. Associations have been found between mental health and neighborhood density (Birtchnell et al. 1988; Coleman 1985), housing typology and space (Newman 1972, 1980), and services within the built environment (Barton et al. 2003).

Some scholars have focused on incivilities within the built environment and their effect on both perceptions and behavior. Although never providing a formal definition of the term, Coleman (1985) describes incivilities as characteristics of the built environment that negatively shape perceptions of neighborhoods and consequently, peoples' actions or behaviors derived from those perceptions. Perhaps the most influential paper on the subject is Wilson and Kelling's (1982) elaboration of their broken windows thesis, in which they argue that physical deterioration, if left unchecked, over time will erode community trust and informal control over public spaces, as well as promoting delinquency and crime (Markowitz et al. 2001; Sampson and Raudenbush 1999; Taylor 2001). Neighborhoods exhibiting high levels of incivilities and disorder may not only promote deleterious behavior, but, because of their lack of effective mechanisms of social control and surveillance, may attract serious offenders to those neighborhoods (Jacobs 1961; Taylor 1988).

Visible physical decay is an indication of the failure of neighborhoods' maintenance and social control mechanisms, which in turn heightens residents' fears. Observed incivilities such as decay that is visible serve as signals of what behaviors are and are not tolerated. As a result, incivilities become self-propagating, with current levels of disorder producing future levels of disorder (Skogan 1990). Physical deterioration may take the form of derelict buildings, vacant lots, unkempt yards, abandoned cars, graffiti, litter, vandalism, and excessive traffic. These features interfere with residents' ability to establish and maintain relations and attachments (Taylor 2001). Fear in this context is an affective state that reflects safety-related concerns about possible victimization (Ferraro 1994). Moreover, individuals who perceive higher numbers of local incivilities, or who are surrounded by less orderly conditions, report higher fear and greater perceived risk (1994). In addition, it can be argued that urban settings, by their very nature, imbue heightened levels of vigilance on the part of their residents, regardless of those residents' prior experiences with victimization. Participants in the National Crime Survey who lived in urban settings reported greater fear of potential victimization than did nonurban dwellers who had been the victims of crime (Cook and Skogan 1984; Dubow et al. 1979).

A number of investigators have found that unfavorable neighborhood conditions are associated with a myriad of negative health outcomes, including infectious disease (Acevedo-Garcia 2000, 2001), mortality (Yen and Kaplan 1999; McCord and Freeman 1990), low birth weight (Morenoff 2003; Roberts 1997; O'Campo et al. 1997), venereal disease (Cohen et al. 2000), smoking (Diez-Roux et al. 2003), physical inactivity (Booth et al. 2001), and depression (Aneshensel and Sucoff 1996). Specific attributes of the built environment have been implicated. Residents of high-rise housing projects, for example, experience more crime than those living in low-rise housing projects, such that the higher the building is, the higher rates of crime experienced (Rand 1984). Houses are more likely to be burglarized if they are in areas with higher speed limits, fewer fences, fewer signs of occupation, and less visual access to neighboring homes (1984). Also, buildings with more than 50 apartments thrust inhabitants into states of anonymity in which they treat each other as strangers, and are less likely to challenge strangers entering the buildings in which they live (Newman 1972).

The availability and quality of resources within the built environment likewise affect health and other outcomes. For example, whereas bars increase crime rates, recreation centers decrease crime rates but only in the most economically deprived communities (Peterson et al. 2000). Poor communities are also at a disadvantage with their lack of access to health-promoting services, such as health-care facilities (McKnight 1995; Hendryx et al. 2002) and grocery stores (Morland et al. 2002, 2006). In addition, levels of pollution and toxic waste are more common in low income than more affluent areas (Anderton et al. 1994; Vrijheid 2000). The same is true for lead paint and pest infestations (Pirkle et al. 1998).

In summary, studies of the built environment suggest factors that intervene between place and health. We know, for example, that the built environment affects health in a number of ways, such as shaping social networks and social interactions and the type and quality of resources available to residents. Yet, although important, this area of inquiry fails to provide an explanation for how the built environment and other features of neighborhoods and communities "get under the skin" to affect health (McClintock et al. 2005).

Culture, Place, and Health

A separate body of literature addresses how conceptions of place affect health beliefs and action and, in so doing, ultimately help to determine health outcomes. Medical geographers suggest that health beliefs and actions are culturally determined and place-based, and must be understood if one is to understand health (Gesler and Kearns 2002). Kearns and Barnett (1998) provides an example in which residents of a remote, predominantly Maori area of New Zealand mobilized against proposed health-care reforms, based on their place-based symbolic ownership of local health services. Under the proposed reform, the community, which had always had local access to health services, faced having to travel for basic services provided by the private sector. Their protest, which successfully resulted in community-run services, concerned "impending intrusions upon local life and sense of place" (Kearns and Barnett 1998).

Although arguments about how conceptions of place affect health through health beliefs and actions are compelling, they are unsatisfying. As was the case with the built environment and health, these arguments tease us by suggesting plausible factors that lie between place and health, yet fail to fully illuminate these factors. We are left with a "black box" between place and health, which further highlights our failure to understand how place "gets under the skin" to affect health.

Place Identity, Behavior, and Health

Environmental psychologists introduced the notion of place identity, a type of self identity connected to place, over three decades ago (Proshansky 1978; Proshansky and Kaminoff 1982; Proshansky et al. 1982; Krupat 1983). According to Proshansky and colleagues (1983), place identity is made up of cognitions about the physical world that occur at the conscious and unconscious levels. These cognitions are personal constructions determined by previous life experiences, which influence how people engage with their social and physical environments and the social roles that they assume (1983:62). Butz and Eyles (1997) have suggested that senses of place are neither purely individually determined nor entirely collectively determined, but instead are the products of social interaction mediated through individuals' subjectivities. In writing about place and the politics of identity, for instance, Hesse (1993) says that the politics of location and dislocation are intimately tied to the identities of blacks in Britain.

One way in which place identity might affect health is through maintaining psychological equilibrium throughout the life cycle. According to Proshansky et al. (1983:73), positive place identities "may function directly as anxiety and defense mechanisms." Physical settings that are congruent with place-identity expectations can protect the individual against low self-esteem. Conversely, incongruent physical settings and place-identity expectations may engender threat and pain. That place identity helps to maintain psychological equilibrium or well-being is bolstered by (Korpela 1989) the notion of active environmental self-regulation, in which the physical environment is used as a means of maintaining the psychic balance of pain and pleasure and the coherence of self and self-esteem. Stedman (2002) suggests that identity salience is based on cognitions of place, and to a lesser extent, on satisfaction with place. Positive identity salience can lead to what Stedman terms place-protective behaviors, such as taking care of one's neighborhood. One could imagine this notion extending to health-protective behaviors, that is to say that positive place identity might lead to health-protective behaviors.

Although compelling, the idea that sense of place might affect health by helping to maintain psychological equilibrium largely remains untested. Also, the concepts used have been criticized for their lack of clarity and the relationships between them have not yet been tested empirically. Nevertheless, the notion that place identity might affect health by helping to maintain equilibrium brings us closer to understanding how place "gets under the skin" to affect health.

The Center for Interdisciplinary Health Disparities Research: A Unique Approach to Linking Place and Biology

The four research projects of the Center for Interdisciplinary Health Disparities Research (CIHDR) provide an ideal mechanism for investigating the pathways through which place shapes biology and health, for two major reasons. First, as will be outlined in the following paragraphs, the team of CIHDR investigators comes from a variety of disciplinary backgrounds, allowing them to consider social, behavioral, and biological aspect of health in the same shared projects and analyses. Second, CIHDR investigators take a multilevel and multifactorial approach to health that considers influences from within the cell to the level of society.

CIHDR is one of eight Centers for Population Health and Health Disparities (CPHHD), funded by the National Institutes of Health (NIH) in 2003 to take a transdisciplinary approach to understanding and ameliorating health disparities. The overarching mission of the CPHHDs is to better understand the determinants of health disparities and devise appropriate multilevel interventions to ameliorate them (Warnecke et al. 2008).

The Black/White Disparity

In their first 6 years of operation, CIHDR investigators focused their investigations on black and white differences in breast cancer mortality. The four mutually informative, multimodal research projects together addressed the same shared research question, namely how factors in women's social environments contribute to the African American and white disparity in breast cancer mortality in the USA. Although white women in the USA are more likely to develop breast cancer than African-American women (130.6 per 100,000 white women and 117.5 per 100,000 for African American), African-American women are 37% more likely to die from the disease (24.4 per 100,000 for white women and 33.5 per 100,000 for African-American women) (Hoyert et al. 2006; Ries et al. 2008). The disparity is even higher in Chicago, with African-American women almost 68% more likely to die from breast cancer than white women (Hirschman et al. 2007).

The black and white disparity in breast cancer mortality cannot solely be due to biological or genetic differences between the two groups; 70–80% of breast cancers are due to sporadic or acquired rather than inherited mutations of breast cancer genes.

Based on the knowledge that breast cancer develops after a series of complex genetic interactions (McClintock et al. 2005), CIHDR investigators sought to understand how these acquired genetic mutations are regulated by the social environment, resulting in the survival of malignant cells, which accumulate to form breast cancer tumors. The process of biological, social, and behavioral scientists working in concert has allowed CIHDR investigators not only to explore the neighborhoods and communities in which women live and the course and outcomes of their breast cancers, but to investigate directly a series of hypothesized pathways between the two. The approach allows the CIHDR team to move beyond forming conclusions based on statistical correlations among variables at different levels to being able to identify causal steps that start with the place in which women live, move to their psychological reactions to those places, and become embodied by specific endocrine, immune, and neural events that regulate cell death (apoptosis), as well as the growth of tumors.

A Working Model

The CIHDR team tests a shared model that has changed as data accrue (Fig. 4.1). This model encompasses forces from the social and physical environment to apoptosis, or the failure of mutated cells to die, and the consequent development of tumors of breast cancer. From this lens, CIHDR's four projects, two animal and

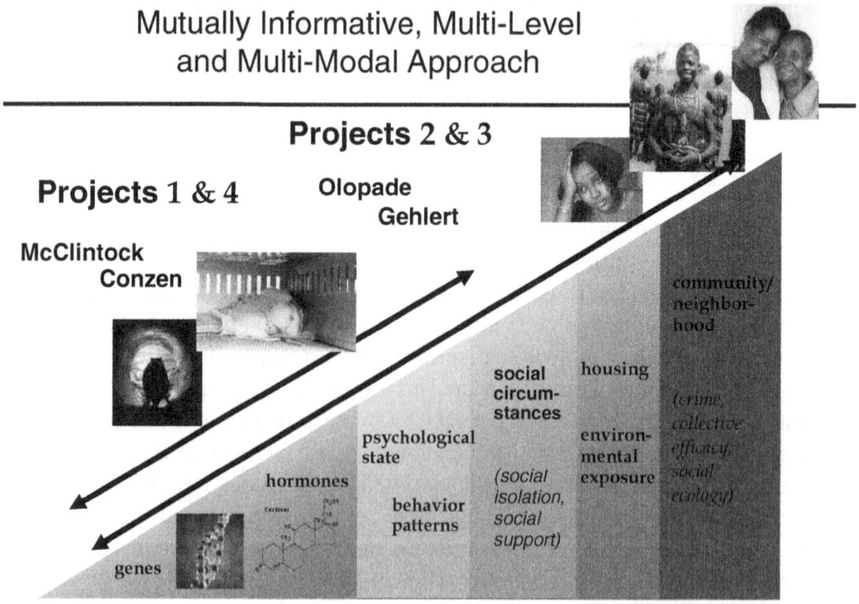

Fig. 4.1 Shared CIHDR model of African-American and white breast cancer health disparities

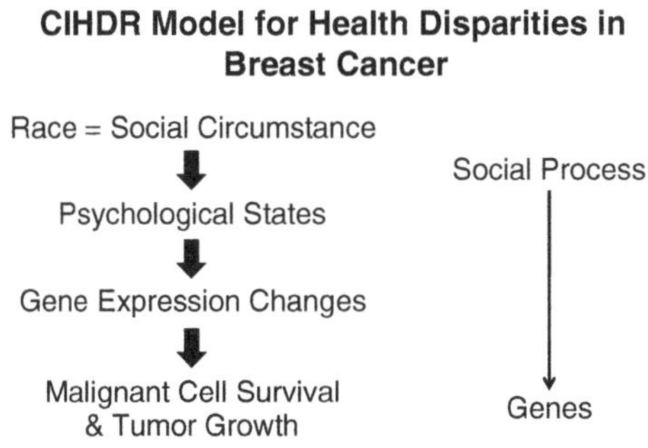

Fig. 4.2 CIHDR approach to understanding African-American and white differences in mortality between African-American and white women in the USA

two human (Fig. 4.2), explore the interactions of genetic mechanisms and neighborhood and community-level factors among a group of African-American women newly diagnosed with breast cancer living in specific neighborhoods on Chicago's South Side.

The Animal Models

Two of the four CIHDR projects use animal models. Sprague–Dawley rats have a genetically undefined predisposition for developing spontaneous mammary gland tumors, while SV40 Tag transgenic mice have a well-defined genetic predisposition for mammary gland cancer. Because mammary cancer in rats and mice mimics human breast cancer, manipulating the social environments of the two animal models allows investigators to explore pathways by which social and psychological factors "get under the skin" to influence disease. This approach has two main benefits. First, it allows social conditions to be manipulated using experiments (and psychological reactions, behavior, and biological processes to be measured). Second, it affords a perspective on gene and environment interactions throughout the life cycle of the organism. Social conditions can, for example, be manipulated at various points in the life cycle, such as during the period of puberty, and the affect on the development and course of mammary cancers can be measured.

McClintock and colleagues, in work on brain aging, identified spontaneous mammary tumors among animals that were socially isolated from the time of weaning. These isolated animals developed larger spontaneous mammary gland tumors at a much earlier age than did their group-housed peers (Hermes et al. 2006). These were also found to have dysregulated stress hormone responses, with higher levels of glucocorticoids from the adrenal cortex, even after a stressor had ended, and slower recovery to baseline (Hermes et al. 2009; Hermes et al. 2006).

The SV40 Tag transgenic mice developed a similar dysregulated glucocorticoid response (GR) to a stressor (Williams et al. 2009).

Findings from the work with animal models suggest that the natural variation in glucocorticoid response to social isolation predicts the timing of mammary tumorigenesis (Cavigelli et al. 2006). In addition, the activation of glucocorticoid receptors initiates a downstream signaling pathway that ultimately results in cell survival through suppression of apoptosis. Thus, higher reactivity to stress may predict earlier tumor development through heightened secretion of glucocorticoids. In addition, socially isolated transgenic mice ate significantly more than their group-housed peers, yet they maintained precisely their body weight, indicating a shift in the energetics of fat and glucose metabolism. This pointed to dysregulation of fat distribution as a second mediating pathway, consistent with the higher prevalence of abdominal adiposity among African-American women. Indeed, isolated mice had differential expression of glycolysis and fatty acid synthesis in the mammary gland, which may be linked to the increased malignant tumor growth in the isolated mice.

The Human Models

The remaining two CIHDR projects followed the same group of 230 African-American women newly diagnosed with breast cancer who were living in 15 predominantly African-American neighborhood areas of Chicago's South Side. One project analyzed the characteristics of their breast tumors while the other followed the women at 6-month intervals for a year and a half after their surgeries with in-home interviews and measurement of the built environments in a four-block area around each woman's home. In addition, publicly available data were obtained on factors such as crime, collective efficacy, services, etc., and geo-coded to each woman's address to form quarter-mile buffer zones. This was done to characterize women's physical and social environments and determine their responses to those environments. In both the human and animal research, a range of environments was measured to create daily stressors (e.g., high crime neighborhoods in humans or a overturned food dish in open-caged rats) or mitigate against them (e.g., collective efficacy in humans or returning an animal that was isolated to its social group), as well as the presence or absence of social support and affiliation in the face of these stressors.

The use of animal models and interviews and observations with women newly diagnosed with breast cancer was mutually informative and allowed the CIHDR team to test hypotheses across models. For example, informed by the findings connecting social isolation to mammary gland tumors, CIHDR investigators explored the issue of social isolation with South Side residents in a series of focus groups. They found that, among some residents, social isolation was associated with lack of desired supports and frequent moves. In response, investigators added measures of the coping styles when rats were moved to new environments. The subsequent findings of this work led to the development of CIHDR's Built Environment Team, to identify factors that impeded or enhanced social interactions and elicited vigilance on the part of residents.

Focus Groups in the Community

In its first year of operation, CIHDR investigators conducted a series of 49 community-based participatory focus groups of residents of the 15 South Side Chicago neighborhood areas that are the locus of their research, in order to ensure that local knowledge was used to understand African-American and white differences in breast cancer. Because no single community agency was well enough positioned to represent South Side concerns about breast cancer and related health issues, CIHDR used a grass-roots recruiting approach to reach community stakeholders.

After reviewing Chicago Department of Public Health data on each of the 15 neighborhood areas to ensure that the composition of focus groups would appropriately reflect their demographics (i.e., age, gender, socioeconomic status, and Muslim vs. Christian religion), CIHDR staff went into neighborhoods to distribute flyers and sent letters of introduction and spoke at community agencies, health clinics, churches, etc., inviting adults over 18 years of age to take part in groups.

Over 1,300 people called the number provided to volunteer. We selected 503 to form two to three groups per neighborhood area that (1) represented the demographics of the area, and (2) would result in groups heterogeneous in terms of age, gender, and socioeconomic status, while avoiding situations in which some person(s) in the group would be dominant over others (e.g., including a participant's work supervisor).

Each group had 10–12 participants and was facilitated by two staff members. The group interviews followed the approach outlined in Balshem's *Cancer in the Community* (1993), in which participants were asked broad questions to stimulate discussion, without biasing its nature and direction. The 2-h interviews were recorded, professionally transcribed, and analyzed using NVivo software (Salant and Gehlert 2008; Masi and Gehlert 2009). At the end of the CBPR focus group interview, participants were asked to review instruments to be used in scientific investigations and comment on their suitability and relevance to their concerns.

Following Newly Diagnosed Women

Informed by the work with animal models and the focus groups, the CIHDR team began recruiting women for the study, namely African-American women newly diagnosed with breast cancer living in 15 neighborhood areas of Chicago's South Side. Women were recruited after receiving a diagnosis of breast cancer at three Chicago hospitals, one that serves those without insurance, one that primarily treats

Medicaid patients, and one whose patient base is largely covered by private insurance. This was done to insure a wide variation in socioeconomic status.

Tumor tissue was collected when women's tumors were excised in surgery and interviews were scheduled for four to six after surgery. African-American social work graduate students interviewed women in their homes over the 1.5-year period to assess a wide variety of psychosocial and other factors, including living situation, social network, perceived stress and discrimination, psychological functioning, health behaviors and history, and life events. Stress hormone regulation was measured using diurnal salivary cortisol levels, which were compared to women's perceptions of stress, daily diaries, and life events. Women provided four saliva samples at prescribed intervals during the day for three consecutive days, every 6 months.

As was mentioned earlier in the chapter, a specially trained Built Environment Team observed and measured the four-block area around each woman's home to assess for features that either impede or enhance social interactions, using metrics devised for the study. Data on crime, services, socioeconomic status, and integrity of individual housing units were obtained from the City of Chicago and geo-coded to women's addresses. Crime statistics were determined for a quarter-mile buffer zone constructed around each participant's home (or, in the case of homeless women, the primary locale).

Results of the Study

Women in the study presented with higher rates of sexual assault and depression than previously reported for African-American women. The National Violence against Women Survey, a large national telephone health survey conducted in 1995 and 1996, reported that 18.8% of African-American women have been sexually assaulted at some time in their lifetimes (Tjaden and Thoennes 2000). Rates for women in the CIHDR study sample, who were interviewed in their homes by African-American research assistants (RAs) with whom they had established rapport, were much higher, with almost 30% reporting prior sexual assault.

Women in the study also exhibited high rates of depression compared to those in prior studies of women with invasive breast cancer, with 30% being clinically depressed at the time of their interview (i.e., 4–6 weeks after breast cancer surgery), based on their scores on the Center for Epidemiological Studies Depression Scale. This compares to 9.6% of women, diagnosed using the Hospital Anxiety and Depression Scale (Zigmond and Snaith 1983), from a mixed-race sample of urban women with early-stage breast cancer conducted at the Memorial Sloan Kettering Cancer Center in New York (Kissane et al. 2004).

CIDHR investigators found a strong correlation between felt loneliness, depression, and sexual assault ($r=0.680$, $p=0.001$ for depression and loneliness; $r=0.410$, $p=0.001$ for sexual assault and loneliness; $r=0.410$, $p=0.001$ for depression and assault), seemingly forming a "psychosocial suite" of social and traumatic variables connecting neighborhood-level variables to stress hormone response.

When women's scores were factor-analyzed using Principal Components Analysis with varimax rotation, two factors emerged, one termed "depression and loneliness" and the other, anomie. In this case, anomie refers not to the group disenfranchisement reported by many African Americans (Massey and Denton 1993), but to individual disenfranchisement, in which women feel they have no place in the world.

Another finding, related to women's need to belong, as measured by scores on the Need to Belong Scale developed by Leary et al. (2001), were higher levels of need to belong among women living in neighborhoods having higher numbers of rental dwellings, as opposed to single family homes ($r=0.276$, $p=0.006$). Lower levels of perceived social support, measured using the Multidimensional Scale of Perceived Social Support (Zimet et al. 1988), were found among women living in neighborhoods with higher percentages of duplexes/townhouses ($r=-0.011$, $p=0.042$).

Need to belong correlated positively with sexual assault ($r=0.650$, $p=0.025$), aggravated assault ($r=0.0677$, $p=0.059$), and robbery ($r=0.0841$, $p=0.033$). The degree of safety that a woman felt in her neighborhood was found to be positively associated with her amount of perceived social support ($r=0.321$, $p=0.032$). Perceived social support, overall, was negatively correlated with total depression, total loneliness, and total stress as the more depressed, lonely, and stressed she was, the lower her perceived social support: for depression ($r=-0.360$, $p=0.00$), for loneliness ($r=-0.0442$, $p=0.00$), and for stress ($r=-0.0304$, $p=0.003$).

The CIHDR team also investigated how sexual assault affects biology. Using ordered logistic regression, associations between sexual assault and increased Her2Neu receptor status ($b=0.209$, $p=0.003$), histological grade of tumor ($b=0.075$, $p=0.013$), and cancer stage at diagnosis ($b=0.075$, $p=0.013$) were found. Other hormone receptor status could be predicted from social and psychological variables. The number of sexual assaults in the neighborhood and age were associated with estrogen-receptor (ER) status ($b=-0.189$, $p<0.05$; $b=0.049$; $p<0.05$) and histological grade of tumor ($b=0.143$, $p<0.05$; $b=-0.061$; $p<0.01$), years of education was associated with progesterone receptor (PR) status ($b=-0.393$, $p<0.01$), and felt loneliness was associated with Her2Neu receptor status ($b=-0.096$, $p<0.05$).

Attempts to connect neighborhood variables to stress hormone response through cluster analysis of the diurnal salivary cortisol data were revealing. Two clusters appeared, one with a typical pattern showing circadian fluctuations (33% of CIHDR women fell into this group (the black line in Fig. 4.3), and one with a flat pattern [67% of women fell into this group (the dark gray line in Fig. 4.3)], similar to that seen among the isolated rodents in CIHDR animal studies. The flat pattern is analogous to what is known as endocrine burnout (Sonnenschein et al. 2007), which is seen in organisms that have experienced severe, chronic stress.

We hypothesized that the women in the group with the flat cortisol pattern were those who had been particularly socially vulnerable for long periods of time and for whom breast cancer was only one of a series of major stressors reported (e.g., the inability to secure safe and affordable housing). We were able to predict into which group the women fall, using logistic regression analysis, with number

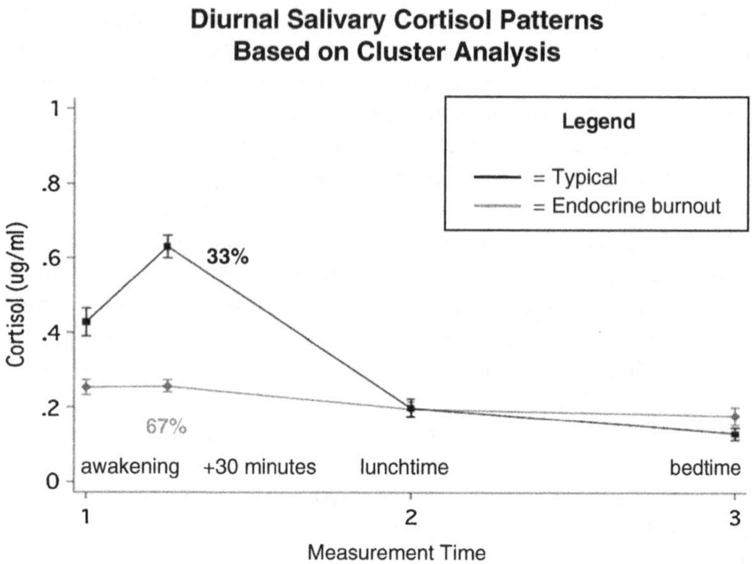

Fig. 4.3 Diurnal salivary cortisol patterns over 3 days for two groups of women, based on cluster analysis. The cortisol was measured at wakeup, 30 min after wakeup, noon time, and bedtime

of crimes (i.e., robberies and homicides) that occurred that year in a quarter-mile buffer zone constructed around each woman's home, and psychological response (i.e., scores on the CES-D depression scale) (*Pseudo* $R^2=0.49$, $Prob>chi^2=0.0315$) as predictors. We hypothesized that salivary cortisol rhythms would be affected by upstream factors. Additional analyses reveal that nighttime rise in salivary cortisol (i.e., the increase between the last collection time of 1 day to 30 min after the first collection of the following day) can be predicted by crimes (sexual assaults, robberies, and aggravated assaults) and depression ($R^2=0.26$; $p<0.01$). Both sexual assaults and robberies were negatively associated with nighttime rise ($b=-0.047$, $p<0.01$; $b=-0.005$, $p<0.05$, respectively), while aggravated assaults were associated with an increase in the nighttime rise of diurnal cortisol ($b=0.007$, $p<0.01$). Interestingly, the effect of depression on nighttime rise disappeared when crime data were added to the models, suggesting the impact of neighborhood-level data such as crimes on physiological functioning.

Conclusions

Based on concomitant work with animal models, and using information gathered from in-home interviews with African-American women newly diagnosed with breast cancer living on Chicago's South Side, investigations of the built environment around each woman's home, and publicly available data geo-coded to their addresses, CIHDR investigators have identified a pathway with significant associations between levels in our multilevel model. This pathway connects the community to inside the nucleus of the cell, in that dilapidated housing, crimes, and generally fractured communities engender isolation and depression, and in so doing, alter stress hormone response (Gehlert et al. 2007).

CIHDR has found links between a woman's psychological state, her neighborhood or "place," and her stress hormone response. Through CIHDR's multiple lens, a clearer, more complete, picture of women's lives emerges and we begin to understand how, as interpretive beings, women's conceptions of place might affect their psychological equilibrium. Women living in very adverse circumstances over which they have little control may exceed their capacities to maintain psychological equilibrium. That is to say that their stress hormone systems might no longer provide the mechanisms by which organisms whose place identities are congruent with the physical settings in which they live maintain psychological equilibrium.

The results of CIHDR investigations to date suggest the importance of considering place in health disparities research. Neighborhood characteristics, as predicted, were associated with a suite of psychosocial factors. Apartment living, as opposed to home ownership, for example, did lead to greater feelings of anomie, vigilance, and social isolation.

The link between neighborhood characteristics and receptor status provide support for the CIHDR model. The increase in hormone receptor status is revealing and supports CIHDR's discoveries of how stress hormone receptors triggered by a psychological "state" can activate biochemical pathways known to increase tumor cell survival. Some women did indeed have a low shallow rhythm, indicating a state of hypocortisolemia typically associated with unrelenting chronic stress (Gehlert, unpublished results). These women might well be those who fail to identify with place, and indeed they have no places of their own.

As Casey (2001) suggests, "there is no place without self, and no self without place." From this working assumption, one supported by Butz and Eyles (1997), we begin to make discoveries at the intersection of place and self; the point at which our natures are altered by the physical environments in which we live, changing our biology or "getting under the skin" to affect stress response, thus creating conditions ripe for disease.

These findings offer a possible explanation for how a woman's altered sense of place affects her feelings of security and control across relationships and interactions. Likening this to what hooks (1999) calls the ability to resist dehumanization, the "construction of a safe-place," one relatively free from the worries of crime and violence, leads to well-being, empowerment, and a strong sense of belonging to and identifying with a "place."

References

Acevedo-Garcia, D. 2000. "Residential segregation and the epidemiology of infectious diseases." *Social Science & Medicine* 51:1143–1161.

Acevedo-Garcia, D. 2001. "Zip code-level risk factors for tuberculosis: neighborhood environment and residential segregation in New Jersey,1985–1992." *American Journal of Public Health* 91:734–741.

Anderton, Douglas L., Andy B. Anderson, John Michael Oakes, and Michael R. Fraser. 1994. "Environmental equity: the demographics of dumping." *Demography* 31:229–248.
Aneshensel, C.S., and C.A. Sucoff. 1996. "The neighborhood context of adolescent mental health." *Journal of Health and Social Behavior* 37:293–310.
Barton, H., M. Grant, and R. Guise. 2003. *Shaping Neighborhoods: A Guide for Health Sustainability and Vitality*. London: Spon.
Balshem, M. 1993. *Cancer in the Community*. Washington, DC: Smithsonian Institute Press.
Birtchnell, J., N. Masters, and M. Deahl. 1988. "Depression and the physical environment: a study of young married women on a London housing estate." *British Journal of Psychiatry* 153:56–64.
Booth, S.L., J.F. Sallis, C. Ritenbaugh, et al. 2001. "Environmental and societal factors affect food choice and physical activity: rationale, influences, and leverage points." *Nutrition Review* 59:S21–S39.
Butz, David, and John Eyles. 1997. "Reconceptualizing senses of place: Social relations, ideology and ecology." *Geografiska Annaler. Series B, Human Geography* 79:1–25.
Casey, E. (2001). "Between geography and philosophy: what does it mean to be in the place-world?" *Annals of the Association of American Geographers* 91:683–93.
Cavigelli, Sonia A., Jason R. Yee, and Martha K. McClintock. 2006. "Infant temperament predicts life span in female rats that develop spontaneous tumors." *Hormones and Behavior* 50:454–462.
Cohen, D., S. Spear, R. Scribner, P. Kissinger, K. Mason, and J. Wildgen. 2000. ""Broken windows" and the risk of gonorrhea." *American Journal of Public Health* 90:230–236.
Coleman, A. 1985. *Utopia on Trial: Vision and Reality in Planned Housing*. London: Fiilary Shipman.
Cook, F.L., and W.G. Skogan (Eds.). 1984. *Evaluating the Changing Definition of a Policy Issue in Congress: Crime Against the Elderly*. Greenwich: JAI Press.
Diez-Roux, A.V., S. Stein, P. Merkin, D.R. Hannan, R. Jacobs, and C.I. Kiefe. 2003. "Area characteristics, individual-level socioeconomic indicators, and smoking in young adults." *American Journal of Epidemiology* 157:315–326.
Dubow, F., F. McCabe, and G. Kaplan. 1979. *Reactions to Crime: A Critical Review of the Literature*. Washington, DC: U.S. Government Printing Office.
Ferraro, K.F. 1994. *Fear of Crime: Interpreting Victimization Risk*. Albany: SUNY Press.
Foucault, M. 1977. *Discipline & Punish: The Birth of Prison*. New York: Random House.
Gehlert, S., et al. 2007. "Cells to Society." Centers for Population Health and Health Disparities, Bethesda.
Gesler, Wilbert M., and Robin A. Kearns. 2002. *Culture/Place/Health*. London: Routledge.
Hendryx, M.S., M.M. Ahern, N.P. Lovrich, and A.H. McCurdy. 2002. "Access to health care and community social capital." *Health Service Research* 37:85–101.
Hermes, G. L., Louis Rosenthal, Anthony Montag, and Martha K. McClintock. 2006. "Social isolation and the inflammatory response: sex differences in the enduring effects of a prior stressor." *American Journal of Physiology. Regulatory, Integrative and Comparative Physiology* 290:R273–R282.
Hermes, G.L., B. Delgado, M. Tsakalis, M. Tretiakova, T. Krausz, S.D. Conzen, et al. 2009. "Social isolation dysregulates endocrine and behavioral stress while increasing malignant burden of spontaneous mammary tumors." *Proceedings of the National Academy of Sciences of the United States of America* 106(52):22393–22398.
Hesse, B. 1993. "Black to front and black again – racialization through contested times and spaces." In M. Keith and S. Pile (Eds.) *Place and the Politics of Identity*. London: Routledge, pp. 162–182.
Hirschman, Jocelyn, Steven Whitman, and David Ansell. 2007. "The black:white disparity in breast cancer mortality: the example of Chicago." *Cancer Causes Control* 18:323–333.
hooks, bell. 1999. *Homeplace: A Site of Resistance*. Cambridge: Southend Press.
Hoyert, D.L., M.P. Heron, S.L. Murphy, and H. Kung. 2006. "Deaths: Final data for 2003." *National Vital Statistics Reports* 54(2):1–116.
Jacobs, J. 1961. *The Death and Life of Great American Cities*. New York: Random House.

Kearns, R.A., and Barnett, J.R. 1998. "To boldly go? Place, metaphor and the marketing of Auckland's Starship Hospital. Environment and Planning D." *Society and Space* 17:201–226.
Kissane, D.W., B. Grabsch, A. Love, D.M. Clarke, S. Bloch, and G.C. Smith. 2004. "Psychiatric disorder in women with early stage and advanced breast cancer: a comparative analysis." *Australian and New Zealand Journal of Psychiatry* 38:320–326.
Korpela, K.M. 1989. "Place-identity as a product of environmental self-regulation." *Journal of Environmental Psychology* 9:241–256.
Krupat, E. 1983. "A place for place identity." *Journal of Environmental Psychology* 3:343–344.
Leary, M.R., K.M. Kelly, and L.S. Schreindorfer. 2001. "Individual differences in the need to belong." Unpublished manuscript.
Markowitz, F.E., P.E. Bellair, A.E. Liska, and J. Liu. 2001. "Extending social disorganization theory." *Criminology* 39:293–319.
Masi, C.M., and S. Gehlert. 2009. "Perceptions of breast cancer and its treatment among African-American women and men: implications for interventions." *Journal of General Internal Medicine* 24(3):408–414.
Massey, D.S., and N.A. Denton. 1993. *American Apartheid*. Cambridge: Harvard University Press.
McClintock, Martha K., Suzanne D. Conzen, Sarah Gehlert, Christopher Masi, and Olufunmilayo I. Olopade. 2005. "Mammary cancer and social interactions: identifying multiple environments that regulate gene expression throughout the life span." *Journals of Gerentology* 60B:32–41.
McCord, C., and H. Freeman. 1990. "Excess mortality in Harlem." *New England Journal of Medicine* 322:173–177.
McKnight, J. 1995. *The Careless Society: Community and Its Counterfeits*. New York: Basic Books.
Morenoff, Jeffrey D. 2003. "Neighborhood mechanisms and the spatial dynamics of birth weight." *American Journal of Sociology* 108:976–1017.
Morland, K., S. Wing, and A.V. Diez-Roux. 2002. "The contextual effect of the local food environment on residents' diets: the atherosclerosis risk in communities study." *American Journal of Public Health* 92:1761–1767.
Morland, K., A.V. Diez-Roux, and S. Wing. 2006. "Supermarkets, other food stores, and obesity-the atherosclerosis risk in communities study." *American Journal of Preventive Medicine* 30:333–339.
Newman, O. 1972. *Defensible Space: Crime Prevention Through Urban Design*. New York: Collier Books.
Newman, O. 1980. *Factors Influencing Crime and Instability in Urban Housing Developments*. Washington, DC: U.S. Government Printing Office.
O'Campo, P., et al. 1997. "Neighborhood risk factors for low birthweight in Baltimore: a multi-level analysis." *American Journal of Public Health* 87:1113–1118.
Perkins, D.P., A. Wandersman, and R.C. Rich. 1993. " The physical environment of street crime: defensible space, territoriality, and incivilities." *Journal of Environmental Psychology* 13:29–49.
Peterson, R.D., J.K. Lauren, and A.H. Mark. 2000. "Disadvantage and neighborhood violent crime: "do local institutions matter?"" *Journal of Research in Crime and Delinquency* 37:31–63.
Pirkle, J.L., R.B. Kaufmann, D.J. Brody, T. Hickman, E.W. Gunter, and D.C. Paschal. 1998. "Exposure of the U.S. population to lead, 1991–1994." *Environmental Health Perspectives* 106:745–750.
Proshansky, H.M. 1978. "The city and self-identity." *Environment and Behavior* 10:147–168.
Proshansky, H.M., and R. Kaminoff. 1982. The built environment of the young adult. In S. Messick (Ed.) *Development in Young Adulthood: Characteristics and Competences in Education, Work and Social Life*. San Francisco: Jossey Bass.
Proshansky, H.M., A.K. Fabian, and R. Kaminoff. 1983. "Place-identity: Physical world socialization of the self." *Journal of Environmental Psychology* 3:57–83.
Rand, G. 1984. "Crime and environment: a review of the literature and its implications for urban architecture and planning." *Journal of Architectural and Planning Research* 1:3–19.

Ries, L.A.G., D. Melbert, M. Krapcho, D.G. Stinchcomb, N. Howlader, M.J. Horner, et al. 2008. *SEER Cancer Statistics Review, 1975–2005*. Bethesda: National Cancer Institute. Available at http://seer.cancer.gov/csr/1975_2002/.

Roberts, E.M. 1997. "Neighborhood social environments and the distribution of low birthweight in Chicago." *American Journal of Public Health* 87:597–603.

Salant, T., and S. Gehlert (2008). "Collective memory, candidacy, and victimization: Community epidemiology of breast cancer risk." *Sociology of Health and Illness* 30(4):599–615.

Sampson, R., and S. Raudenbush. 1999. "Systematic social observations of public spaces: A new look at disorder in urban neighborhoods." *American Journal of Sociology* 105:603–651.

Sampson, Robert J., Stephen W. Raudenbush, and Felton Earls. 1997. "Neighborhoods and violent crime: A multilevel study of collective efficacy." *Science* 277:918–924.

Skogan, W. 1990. *Disorder and Decline: Crime and the Spiral of Decay in American Cities*. New York: Free Press.

Sonnenschein, M., P.M.C. Mommersteeg, J.H. Houtveen, M.J. Sorbi, M.B. Schaufeli, and L.J.P. van Doornen (2007). Exhaustion and endocrine functioning in clinical burnout: An in-depth study using the experience sampling method. *Biological Psychiatry* 75:176–184.

Stedman, R.C. 2002. "Toward a social psychology of place: Predicting behavior from place-based cognitions, attitude and identity." *Environment and Behavior* 34(5):561–581.

Taylor, R.B. 1988. *Human Territorial Functioning*. Cambridge: Cambridge University Press.

Taylor, R.B. 2001. *Breaking Away from Broken Windows: Baltimore Evidence and Implications for the Nationwide Fight Against Crime, Grime, Fear and Decline*. New York: Westview Press.

Taylor, R.B., S.A. Shumaker, and S.D. Gottfredson. 1985. "Neighborhood-level links between physical features and local sentiments: Deterioration, fear of crime, and confidence." *Journal of Architectural and Planning Research* 2:261–275.

Tjaden, Patricia, and N. Thoennes. 2000. "Full report of the prevalence, incidence, and consequences of violence against women." Washington, DC: U.S. Department of Justice.

Vrijheid, M. 2000. "Health effects of residence near hazardous waste landfill sites: a review of epidemiologic literature." *Environmental Health Perspectives* 108(Suppl 1):101–112.

Warnecke, Richard B., April Oh, Nancy Breen, Sarah Gehlert, Electra Paskett, Katherine L. Tucker, Nicole Lurie, Timothy Rebbeck, James Goodwin, John Flack, Shobha Srinivasan, Jon Kerner, Suzanne Heurtin-Roberts, Ronald Abeles, Frederick L. Tyson, Georgeanne Patmios, and Robert A. Hiatt. 2008. "Approaching health disparities from a population perspective: The National Institutes of Health Centers for Population Health and Health Disparities." *American Journal of Public Health* 98:1608–1615.

Williams, J.B., D. Pang, B. Delgado, M. Kocherginsky, M. Tretiakova, T. Krausz, D. Pan, J. He, M.K. McClintock, and S.D. Conzen. 2009. "A Model of Gene-Expression Interaction Reveals Altered Mammary Gland Gene Expression and Increased Tumor Growth Following Social Isolation." *Cancer Prevention Research* 2(10):850–861.

Wilson, J.Q., and G. Kelling. 1982. "Broken Windows: The police and neighborhood safety." *Atlantic Monthly*.

Yen, Irene H., and George A. Kaplan. 1999. "Neighborhood social environment and risk of death: A multilevel evidence from the Alameda County study." *American Journal of Epidemiology* 149:898–907.

Zigmond, A.S., and R.P. Snaith. 1983. "The hospital anxiety and depression scale." *Acta Psychiatrica Scandinavia* 56:250–269.

Zimet, G.D., N.W. Dahlem, S.G. Zimet, and G.K. Farley. 1988. "The multidimensional scale of perceived social support." *Journal of Personality Assessment* 52:30–41.

Chapter 5
Race, Place, and Health

ManChui Leung and David T. Takeuchi

Introduction

Medical technologies and innovative public health strategies have improved screening, prevention, clinical care, and treatment for a wide range of health conditions. These improvements have greatly enhanced the quality of life of people around the world, especially in the USA. From 1960 to 2010, life expectancy for the entire population in the USA has steadily increased by 9.8 years (UN Human Development Programme 2010). Despite improvements on some health indicators and a wealth of resources invested in health care, the USA continues to have poorer outcomes on critical health dimensions when compared with other countries. Using the same United Nations data, the USA in 1960 had a life expectancy of 69.8 years and ranked 16th among all countries. In 2010, life expectancy had increased to 79.60 years but the USA slipped in the ranks, falling to 29th among comparison countries (UN Human Development Programme 2009). This decline in rank, an important measure of human development, is partially due to persistent social and economic inequalities, and a rapidly increasing rate of obesity and obesity related health problems (OECD 2010).

Empirical studies over the past three decades have consistently found that health and illness are unevenly distributed within the US society. The relative decline in population health gains has been found to be associated with social and environmental factors including race and ethnicity (Smedley et al. 2003; Bezruchka and Mercer 2004). While evidence accumulates about health inequities among racial and ethnic groups, the study of race and ethnicity has become more complex and nuanced. Immigration has transformed the demographic profile of the USA to include multiple racial and ethnic categories leading to a growing diversity across

M. Leung (✉)
Department of Sociology, University of Washington, 211 Savery Hall, Box 353340, Seattle, WA 98195, USA
e-mail: mleung8@u.washington.edu

L.M. Burton et al. (eds.), *Communities, Neighborhoods, and Health*, Social Disparities in Health and Health Care 1, DOI 10.1007/978-1-4419-7482-2_5,

and within racial and ethnic groups. As a result, dominant theories about race and ethnicity are being contested and reconsidered, and the very meaning of race and racial categories continues to be challenged and debated (Hune 1995; Omi and Winant 1994). However, the shifts in racial categorization and meaning do not minimize the salience of race and ethnicity as a central tool to organize society. Race and ethnicity continue to structure social hierarchy, which determines who has access to social, political, economic, and health resources (Smelser et al. 2001). Racial categories carry with them implicit and explicit images and beliefs about phenotypes that provide rationale for societal and individual hierarchical treatment of specific groups. The conceptualization and meaning of race speaks racist and discriminatory ideologies that have historically stratified society (LaVeist 1994; Takeuchi and Gage 2003). Since the formation of the USA, efforts to control national racial and ethnic composition and maintain racial hierachies remain a key concern for health policy as much as for immigration, education, and economic policies (Zolberg 2006).

This chapter focuses on one facet of race and health by describing the geographic, social and psychological processes of place. The interaction of race, ethnicity, and place in health research allows for a rethinking of "risk groups" into "spaces and landscapes" of challenges and opportunities. Place considers how different health determinants and processes come together and interact, resulting in a variation of health outcomes across population groups and spaces. The effects of racial and ethnic hierarchies and discriminatory practices are particularly critical and meaningful in analyzing location, landscape, and awareness of place. For example, in racially and economically segregated neighborhoods, individuals have additional difficulties in obtaining health resources and services because of their group membership, socioeconomic position, and environmental limitations (Williams and Williams-Morris 2000). Moreover, the place-based experiences of displacement, colonization, and forced relocation shared among racial and ethnic minorities have been found to have long-term detrimental effects on individual and collective social capital accumulation and psychological well-being. These effects, in turn, influence health behaviors and increase health risks across generations (Fullilove 2004; Brave Heart 1998; Walters et al. 2002).

Racial stratification and racial inequities are also formed and reified by and through place. Places are often melded with racial characteristics just as some stereotypes are ascribed to groups (Goldberg 2005; Omi and Winant 1994). This racialization of place acts to reinforce racial discrimination and social hierarchies of its inhabitants. For example, "urban" and "inner-city" are used synonymously as a geographic and a racial demarcation. Dominant society attaches terms to immigrant enclaves that omit the central presence of its residents (Chinatown), and as a reminder of relative power (Little Tokyo). These dominant and dominating place-names remain even though its inhabitants have very different naming orientations. For example, Chinatown is referred to as "Chinese people street," by the Chinese, and indigenous place-names (*Denali*) are systematically replaced by the names of colonial explorers, prospectors, or business leaders (Mount McKinley).

Why Does Place Matter in Health?

Place allows for a wide and multi-dimensional framework which encompasses the complexity of spatial, psychological, social and ecological analysis. The concept of place and health has traditionally been built on geographic frameworks that emphasize the locations or spaces where people live, work, and play. A location pinpoints an individual or population within a specific area to measure health risk exposure or describe how diseases spread or cumulate. A spatial analysis helps to identify the origin and routes of infectious diseases, measure the degree of exposure from a pollution source, and understand the distribution of disease in association with other factors such as socioeconomic status, and race and ethnicity. Moreover, the built environment, the physical structures and infrastructure that are designed to make a place, are increasingly being acknowledged as a significant influence on health. For example, more physical activity and healthier diets may be attributed to convenient, safe walking paths and accessible sources of fresh food groceries. Poorer mental and physical health indicators may be attributed to high crime rates, few parks, disproportionate number of alcohol and tobacco outlets and limited access to fresh produce.

Socioecological and landscape perspectives emphasize how place contributes to health processes by constraining action, confining resources, and imposing norms and behaviors. The effects of these processes can be seen in deleterious health outcomes associated with the prevalence of violence and the availability of jobs (Macintyre et al. 2002; Krieger 2001; Morenoff 2003), as well as salutary health outcomes associated with the use of neighborhood and/or ethnic social networks and the prevalence of civic participation (Portes and Rumbaut 2006). Landscape perspectives of place also employ the concept of therapeutic layers that achieve lasting reputations for providing physical, mental, and spiritual healing (Gesler 1992). Different types of places, such as home places, spiritual places, natural places, and healing places, can contribute to better individual and group health by fostering a sense of belonging and being valued by a social group (Curtis 2004).

The "sense of place" or psychological perspective of place is often overlooked in the analysis of health risk and benefits. The "sense of place" describes how physical and mental health is associated with the bonds people have with places and with people in those places (Tuan 1974; Meade et al. 1988). The sense of place gives insight into analyzing the health effects connected to experiences of place, attachment or detachment to place, and the influence of place onto real or perceived opportunities and investments (Gieryn 2000; Kearns 1993; Relph 1976, 2007). The psychology of place posits that individuals require an environment where needs are satisfied and people experience emotional ties. Tuan (1974) links people to their environment through three key psychological and social processes: attachment, familiarity, and identity. Tuan is especially concerned with how place relates to perceptions of shared identity, group belonging, and cultural reproduction across time, and emphasizes that experiences are dependent on social *and* spatial contexts (Tuan 1974). For example, the mere presence of a neighborhood health clinic does not automatically increase access. Health access increases when trust, in the form of outreach, collaborative partnerships and cultural and linguistic competent services, is built between the community members and service providers. Then, a *place* like a neighborhood health clinic is no longer a passive and depersonalized container but is an active contributor to community life and social processes.

The socioecological and psychological characteristics of place such as intimacy, domesticity, and refuge can be vital dimensions for health and well-being among racial and ethnic minority groups. Among African-Americans, the construction of home as a permissible and liberating place has radical political salience given the history of enslavement, racial discrimination, and residential segregation. hooks (1990) writes about how "homeplace" for African-Americans was vital because of the need to have a site, no matter how vulnerable or tenuous, where one could be a subject instead of an object. Even though home could also be a place of fear, conflict, and oppression, hooks emphasizes that the homeplace may have been the *only* place where some African-Americans could be affirmed of their humanity despite overwhelming poverty, hardship, and depravation. According to hooks, homeplace was more than a refuge that provided protection; it was a site of resistance and political solidarity that interwove therapeutic properties and healing.

Place is one concept in which health research can be used to understand the complex and shifting processes that effect social life and health outcomes across and between racial and ethnic groups. Place, as a geographic and social location, has been paramount in public health research findings (Broad Street cholera outbreak). The theoretical and analytical expansion of spatial analysis to include the socioecological and psychological perspectives of place allows for a much deeper and interdisciplinary investigation that reveals important underlying mechanisms associated with the unequal distribution of health outcomes (Cummins et al. 2007).

Place Inequalities

Racial Residential Segregation

In the USA, place and race are highly associated with each other as evidenced by the long history of racial residential segregation and geographic isolation of indigenous, African-American and immigrant groups. Residents in racially segregated neighborhoods attach different meanings to their neighborhood and community that can have positive (place as cultural resource) and detrimental (place as disrepair) effects on health and well-being. Although some health protective factors have been found among residents in some ethnic enclaves, the residential segregation of racial and ethnic groups, especially among the poor, has contributed to compromised health behaviors and outcomes.

Racial residential segregation creates distinctive and hierarchical ecological environments. This interaction of race and place determines which racial and ethnic groups have access to resources, opportunities, and services. Poor housing, few living wage jobs, substandard schools, and limited access to health and human service institutions characterize these segregated and isolated environments (Massey and Denton 1993; Wilson 1996). Socially and economically isolated residents have fewer social network ties that facilitate social mobility and educational opportunities (Berkman and Clark 2003). Moreover, the disproportionate distribution of liquor stores, environmental pollutants and hazards, payday loan businesses, and fast food restaurants can contribute to ill health and inhibit intentions to change health behaviors (LaVeist and Wallace 2000). These forms of structural disadvantage and discrimination concentrate poverty, reinforce inequality, and perpetuate a cycle of political and economic divestment that has direct and indirect effects on health.

African-Americans and other racial and ethnic minorities have been historically exposed to disadvantaged segregated environments such as inner-city ghettos and slums, and rural reservations and plantations. The socioeconomic conditions of racial residential segregation at the individual, household, neighborhood, and community levels have been a primary cause for racial and ethnic disparities in health status. Williams and Collins (2001) highlight how segregation of African-Americans in the USA limits opportunities for social mobility and constrains health access to services and information that pervade across the lifespan and across generations. Racial residential segregation has produced a distinctive geographic and social ecology for African-Americans compared with whites and some immigrant groups. It consists of a higher concentration of African-Americans in disadvantaged neighborhoods shaped by historical and current discriminatory practices which disadvantage the average African-American, regardless of zip code or socioeconomic status (Williams and Collins 2001). Empirical data show that the unabated stressful and isolating conditions of racially segregated neighborhoods have been linked to poorer health outcomes, higher mortality, and lower life expectancy among African-American adults and infants (Massey and Denton 1993; Massey and Fischer 2000; Schulz et al. 2002; Williams and Collins 2001). Segregated neighborhoods often provide greater exposure to interpersonal and community violence that may be tied to higher levels of psychological distress and mental disorders (Morenoff 2003; Ross and Jang 2000; Warr and Ellison 2000). Residential segregation also concentrates and perpetuates the conditions of disadvantage such as drug use, joblessness, welfare dependency, unwed teenage childbearing, and community-level violence, producing a social context which normalizes these conditions and makes individual behavior change difficult (Massey and Denton 1993; Wilson 1996).

A similar disadvantaged ecology also affects Native Americans, especially those residing in rural reservations. The ecological constraints result in higher rates of poverty chronic alcohol and drug use, diabetes, depression and trauma, and a lower life expectancy compared with all other racial and ethnic groups. The high and persistent levels of poor physical and mental health conditions that span across multiple generations of Native Americans are found to be indirectly and directly linked to social determinants of health that interact with place – education, employment, socioeconomic status, housing quality, and individual, and household behaviors (Beals et al. 2005; Brave Heart 2003; Gracey and King 2009; Whitbeck et al. 1998).

Direct and Indirect Place Effects

While health outcomes are complex to measure given biomedical, behavioral, social, and environmental pathways, there have been numerous studies that continue to find direct and indirect place and neighborhood effects. In their study of four cities and suburbs in the USA, Diez-Roux et al. (2001) found that after controlling for education, income, occupational status, and common biomedical and individual behavioral risk factors for coronary heart disease, people residing in segregated and disadvantaged neighborhoods continued to have a higher incidence of heart disease than those who lived in more integrated and middle class neighborhoods. In a tuberculosis study of four racial and ethnic groups in New Jersey, Acevedo-Garcia (2001) found indirect and direct effects of racial residential segregation on the transmission of tuberculosis. The direct effects were overcrowding and isolation among coresidents with similar susceptibility to health risks. The indirect effects were the lower quality of segregated neighborhoods exemplified by the concentration of poverty, dilapidated housing, and limited access to health services. All these socioecological factors made residents in racially segregated neighborhoods more at risk for infectious and noncommunicable diseases, and less likely to seek immediate medical care (Acevedo-Garcia 2000).

High rates of violence, economic instability, isolation, and discrimination – all of which are disproportionately concentrated in racially segregated neighborhoods – have direct effects on ill health, especially disability, mental disorders, and early mortality (Morenoff 2001). Segregated residents, especially among the US born, also have fewer protective health factors due to less accumulation of social capital, more constrained social networks, and fewer opportunities for social mobility. Massey (2004) further argues that the biosocial mechanisms underlying environmental stressors lead to increased health risk. Massey's biosocial model empirically links the structure of social stratification such as racial residential segregation and discrimination to chronic stress indictors like high allostatic load and cortisone levels. These high and persistent levels of stress reaction have been found to be associated with elevated risk of coronary heart disease, hypertension, diabetes, obesity, asthma, as well as mental disorders and memory dysfunctions.

Psychological factors such as chronic stress and fear also have indirect effects on health by decreasing physical activities for pleasure, exercise, and transportation (Ross and Mirowsky 2001; Sampson and Raudenbush 1999). Aneshensel and Sucoff (1996) in their study of adolescents in Los Angeles neighborhoods found that adolescent perceptions of their neighborhood as dangerous influenced their mental health and behaviors. This perception of neighborhoods as threatening which also indicates a detachment from place, was associated with a higher prevalence of depression, anxiety, oppositional defiant disorder, and conduct disorder among adolescents.

Immigrant Ethnic Enclaves

Similar racial residential segregated conditions exist among immigrants who live in ethnic enclaves, but additional facets of place may be associated with a wider variation in health outcomes among immigrants that differ from African-Americans. Among some Latinos and Asians, living among coethnics, especially upon arrival to the USA, has been found to be more protective for health than detrimental. The immigrant enclave may provide protection by supporting conditions of ethnic solidarity, community building, economic support, and access to established social networks (Kasinitz et al. 2008; Logan et al. 2002; Zhou 1992). The health impacts of residential segregation among immigrant groups paint a more complex and nuanced picture of how race, ethnicity, and place interact to govern health behavior and disease ecology. Some compositional and contextual factors of place in immigrant enclaves are similar to segregated African-American neighborhoods. Substandard housing, overcrowding, dead-end jobs, and a high concentration of coethnic residents with low socioeconomic status also limits upward mobility and health for many immigrants. Yet the concentration of coethnic and colinguistic neighbors and the presence of immigrant social networks may structurally buffer negative encounters with whites and the larger US society, thus reducing the acculturative stress and social strains caused by exposure to individual and interpersonal discrimination. Moreover, immigrant networks provide important and timely resources that aid in the adaptation to new environments and enhance the knowledge attainment needed to take advantage of opportunities. Immigrant networks and community based institutions have been found to connect coethnics to jobs inside and outside the enclave, provide financial resources, and create informal lending and apprenticeship opportunities to develop ethnic businesses and job niches (Bashi 2007; Menjívar 2000; Portes and Rumbaut 2006).

The segregated immigrant enclave also differs because of the presence of immigrant entrepreneurs within a distinct ethnic economy. Although the businesses are often small, informal, and serve mainly low-income customers, their growing presence builds political and economic infrastructure, and capital for its residents (Portes 1995). Strong ethnic and linguistic networks are instrumental in assisting with financial needs, finding employment opportunities, connecting to health and human services, aiding in the adjustment to new routines and institutions, and providing informal health care and family assistance (Berkman and Glass 2000; Weiss et al. 2005). While enclaves may be prone to isolation and unequal treatment, the internal community development of resources has been found to improve health outcomes. Formal and informal community institutions foster increased opportunities for social mobility inside and outside the immigrant enclave, and are associated higher levels of collective efficacy and engagement, an indicator of attachment to place (Menjívar 2000; Morenoff et al. 2001; Portes 1995).

Examining the temporal processes of place can uncover some of the mechanisms that explain the differences in health outcomes between segregated racial and ethnic groups. Jacobs' (1961) work continues to provide insight into how differences in health determinants among racial and ethnic groups may manifest in similar isolated environments. She distinguishes two types of poor neighborhoods, perpetual slums and "unslumming" neighborhoods, in order to highlight how these environments may look the same, cross-sectionally, but are on distinctly different time trajectories based on historical origins, residential attachment, and investment to place. A perpetual slum endures if people with the most socioeconomic mobility leave quickly and steadily, with minimal replacement. For example, in the post Jim Crow era, the African-American middle class moved to white and suburban neighborhoods from inner-city neighborhoods. This outflow of African-American middle class professionals, their businesses, and people of working age, coupled with little inflow of equivalent residential resources, left a neighborhood and its remaining residents in a perpetual cycle of economic instability and isolation (Wilson 1987).

While many immigrant enclaves and non-immigrant communities share similar conditions of socioeconomic and political isolation, Jacobs emphasizes that the difference stems from the constant multigenerational and diverse socioeconomic flow of residents leaving, staying, and arriving in the immigrant enclave. New immigrant arrivals bring their willingness to invest their limited resources, those who stay contribute by connecting others with their human and social capital, and those who leave often maintain family, cultural, and economic ties to the immigrant enclave (Jacobs 1961; Portes 1995; Portes and Zhou 1993). Although immigrant enclaves are not always places of positive collective engagement and social support, the strong attachment to place and interaction with coethnics across generations may play a key role in providing more dynamic and diverse routes of social mobility associated with better health and wellness outcomes (Fullilove 2004; Osypuk et al. 2009; Portes and Zhou 1993).

Despite increasing variation in health outcomes associated with neighborhood segregation, racial residential segregation continues to be a robust determinant of racial and ethnic group access to resources, accumulation of social and economic capital, and sense of place. The health disparities among the racially segregated urban and rural poor, who have less choice of where they live and with whom they live, will continue to manifest as long as the effects of concentrated poverty, stress, and inadequate services and housing persist. Without structural changes to racially segregated neighborhoods, places like the urban ghetto, immigrant enclave, and the rural reservation will continue to perpetuate disadvantage for its residents.

Displacement and Loss of Place

Place attachment, place identity, and sense of place are main constructs of the sociopsychology of place. Moving beyond location mapping and ecological descriptions, the sociopsychological approach conceptually expands place to underscore how attachment and identity to place can effect mental and physical health. A diminished sense of place, self-esteem, and belonging resulting from individual and collective experiences of loss, forced removal and displacement can produce anxiety, depression, and negatively influence behaviors that are relevant for a healthy, meaningful and engaged community life. Displacement also disrupts and dismantles social support networks, which are often place based, thus furthering isolation and vulnerability (Fullilove 1996; Gieryn 2000; Mollica 2000).

Among the displaced, racial and ethnic minorities are disproportionately represented in place-detachment processes of migration (immigrants), forced migration and removal (refugees, slaves, and indigenous populations), confinement and isolation (incarcerated and interned populations, residents of central city ghettos, and rural reservations), and place-lessness (homeless adults and children, and foster children). Fullilove (2004) has named this process of displacement "root shock," a traumatic stress reaction related to the destruction of emotional and social ecosystems. Tightly weaving trauma of the body with trauma of place, Fullilove examines three urban settings in which African-Americans and their neighborhoods have been systematically and chronically uprooted and disrupted. To measure the impact of loss and displacement, Fullilove constructs a "community burn index" which measures the feasibility of community recovery by calculating the ratio of the number of blocks with "third degree burns" per neighborhood. "Third degree burns" are equivalent to total demolition of a block without replacement. Root shock can be illustrated with the following examples among Native Americans in reservations, foster care youth and homeless adults, immigrants, and the formerly incarcerated.

Native Americans have experienced forms of root shock when they were displaced from their homelands, segregated onto reservations, and limited in their ability to exercise their sovereignty. Colonial efforts to eliminate their population, culture, language, and homelands have caused multiple forms of loss that manifest in various poor health outcomes including high rates of historical and intergenerational trauma. Root shock can be found in the politics and history of indigenous place-names. Place-names hold significant historical and cultural meaning among some indigenous populations. Place-names for landmarks are not just mapping references but are meant to summon a wide range of mental, emotional, cultural, and spiritual associations with the people who live and have lived in a specific location. The symbolic meaning of a place and its place-name is closely interconnected with its ecology, historical imagination, and mental, physical, and spiritual health of its inhabitants. This interconnection underscores the traumatic reaction to the systematic efforts of replacing indigenous place-names with Christian, English, or colonial names (Basso 1996; Walters 1999). Therefore, ongoing colonial name references act to re-traumatize, hinder connection, and deepening the "third degree burn" into an indigenous community's ability to achieve a high level of health.

Foster care youth, homeless adults and children, the prison re-entry (formerly incarcerated) population, and immigrants were identified in a needs assessment of low-income uninsured residents of Alameda County, CA who consistently experienced barriers to health care despite the availability of safety net services (Penserga and Newell 2009). Disproportionately represented by racial and ethnic minorities, these groups share common characteristics of displacement and detachment to place that affect their access to health services and their overall mental and physical health. Among these groups, being permanently or temporarily homeless was not simply an absence of a physical domicile, but the experience of reduced social ties and networks. Without a place to call home with others, future expectations and planning are minimized, connections and associations to jobs and education are truncated, and social and emotional support ties are difficult to forge. More importantly, these marginalized and stigmatized groups lacked a "homeplace" – a place to rest and pause in order to build resistance and recovery (hooks 1990). These experiences of re-occurring place-lessness thrust marginalized groups into a revolving cycle of loss and despair further eroding their mental and physical well-being (Vandemark 2007).

The revolving cycle of loss associated with root shock is evident in the findings of Cahill and LaVigne's (2008) study on the spatial clusters and mobility patterns among parolees released in San Diego, CA. They found an association between high rates of drug use and mobility among parolees in disadvantaged neighborhoods because attempts to change stressful environmental influences usually meant a move to a similar or even more disadvantaged neighborhood. Cahill and LaVigne found that these lateral and downward moves stemmed more from the restrictions resulting from racial, social and economic segregation than from individual choice. These restrictions limited the parolee's chances for successful employment and quality housing, thus continuing their exposure to drug use and criminal networks. As found in other studies neighborhood distress, lack of opportunity, and the geographic clustering of other parolees increased the risk for high recidivism and reconviction (LaVigne et al. 2006; Morenoff et al. 2001).

The health of racial and ethnic minorities continues to be disproportionately impacted by place loss and displacement associated with social stratification and discrimination. To further uncover how different forms of "root shock" produce health inequity across groups and generations health research should consider measuring place based and structurally processes along with social demographic characteristics.

Future Directions: Building Healthy Places by Creating Place Attachment, Meaning, and Value

> Attachment to place… is central to self identity, the sense of belonging, and self-efficacy – the ability to be and do in the world.
>
> (Tuan 1977)

Despite significant structural barriers to developing healthy communities, the drive to make place – to establish attachment, familiarity, and identity – has been the main force for collective action and community building. Place-based measures that include social, economic, psychological, biological, and geographical pathways can further the understanding of health inequality, especially among racial and ethnic minorities. The prioritization of health and social justice goals in many racial and ethnic social movements have directly connected place to wellness and power. In addition to measuring the accessibility to health resources such as medical services, these movements have included the presence of social cohesion, access to social and economic resources, and the improvement of the physical and built environment (Minkler and Wallerstein 2003). This section proposes three approaches that can be used to guide future theoretical and empirical research on place, race and health. First, Robert's socially expected durations and the process of immigrant settlement and transnationalism provides useful insight to explain the mechanisms associated with socioeconomic and health variation within racial and ethnic groups. Second, the Healthy Cities Project provides a comprehensive example of how place-based measures can be developed and implemented to improve health program and policy. Third, the Health Environments Partnership provides an effective local example of a place-based health intervention that can inform projects and collaborations in other locales.

Attachment to place and community building often involves varying levels of resources, group cohesion and social capital. To explain immigrant adjustment and identity formation, Robert (1995) adapted Merton's concept of socially expected durations to examine the effect of immigrant attachment and meaning to place. Socially expected durations explore relationships embedded in spatial and temporal dimensions, and are distinguished by three types of durations: prescribed durations of institutions and society (immigration laws); collectively expected durations among coethnic community members (promotion of ethnic and cultural identity through institutions); and patterned expected durations among family and friend networks (building a sense of a common future and shared values). Robert highlights how each of these socially expected duration types work both independently and interdependently to explain the behavioral variations among immigrant groups that reflect their attachment to place and their embeddedness in social networks.

Temporal and spatial processes may be a vital factor in analyzing and comparing the effects of place and health among immigrants and US born residents of neighborhoods undergoing development or change. For example, a framework of socially expected durations may help explain how both positive and negative adjustments among immigrants are associated with differing health outcomes and may produce protection against poor health despite sharing similar socioeconomic and residential segregation profiles with African-Americans. Place-based concepts such as citizenship, ethnic identity and family integration can highlight how socially expected durations among immigrants are especially important for understanding adjustment and attachment during an immigrant's migration and settlement career. Attachment to place is often demonstrated by acts of permanence and investment such as purchasing a house, getting naturalized, voting, or establishing a business with a longer return in assets. These actions have been found to positively affect health (Portes and Rumbaut 2006; Robert 1995). Strongly shared temporal expectations of return to the homeland and the maintaining of transnational ties can strengthen racial and ethnic group identity and belonging, acting as a form of health protection theorized by scholars such as Portes and Rumbaut (2006) and Zhou (1992, 2007). Moreover, the temporal and social aspects of patterned expectations among family and friend networks becomes an essential element for immigrant adjustment to a new environment and culture because it allows immigrants to identify which relationships can be counted on for different needs and at different times. These limits to the immigrant social network has been illustrated by the gendered patterns of reciprocation in Menjívar's (2000) study of Salvadorian immigrant networks. Menjívar found that women, especially those who were recent immigrants and single, were limited in cross-gender exchanges involving service, money, or monetized exchanges of child care and transportation. This left them less advantaged compared to men and married women in accessing the full array of immigrant network resources.

In the Healthy Cities Project, Kegler et al. (2000) highlight the importance of adopting a broad definition of a "healthy city" to guide their assessment of health and wellness in racially and ethnically diverse urban populations. Using a definition from the World Health Organization, the Healthy Cities Project refers to a healthy city as "one that is continually creating and improving those physical and social environments and strengthening those community resources which enable people to mutually support each other in performing all the functions of life and achieving their maximum potential" (Hancock and Duhl 1986). In their evaluation, Kegler et al. focused on 16 indicators that addressed the link between place and health such as empowerment, sense of community, resident involvement, availability of programs and services, social capital, organizational practices and policies, and the physical environment. Orienting their measurements around socioepidemiological, community capacity building, and urban planning disciplines, Kegler et al. were able to measure multilevel change at the individual, civic participation, organizational, interorganizational, and community levels. They approached methodological challenges of evaluating community change and the presence of health through the combination of mixed and participatory methods with more traditional measures of individual and group health behavior and self-rated health (Kegler et al. 2000).

With the aim to improve and control their quality of life and health, racial and ethnic minorities, immigrants, and poor communities have also made the places in which they live, work, and play into sites for mobilization and collective action. Community-based participatory research methods have provided a compelling model for communities to collaborate with research and government agencies in order to directly investigate and combat the sources of health problems in their neighborhoods. One example is the "Health Environments Partnership" with Black, Latino, and white residents of three disadvantaged and racially segregated neighborhoods in Detroit. Schulz et al. (2005) formed a collaborative research project which included a wide range of health measures and data collection methods over a 3-year period. This included collection of airborne particulate matter, a neighborhood observation checklist, a household survey with a focus on perceived stressors, access to social support and health-related behaviors, and a collection of anthropometric, biomarker, and self-rated cardiovascular health data. Using a participatory methodology, these measures were collected by researchers and community members and analyzed collaboratively. In addition to scientific aims, the project's goals included aims directly addressing the found causes of neighborhood pollution and health disparities. These issues were addressed through collective action, service provision, and policy change. The community-based participatory research methodology which increased community resources and skills through the development of research oriented jobs and training fostered a new way for research to engage with place and people. The collaborative methodology also extended academic and community awareness of the complex ecological and social influences of cardiovascular health. This broad awareness increased their effectiveness in civic engagement and promoted more community–academic–public sector collaborations (Schulz et al. 2005). These outcomes mirrored many of the key indicators outlined in the earlier research of Kegler et al. in the Healthy Cities Project. Furthermore, this type of participatory engagement and multisector collaboration also allows for the affected local community to take quicker and more direct action in addressing the sources of ill health through service, policy, advocacy, and education.

This chapter has reviewed different approaches to understanding how place interacts with race to affect health and well-being. Racial residential segregation and displacement are two key historical and social processes that exemplify how racial and socioeconomic stratification are created, reinforced, and maintained by place dynamics. Place-based social, geographic, and physical processes are racialized to reflect and reinforce social advantages and disadvantages to certain groups and locales. These processes converge and interact to perpetuate health disparities at the individual, neighborhood, and community level. Conversely, the drive to make attachment, meaning, and value within geographic spaces highlights how the dynamics of place, race, and health can be used to produce social, economic, and political processes for research, social movements, healthy communities, and political empowerment.

References

Acevedo-Garcia, Dolores. 2000. "Conceptual framework of the role of residential segregation in the epidemiology of infectious diseases." *Social Science & Medicine* 51(8):1143–1161.

Acevedo-Garcia, Dolores. 2001. "Zip code-level risk factors for tuberculosis: Neighborhood environment and residential segregation in New Jersey, 1985–1992." *American Journal of Public Health* 91:734–741.

Aneshensel, C.S. and C.A. Sucoff. 1996. The neighborhood context of adolescent mental health. *Journal of Health and Social Behavior* 37:293–310.

Bashi, Vilna Francine. 2007. *Survival of the Knitted: Immigrant Social Networks in a Stratified World.* Palo Alto, CA: Stanford University Press.

Basso, Keith H. 1996. *Wisdom Sits in Places: Landscape and Language Among the Western Apache*. Albuquerque, NM: University of New Mexico Press.

Beals, Janette, Douglas K. Novins, Nancy R. Whitesell, Paul Spicer, Christina M. Mitchell, and Spero M. Manson. 2005. "Prevalence of mental disorders and utilization of mental health services in two American Indian reservation populations: Mental health disparities in a national context." *American Journal of Psychiatry* 162:1723–1732.

Berkman, Lisa F. and Cheryl Clark. 2003. "Neighborhoods and Networks: The Construction of Safe Places and Bridges." In *Neighborhoods and Health,* edited by Ichiro Kawachi and Lisa F. Berkman. New York, NY: Oxford Press.

Berkman, Lisa F. and Thomas Glass. 2000. "Social Integration, Social Networks, Social Support, and Health." pp: 137–173 In *Social Epidemiology*, edited by L.F. Berkman and I. Kawachi. New York, NY: Oxford University Press.

Bezruchka, S. and M.A. Mercer 2004. "The Lethal Divide: How Economic Inequality Affects Health." pp: 11–18 In *Sickness and Wealth: The Corporate Assault on Global Health*, edited by M. Fort, M.A. Mercer, and O. Gish. Boston, MA: South End Press.

Brave Heart, Marie Yellow Horse. 1998. "The American Indian holocaust: Healing historical unresolved grief." *American Indian and Alaskan Native Mental Health Research: The Journal of the National Center* 33(3/4):60–82.

Brave Heart, Marie Yellow Horse. 2003. "The historical trauma response among natives and its relationship with substance abuse: A Lakota illustration." *Journal of Psychoactive Drugs* 35:7–13.

Cahill, Meagan and Nancy LaVigne. 2008. "Residential Mobility and Drug Use Among Parolees in San Diego, California and Implications for Policy." pp: 85–116 In *Geography and Drug Addiction*, edited by Yonette F. Thomas, Douglas Richardson, and Ivan Cheung. The Netherlands: Springer.

Cummins S., S. Curtis, A.V. Diez-Roux, and S. Macintyre. 2007. "Understanding and representing 'place' in health research: A relational approach." *Social Science and Medicine* 65:1825–1838.

Curtis, Sarah. 2004. *Health and Inequality: Geographical Perspectives.* London: Sage.

Diez-Roux, A., S.S. Merkin, D. Arnett, L. Chambless, M. Massing, F. Nieto, P. Sorlie, M. Szklo, H. Tyroler, and R. Watson. 2001. "Neighborhood of residence and incidence of coronary heart disease." *New England Journal of Medicine* 345:94–105.

Fullilove, Mindy T. 1996. "Psychiatric implications of displacement: Contributions from the psychology of place." *The American Journal of Psychiatry* 153:1516–1523.

Fullilove, Mindy T. 2004. *Root Shock: How Tearing Up City Neighborhoods Hurts America, and What We Can Do About It.* New York, NY: Ballantine Books.

Gesler, W. 1992. "Therapeutic landscapes: Medical geographic research in light of the new cultural geography." *Social Science and Medicine* 34(7):735–746

Gieryn, Thomas F. 2000. "A space for place in sociology." *Annual Review of Sociology* 26:463–493.

Goldberg, David Theo. 2005. "Racial Americanization." pp: 87–102 In *Racialization: Studies of Theory and Practice*, edited by Karin Murji and John Solomos. Oxford: Oxford University Press.

Gracey, Michael and Malcolm King. 2009. "Indigenous health – Part 1: Determinants and disease patterns." *The Lancet* 374(9683):65–75.

Hancock T. and L. Duhl. 1986. *Healthy Cities: Promoting Health in the Urban Context.* Copenhagen: WHO Europe.

hooks, b. 1990. "Homeplace: A Site of Resistance." pp: 41–49 In *Yearning: Race, Gender and Cultural Politics*. Boston, MA: South End Press.

Hune, S. 1995. "Rethinking race: Paradigms and policy formation." *Amerasia Journal* 21:29–40.

Jacobs, Jane. 1961. *The Death and Life of Great American Cities.* New York, NY: Random House.

Kasinitz, Philip, John H. Mollenkopf, Mary C. Waters, and Jennifer Holdway. 2008. *Inheriting the City: The Children of Immigrants Come of Age*. New York, NY: Russell Sage Foundation; and Cambridge, MA: Harvard University Press.

Kearns, R. 1993. "Place and health: Toward a reformed medical geography." *Professional Geographer* 45:139–147.

Kegler, M.C., J.M. Twiss, and V. Look. 2000. "Assessing community change at multiple levels: The genesis of an evaluation framework for the California Healthy Cities Project." *Health Education & Behavior* 27:760–779.

Krieger, Nancy. 2001. "Theories for social epidemiology in the 21st century." *International Journal of Epidemiology* 30:668–677.

LaVeist, T.A. 1994. "Beyond dummy variables and sample selection: What health services researchers ought to know about race as a variable." *Health Services Research* 29:1–16.
LaVeist, T.A. and J.M. Wallace. 2000. "Health risk and inequitable distribution of liquor stores in African American neighborhood." *Social Science and Medicine* 51(4):613–617.
LaVigne, N.G., J. Cowan, and D. Brazzell. 2006. *Mapping Prison Reentry: An Action Research Guidebook.* Washington, DC: Urban Institute.
Logan, J., W. Zhang, and R.D. Alba. 2002. "Immigrant enclaves and ethnic communities." *American Sociological Review* 67(2):299–322.
Macintyre, S., A. Ellaway, and S. Cummins. 2002. "Place effects on health; how can we conceptualize and measure them?" *Social Science and Medicine* 55:125–139.
Massey, Douglas S. 2004. "Segregation and stratification: A biosocial perspective." *Du Bois Review* 1(1):7–25.
Massey, Douglas S. and Nancy A. Denton. 1993. *American Apartheid: Segregation and the Making of the Underclass.* Cambridge, MA: Harvard University Press.
Massey, Douglas S. and Mary J. Fischer. 2000. "How segregation concentrates poverty." *Ethnic & Racial Studies* 23:670–691.
Meade, M., J. Florin, and W. Gesler. 1988. *Medical Geography.* New York, NY: The Guilford Press.
Menjívar, Cecilia. 2000. *Fragmented Ties: Salvadoran Immigrant Networks in America.* Berkeley, CA: University of California Press.
Minkler, Meredith and Nina Wallerstein, eds. 2003. *Community Based Participatory Research for Health.* San Francisco, CA: Jossey Bass.
Mollica, R.F. 2000 "Waging a new kind of war. Invisible wounds." *Scientific American* 282(6):54–57.
Morenoff, Jeffrey D. 2003. "Neighborhood mechanisms and the spatial dynamics of birth weight." *The American Journal of Sociology* 108:976–1017.
Morenoff, Jeffery D., R.J. Sampson, and S.W. Raudenbush. 2001. "Neighborhood inequality, collective efficacy, and the spatial dynamics of urban violence." *Criminology* 39:517–559.
Omi, Michael and Howard Winant. 1994. *Racial Formation in the United States: From the 1960s to the 1990s.* New York, NY: Routledge.
Organization for Economic Cooperation and Development (OECD). 2010. *OECD Health Data 2010: Statistics and Indicators for 30 Countries.* France: OECD Health Division.
Osypuk, T., A.V. Diez Roux, C. Hadley, and N. Kandula. 2009. "Are immigrant enclaves healthy places to live? The Multi-ethnic Study of Atherosclerosis." *Social Science and Medicine* 69(1):110–120.
Penserga, Luella and Beth Newell. 2009. *Increasing Access to Health Care for Low-Income Uninsured Residents of Alameda, County, California; Baseline Assessment 2007.* Alameda, CA: Alameda County Assess to Care Collaborative.
Portes, Alejandro. 1995. "Economic Sociology and the Sociology of Immigration." pp: 1–41 In *The Economic Sociology of Immigration: Essays on Networks, Ethnicity, and Entrepreneurship,* edited by Alejandro Portes. New York, NY: Russell Sage Foundation.
Portes, Alejandro and Ruben G. Rumbaut. 2006. *Immigrant American: A Portrait.* Berkeley and Los Angeles, CA: University of California Press.
Portes, Alejandro and Min Zhou. 1993. "The new second generation: Segmented assimilation and its variants." *The Annals of the American Academy* 530:74–96.
Relph, E. 1976. *The Placelessness of Place.* London: Pion.
Relph, Edward. 2007. "Senses of Place and Emerging Social and Environmental Challenges." pp: 31–44 In *Sense of Place, Health and Quality of Life,* edited by John Eyles and Allison Willams. Burlington, VT: Ashgate Publishing Company.
Robert, Bryan. 1995. "Socially Expected Durations and the Economic Adjustment of Immigrants." In *The Economic Sociology of Immigration: Essays on Networks, Ethnicity, and Entrepreneurship,* edited by Alejandro Portes. New York, NY: Russell Sage Foundation.
Ross, Catherine E. and Sung Joon Jang. 2000. "Neighborhood disorder, fear, and mistrust: The buffering Role of Social Ties with Neighbors." *American Journal of Community Psychology* 28:401–420.
Ross, Catherine E. and John Mirowsky. 2001. "Ncighborhood disadvantage, disorder, and health." *Journal of Health and Social Behavior* 42:258–276.

Sampson, Robert J. and Stephen W. Raudenbush. 1999. "Systematic social observation of public spaces: A new look at disorder in urban neighborhoods." *American Journal of Sociology* 105:603–651.

Schulz, A.J., S. Kannan, J.T. Dvonch, B.A. Israel, A. Allen, S.A. James, J.S. House, and J.M. Lepkowski. 2005. "Social and physical environments and disparities in risk for cardiovascular disease: The Healthy Environments Partnership conceptual model." *Environmental Health Perspectives* 113(12):817–825.

Schulz, Amy J., David R. Williams, Barbara A. Israel, and Lora Bex Lempert. 2002. "Racial and spatial relations as fundamental determinants of health in Detroit." *The Milbank Quarterly* 80:677–707.

Smedley, Brian D., Adrienne Y. Stith, and Alan R. Nelson, eds. 2003. *Unequal Treatment: Confronting Racial and Ethnic Disparities in Health Care*. Washington, DC: National Academy of Science.

Smelser, N., W. Wilson, and F. Mitchell. 2001. "Introduction." In *America Becoming: Racial Trends and Their Consequences, Volume 1*, edited by Neil J. Smelser, William Julius Wilson, and Faith Mitchell. Washington, DC: Commission on Behavioral and Social Sciences and Education, National Academy Press.

Takeuchi, David T. and Sue-Je L. Gage. 2003. "What to do with race? Changing notions of race in the social sciences." *Culture, Medicine and Psychiatry* 27:435–445.

Tuan, Yi-Fu. 1974. *Topophilia: A Study of Environmental Perception, Attitudes, and Values.* Englewood Cliffs, NJ: Prentice-Hall.

Tuan, Yi-Fu. 1977. *Space and Place: The Perspective of Experience*. Minneapolis, MN: University of Minnesota Press.

UN Human Development Programme. 2010. *The Real Wealth of Nations: Pathways to Human Development.* New York, NY: United Nations Human Development Programme.

Vandemark, Lisa M. 2007. "Promoting the sense of self, place, and belonging in displaced persons: The example of homelessness." *Archives of Psychiatric Nursing* 21(5):241–248.

Walters, K.L. 1999. "Urban American Indian identity attitudes and acculturative styles." *Journal of Human Behavior and the Social Environment* 2(1/2):163–178.

Walters, Karina L., Jane M. Simoni, and Teresa Evans-Campbell. 2002. "Substance use among American Indians and Alaskan Natives: Incorporating culture in a 'indigenist' stress-coping paradigm." *Public Health Reports* 117:S104–S117.

Warr, Mark and Christopher G. Ellison. 2000. "Rethinking social reactions to crime: Personal and altruistic fear in family households." *American Journal of Sociology* 106:551–578.

Weiss, Carlos O., Hector M. Gonzalez, Mohammed U. Kabeto, and Kenneth M. Langa. 2005. "Differences in amount of informal care received by non-Hispanic Whites and Latinos in a nationally representative sample of older Americans." *Journal of the American Geriatrics Society* 53:146–151.

Whitbeck, L.B., G. Adams, D. Hoyt, and X. Chen. 1998. "Conceptualizing and measuring historical trauma." *American Journal of Community Psychology* 33(3/4):199–130.

Williams, David R. and Chiquita Collins. 2001. "Racial residential segregation: A fundamental cause of racial disparities in health." *Public Health Reports* 116:404–416.

Williams, David R. and R. Williams-Morris. 2000. Racism and mental health: The African American experience. *Ethnicity & Health* 5(3/4):243–268.

Wilson, William Julius. 1987. *The Truly Disadvantaged.* Chicago, IL: University of Chicago Press.

Wilson, William Julius. 1996. *When Work Disappears: The World of the New Urban Poor*. New York, NY: Vintage Books.

Zhou, Min. 1992. *Chinatown: The Socioeconomic Potential of an Urban Enclave*. Philadelphia, PA: Temple University Press.

Zolberg, Aristide R. 2006. *A Nation by Design; Immigration Policy in the Fashioning of America.* New York, NY: Russell Sage Foundation.

Part II
Missing Places, Invisible Places

Chapter 6
Morality, Identity, and Mental Health in Rural Ghettos

Linda M. Burton, Raymond Garrett-Peters, and John Major Eason

> It makes me sick and crazy to see how our beautiful and oh so peaceful community has changed. The city influence is ruining us. We are losing our impeccable morals and our sense of who we are as strong, hard-working, law-abiding American citizens who care about others. Those poor Blacks [from Philadelphia and New York City] and Mexicans [from across the border] are moving into our community by the hundreds [because of new prisons, migrant farm work, new drug rehabilitation centers, and low-income housing]. Those people are degenerates and are ruining this place. I'm ashamed to say I am from here anymore. When we have concerts in the park, I see and hear them with their music blaring and their ghetto talk that nobody but them understands. When they sit down anywhere in my vicinity I move my picnic blanket away from them as fast as I can. I don't want my children to sit close to them and *catch* what they have. Those people are stressing me out. They give me migraines. My family and friends feel the same way. We are losing our minds with them here and all these changes in our precious community. I wish the people who don't belong here would die or leave! They have turned our community into a smutty ghetto cesspool with no morals, no pride, [and] no hope of sanity or salvation (Samantha, a semirural small town resident).

Samantha is a 32-year-old White Catholic social worker for a local religious-based charity in a small semirural town in Pennsylvania. She shared these comments with us when we asked how her views of her community and the surrounding rural landscape had changed in the last 10 years. Her words spoke for themselves. In angry and bitter tones she chronicled the rise of "smutty ghetto cesspools" in her community and what she perceived to be declines in morality and residents' historical pride in personal identities anchored in place. As Samantha shared her thoughts with us in the presence of a towering statue of the Blessed Mother, boxes piled high with food and clothing for the poor on either side of her, and a silver cross on a delicate chain around her neck, her face showed both contempt and fear as she relished in her tirade. She was seemingly unaware of the stark contradictions of her opinions and the "pulpit" from which she delivered them. Samantha, like many native residents of this once, in her opinion, bucolic community, was, at that moment in time, a Paul Revere doppelganger. With a rosary in one hand and epitaphs

L.M. Burton (✉)
Department of Sociology, Duke University, Durham, NC 27708-0088, USA
e-mail: lburton@soc.duke.edu

L.M. Burton et al. (eds.), *Communities, Neighborhoods, and Health*,
Social Disparities in Health and Health Care 1, DOI 10.1007/978-1-4419-7482-2_6,

of the disparaged in another (e.g., temporary housing vouchers for displaced poor families), she figuratively harkened to all who would listen, "the ghettos are coming, the ghettos are coming, and our sanity will never be the same."

Samantha's opinions are not rare or isolated sentiments in rural America. Although social scientists have not explored these issues extensively, there are several who have uncovered similar attitudes within US rural populations in the Northeast (Fitchen 1991; Nelson 2005; Schafft 2006), South (Duncan 1999; Falk 2004; Stack 1996), Midwest (Harvey 1993; MacTavish et al. 2006; Salamon 2003) and the West (Sherman 2009). The classic ethnographic work of Naples (1994) is a case in point. In her study of rural Iowa, she described how poor Mexican American migrants to the area changed the social and psychological landscape of the town in which they settled and "posed a significant challenge to the community identity of the town's White European American residents" (Naples 1994:129). Moreover, these White residents saw their moral standards, values, and, their "neat little community" being threatened by the mere presence of new arrivals as one long-time native resident remarked (p. 121):

> [M]y values are just different. [You] see that our school is [increasingly comprised of] people that do not have strong values…now parents with strong values are the underdogs and this other group is taking over. And, I do not like to see that in this community. That bothers me terrifically!

In this essay, we explore these characterizations of rural America focusing on the emergence of rural ghettos and their roles in shaping the well-being and mental health of their residents and those who live in close proximity. We discuss two dimensions of place that are endemic to understanding the influence of rural ghettos on old and new residents' well-being – morality and identity. We argue that, as Samantha so clearly articulated, emerging ghettoized sections of rural communities, particularly those comprised of poor urban and migrant racial/ethnic minority newcomers, have presented challenges to native residents' perceptions, beliefs, and practices about their "moral codes" and their "place identities" in ways that, as one ethnographic informant stated, "rattles their mental health cages."

We explore the concept of rural ghettos in the context of broader changes in rural America and we define them as residentially bounded segregated places with high concentrations of poverty, disadvantage, marginalized populations, and contextual stigma (Eason 2010). The core of rural ghettos can take different forms: dilapidated tracts of housing in small rural towns, subsidized housing projects, and even run-down trailer parks on the outskirts of town (MacTavish and Salamon 2001; Twiss and Mueller 2004). While the term "ghetto" has traditionally been used in the US to identify urban and largely *Black* areas of spatial segregation and disadvantage, we employ the term more broadly here and consider racially homogeneous and segregated areas populated by poor Hispanics or Whites as well. We expand the concept even further by considering the larger ecologies of local residents who reside in protected and affluent spaces on the geographic peripheries of these ghettos (Eason 2010; Pattillo 2003).

To address this topic, we synthesize and draw conceptual connections between the extant literature on rural communities, ghettos, morality, identity, and the impact of place on mental health and well-being. Where appropriate, we integrate into the discussion illustrative exemplar case study information from our own ethnographic work on the *Family Life Project*. The *Family Life Project* is a longitudinal interdisciplinary program project designed to investigate the ways in which community and family contexts influence child development among Black and White families residing in six poor rural counties in Pennsylvania and North Carolina. The project comprises five interrelated interview studies, each of which addressed a unique aspect of family and child development. The project also includes an ethnographic study of the six counties. The ethnographic study intently focused on discerning the contextual meanings and shared understandings of local norms, beliefs, and practices as they were manifested in community relations and family processes within the study sites. Additionally, it explored, in great detail, the daily lives of 101 African American, White, and Hispanic families in these communities as well as recent migrants to these locales from neighboring and out-of-state metropolitan areas. In this chapter, we draw specifically on ethnographic data about the Pennsylvania sites.

We acknowledge that our current thinking about this topic is still under construction and that, at this point, our work is fairly focused on predominately White rural communities with recent racial/ethnic minority migrants. Nonetheless, we are at a place in our thinking in which we feel that we can humbly take it out for an intellectual walk in this chapter. To contextualize our walk, we begin with a brief overview of recent broad-based economic and social changes in rural America. Next, we discuss the emergence of rural ghettos, the contextual and conceptual frame we use for exploring how morality, identity, and residents' well-being are shaped by changing rural landscapes. We conclude with a discussion of the implications of our "intellectual" walk for future research.

The Changing Landscapes of Rural America

> Rural America is, in the country's imagination, still a bastion of traditional values and traditional families. While certain aspects of that vision remain true, a number of things have decidedly changed (Smith, 2008:1).

As Smith (2008) and others have clearly documented, the face of traditional rural communities has undergone considerable changes in recent decades (Brown et al. 2003; Conger and Elder 1994; Cromartie and Swanson 1996; Dill 1999; Lichter and Brown in press). These changes are owing to several trends including the restructuring of rural economies (Fitchen 1991; Naples 1994; Sherman 2006), a recent rise in the migration of low-income racial/ethnic minorities to largely White small-town and pastoral communities (Fitchen 1994; Foulkes and Newbold 2008; Hamilton et al. 2008; Lawson Clark 2008; Salamon 2003), and a redistribution in the spatial concentration of rural poverty (Flora et al. 2004; Lichter et al. 2008; Tickamyer and Duncan 1990). We briefly discuss these trends below.

Economic Restructuring

Economic restructuring in the rural US is represented by shifts away from stable, family-sustaining production jobs to low-wage service employment (Brown et al. 2003; Naples 1994; Tickamyer 1992). These shifts were kindled by contractions in the agricultural sector of rural economies which sent ripple effects through communities that had direct and indirect associations with farming. Advances in global and technology markets ensued and resulted in many higher paying manufacturing and mining jobs moving offshore or being closed out all together (Knapp 1995; McGranahan 1994). Meanwhile, the portion of jobs in lower-paying sectors of the economy (e.g., Walmart) grew dramatically and differentially transformed the availability of jobs for men and for women.

There have been significant declines in job opportunities for men in rural areas while women's employment has markedly increased. In some communities, the majority of women with children have become primary and/or sole providers for their families (Nelson 2005; Smith 2008; Snyder and McLaughlin 2004; Tickamyer and Henderson 2003). Thus, not only have good-paying jobs become more scarce in rural America, but the increased work opportunities actually available have arguably added stress to the lives of women and men as women supplant men as the traditional income-earners in many homes (see for example Harvey 1993). The physical and mental well-being of all concerned in these situations has suffered. Men are more likely to commit suicide (Gessert 2003; Singh and Siahpush 2002). Women have depressive symptoms that are double those in urban areas, and are more likely than urban women to suffer a number of health and mental health problems (Bushy 1997). And children are increasingly turning to drug and alcohol use during adolescence (Scaramella and Keyes 2001; Van Gundy 2006).

Futhermore, several studies have examined the effects of economic restructuring on the values and identities of rural Americans (Fitchen 1991; Greenhouse 1986). Nelson and Smith (1999), for example, found that rural working families had strong values of independence, self-sufficiency, and hard work but almost to the detriment of their well-being. These families often positioned themselves as different from families who were unemployed or who they characterized as not wanting to work and willing to take government handouts – assistance that upstanding employed families saw coming out of their pockets. Adherence to these values and identities may be a partial explanation for the pattern described by Hirschl and Rank (1991) of lower rates of welfare participation among rural poor than urban poor. This resistance to seeking assistance and the negative characterizations of others around the morality of work appears to be part of contemporary rural landscapes that has spawned the polarization of working and nonworking families within rural communities (Sherman 2009).

Migration of Low-income Ethnic/Racial Minorities to Rural Communities

Evidence of the polarizations among groups has increasingly come to light in rural areas as low-income racial/and ethnic minority migrants from urban areas move to these places in search of housing and low-wage jobs (Naples 1994; Lichter and Brown in press). Fitchen (1991), for example, was among the first social scientists to identify this trend in her ethnography of rural New York. In doing so, she cautioned researchers to monitor migration to rural locales in terms of what it meant for social relations between newcomers to and long-time residents of these communities. Indeed, Fitchen's insightful admonitions were borne out as researchers in the millennium are now observing the challenges rural residents and new arrivals face in sharing the same space and place (Johnson 2003). These challenges are typically around perceived differences in morals, values, and place identities.

It is important to note that at the core of these challenges, in some communities, is racism. Naples (1994) hit the proverbial nail on the head when she described the covert and complex ways in which race operated in a rural Iowa community. She reported that even though Whites would not necessarily own their racists' attitudes outright, they shared sentiments with her that suggested that their quality of life was severely undermined by racial/ethnic minorities moving into their communities. Naples (1994) argued that for Whites, the once racial/ethnic homogeneity of their communities had masked, for them, the extent to which whiteness was a component of their rural identity – an identity that poor families of colors now threatened by just "being there."

The Redistribution of Poverty

Along with economic restructuring and the migration of urbanites to rural locales, the redistribution of poverty in these communities had a prominent impact on rural landscapes (Dill and Williams 1992; Duncan and Lamborghini 1994; Weber et al. 2005). Lichter et al. (2008) pointed out that while many rural areas experienced large declines in poverty during the 1990s despite economic restructuring, over half of the rural poor were located in high-poverty areas that were segregated from Whites and nonpoor populations. What this means is that poor racial/ethnic minorities were geographically concentrated and segregated from low-income, as well as affluent Whites. Duncan's (1999) ethnography of three rural communities clearly demonstrated this pattern as she found that the lower class in one of the communities she studied almost exclusively comprised Blacks. It is believed that this type of separation among rural residents by race and poverty has led to the tensions that surround proclamations of the demise of rural morality and identity in ways that create the "craziness and migraines" that White native rural residents like Samantha talk about. These forces are also complicit in the creation of what Davidson (1990) described as rural ghettos. Davidson (1990:157–158) wrote that

> Conditions in America's rural communities are far worse than is generally recognized. Contrary to national assumptions of rural tranquility, many small towns today warrant the label "ghetto." The word "ghetto" speaks of rising poverty rates, the chronic unemployment, and the recent spread of low-wage dead end jobs. It speaks of the relentless deterioration of health-care systems, schools, roads, buildings, and of the emergence of homelessness, hunger, and poverty. It speaks of the inevitable out-migration of the best and brightest youths. Above all, the word "ghetto" speaks of the bitter stew of resentment, anger, and despair that simmers silently in those left behind. The hard and ugly truth is not only that we have failed to solve the problems of our urban ghettos, but that we have replicated them in miniature a thousand times across the American countryside.

Although Davidson's comments are on target in many ways, what it is missing in his description is fuller attention to the role of race relations in the emergence of these ghettos. Race relations are clearly a powerful social force in rural ghettos and one that a number of scholars have hastened social scientists to take seriously (see for example Lichter et al. 2008; Naples 1994).

The Making of Rural Ghettos

> Even though we were poor and growing up in a broken down trailer park, my father forbid me to talk to or socialize with Blacks on Gospel Hill [Black ghetto in a rural Pennsylvania community]. He said they were turning our town into a ghetto and that they were no better than monkeys swinging from trees. He said they come together like roaches, are violent, and don't have any home training or values. They are not like us...they are not made of good country stock (Haley, a 32-year-old White rural community resident).

When one considers the themes we address in this paper – ghettos, morality, identity, and mental health – one's thoughts may initially travel to images of Northeastern and Midwestern urban Black ghettos comparable to the hyperboles of Haley's father. The emergence, prevalence, and images of ghettos, however, are not restricted to a focus on Blacks who reside in urban areas. In fact, the study of poor Blacks in the rural South is what launched the study of *rural* ghettos.

Nearly 20 years ago, geographer Charles Aiken claimed a new form of Black ghetto was emerging in the Yazoo Mississippi Delta (1990; 1998). This ghetto was the result of several social forces including the mechanization of agriculture, the response of "unbounding" to the Civil Rights movement, and the War on Poverty which led to the construction of public housing units in rural areas (Aiken 1987, 1998). The key structural elements of these ghettos included residential segregation, concentrated poverty, relative population density, and minority populations concentrated in public or subsidized housing (Sampson and Morenoff 2006; Small 2007). Independent of size, a town with high poverty and a 75% Black population could be considered a rural ghetto (Aiken 1998). Rural ghettos were argued to emerge when poor Blacks from the most rural areas moved into public housing, compounding White flight in already racially segregated towns (Aiken 1998). Aiken concluded that most towns in the Mississippi Delta with failing economies would inevitability become completely poor, Black, and hopeless.

Recently, geographers, rural sociologists, and demographers have revisited the work of Charles Aiken, finding that rural Blacks, like urban Blacks, live in the most residentially segregated census blocks in the US (Wahl and Gunkel 2007; Lichter et al. 2007a, 2008). Other studies reexamined Aiken's notion of "unbounding," finding that this political strategy of not incorporating Black populations surrounding a White town is still used as a form of racial exclusion (Lichter et al. 2007b). Additionally, research has found that Black and Hispanic housing patterns are linked to concentrated poverty (Lichter et al. 2008; Lichter and Johnson 2007). And, several scholars have expanded the original concept of the ghetto beyond the Yazoo Mississippi Delta suggesting that many rural areas now have areas that resemble ghettos (Cromartie and Beale 1996) or poverty catchments (Foulkes and Newbold 2008).

Stigma and the Rural Ghetto

A critical factor in the development of rural ghettos involves the dynamics of stigma (Wacquant 2001; Wirth 1956[1928]). Knowing how stigma is used to frame a ghetto is critical for understanding the ecological role of disadvantage in shaping morality, identity, and mental health for those residing within ghettos (typically ethnic/racial minorities or extremely poor Whites) as well as those living outside of them (usually working-class to affluent Whites). While spatial concentration by race, class, or ethnicity can define the ghetto conceptually, the ghetto is perceived as a stigmatized space that a "respectable" person would not inhabit or visit (Anderson 1999). This stigmatization occurs, in part, through a process of social isolation. The process begins with a disadvantaged group clustering in a defined space usually because of racial/ethnic affinity and constrained social and economic resources and opportunities. Because a clustering of disadvantaged people is often characterized as a ghetto, the attributes of people residing within these areas are frequently stigmatized as "subpar" or "underclass" by those outside of the group (Wilson 1987). Heightened stigmatization and discrimination by privileged outsiders against ghetto residents follow, resulting in mounting social isolation between the groups (Hirsch 1998; Massey and Denton 1993; Wilson 1987; Wacquant 2002). That social distancing coupled with the stigmatization process, we argue, does much in the way of reconfiguring morality and identity in rural places as well as challenging peoples' well-being. We will speak directly to these issues momentarily, but before doing so we will briefly describe some contextual features of rural ghettos that are relevant to this discussion.

Contextual Features of Rural Ghettos

What does a rural ghetto look like and how does it compare to an urban one? The use of social and physical space in rural ghettos differs somewhat from urban ghettos.

The rural ghetto may be marked by the absence of certain public characters that are endemic to urban ghettos such as the squeegee man, performance artist, or panhandler (Anderson 1999; Bourgois 1996; Duneier 1999). For all practical purposes, signs of homelessness normally associated with urban homelessness do not exist in rural spaces. [The invisibility of homelessness in rural areas does not necessarily mean an absence of homelessness (see MacTavish et al. 2006).] Instead, clusterings of badly worn mobile homes, nearly dilapidated houses, and “the projects” (low-income public housing) serve as structural representations of poverty across various ghetto enclaves.

Rural ghettos are typically racially and socioeconomically homogeneous such that poor Black, Hispanic, White, or other racial/ethnic clusters are easily recognizable in small rural towns, particularly when the majority population is working- to middle-class White. What is more, the designation of a rural ghetto can also be ascribed according to its population’s sexual orientation. For example, in our *Family Life Project* ethnography, we identified pockets of gay and lesbian “ghettos” that don’t correspond to the usual socioeconomic ghetto prototype, but were named as such by native White community residents who saw these enclaves as representing “morally indecent areas comprised of people with confused identities.”

Public displays of social relations and interactions in these areas are also not as animated as they are in some urban ghettos. There is little public activity in “rural hoods” regardless of the time of day or night one visits them. Most socializing occurs behind closed doors. Thus, Eason (2010) writes that rural ghettos are like urban ones, only quieter.

Although there are stark differences between rural and urban ghettos (e.g., relatively smaller clusters of population density among the poor), elements of an underground economy do exist in some places. For example, you may get your car repaired in what otherwise appears to be a residential zoned neighborhood. This type of untaxed, normalized commercial activity is akin to street vending, a form of hustling. Although rural street hustling is not performed quite the same way as urban street hustling, it may have the same substantive value or meaning (Anderson 1990; Duneier 1999; Venkatesh 2009).

Lastly, contrary to what most people believe, rural America has for decades had higher rates of drug and alcohol abuse than any of the nation’s urban areas (Van Gundy 2006; Moore 2001). A recent treatise on the topic by Nick Reding (2009) chronicled the crystal methamphetamine (crystal meth) economy in rural and small-town America, highlighting its notable presence and destructive impact on users of all ages. Other types of drug trafficking (e.g., crack and cocaine), as well as related violent crimes (e.g., murder), also occur at high rates in these environments. As Van Gundy (2006) noted in a report on substance abuse in rural and small town America, rural America is not immune to the drug economies that plague urban ghettos. With this contextual backdrop, we now turn our attention to a discussion of how changes in rural America, specifically the rise of rural ghettos, influence the morality, identity, and mental health of its residents.

Rural Morality and the "Crazy-Making" Attributes of Rural Ghettos

> The [White] police chief told me that he thought it was a moral travesty that those Black boys from the city who moved to town were "getting with" the local White girls. "It is just morally wrong, a violation of our way of life," he said. "The only reason why they are getting our women is because they can dance…and being able to dance is not a sign of character. I thought, jokingly, as he talked, that perhaps the town could fix this moral quagmire by teaching White boys to dance. Then they could get their women back and all would be right with the world again" (Cynthia, a *Family Life Project* ethnographer).

Cynthia's comments raise challenging questions concerning the link between rural ghettos, morality, and mental health. How do we interpret the relationship between place and morality in rural America? Why does morality seem so laden with contradictions to the point of making people, like the police chief and Samantha, "crazy"? Is there a "rural morality" that we can identify and relate to current transformations and processes, particularly around ghettos, in rural America?

To answer these questions we queried the sociological literature and found that there was hardly any cultural commentary on the concept of "rural morality," at least no full treatments of the topic. We did find an occasional mention of it as particular researchers highlighted the moral problems that people in their studies confronted in specific rural contexts (e.g., Falk 2004; Sherman 2006, 2009). With that in mind, our initial response to the question of whether there is such a thing as a "rural morality" is "yes and no." Yes, to the extent there are still some examples of the prototypical rural community and people within it that most commentators would recognize as traditionally rural – i.e., agrarian or small-town locales sparsely populated by hard-working, self-sufficient, and family-oriented types of people who go to church every Sunday. No, because such areas typically do not pervasively exist in contemporary rural America at least not in any coherent and dominating way. Thus, without being able to distinguish a prominent and pervasive cultural rural morality in this discussion, we define and discuss morality in the universal sense of the word.

By "morality," we are referring to both the particular doctrine of thought, feeling, and action that most people in a given social world agree upon and consider proper and those individuals' conformity to such rules of conduct. People in every social setting learn to evaluate themselves and others based on learned notions of morality and cultural competence. This is true for any social world, whether rural, urban, suburban, or otherwise. Thus, moral characteristics, such as lazy, hard-working, trustworthy, and criminal are often used as criteria for distinguishing one individual or group of people from others as a basis for liking, assessing social worth, giving support, and relegating rewards (see Gans 1972). Lamont and Fournier (1992) have discussed this differentiation process as a core behavior for all human beings, and we argue that it has forcefully taken hold in rural contexts that are experiencing changes such as the emergence of ghettos in formerly homogeneous White rural communities.

With these thoughts in mind, then, we can talk about morality in the sense of: (a) the dominant moral code that characterizes a whole community or region, or (b) the specific moral rules-in-use that people apply in specific settings. To further complicate things, the latter, more situated kind of morality may or may not map onto that which holds sway in the larger community (see, e.g., Jackall 1988). There is always some potential mismatch of the two types of morality, particularly when you look at rural areas – or pockets of rural areas – characterized by isolation, extreme poverty, and/or economic desperation (cf. Bageant 2007; Duncan 1999; Reding 2009), places where largely invisible and desperate populations of people operate covertly, often taking advantage of one another in ways that are morally questionable by the larger population (see Schwalbe et al. 2000 on "defensive othering"). So ultimately, we think the answer to our question is one that depends on both the type of morality you are talking about and the particular slice of social life – macro or micro – you are focusing on.

Having said all that, if we are considering how people use morality in contemporary rural environments we must account for the ways in which they, specifically Whites, "borrow" the broad regional sense of morality from days gone by and believe that they are enacting it in their current social relations. We are talking about the traditional type of moral behavior recognized and adhered to by the majority of rural residents, in the past, who were in relatively stable and cohesive rural communities characterized by strong family ties, the willingness to help neighbors, a strong work ethic, and belief in God. Key here is the relative social and economic stability of such places, stasis that provided both a coherent worldview – including the moral guidelines for thinking and acting that go along with it – and some measure of social control older generations have over younger ones (see Falk 2004:42–44). This is social control and social order based on: (a) a common way of looking at the world, (b) the power of individuals to police themselves according to a well-defined moral code, and (c) with the power of community members to successfully enforce penalties against moral transgressions, if necessary.

Given the changes in rural contexts that we have already outlined, we suggest that the traditional moral order described above is what some native White rural people still believe themselves to have while in fact their vision of their moral toolkit is quite distinct from the on-the-ground moral realities they execute in their daily lives. In reality, their on-the-ground moralities may have been transformed because of the loss of family-sustaining jobs and industries, the influx of new populations, the rise of rural ghettos, and people's altered sense of community.

Moreover, we have seen in our own work on the *Family Life Project* the emergence of what Reding (2009) calls the "morality play." In changing rural communities, especially those with rural ghettos and an influx or poor racial/ethnic minorities to homogeneously White towns, native residents may create dramaturgical processes around their beliefs and enactments of morality (see Goffman 1959). Essentially, residents create moral dramas or "theatrical stage acts" that appear to be anchored in moralities of the past, but that are actually desperate attempts to create and sustain a strong sense of self that is distinct from those in their changing communities whom they see as morally inferior. On these residents' parts, an elevated form of morality emerges that is characterized by illusions and contradictions about how they, as "good" White native economically stable ruralites, are compared to "bad" underclass newcomers or those who have declined in favor because of job loss or other economic down turns (see Sherman 2009). So, it is through this process that we witnessed Samantha's emotion-laden tirade and the police chief's homily as they shared disparaging remarks about the morality of ghetto Blacks, while morally elevating themselves as representatives of traditional rural virtues. Hazel, a 51-year-old African American woman and one of the *Family Life Project's* key community informants characterized this process best. She said:

> There are two kinds of morality in this town, one for Whites and one for Blacks. Whites go to church every Sunday, and talk the talk about helping Blacks in Gospel Hill to cultivate a higher standard of living, strong morals, and faith in the right God. That's the way they did it back in the day, or so they say. That sounds good, but it didn't stop them for killing my Black brother for dating a White woman. So what's the 411 [the real story]? Whose morality are they using anyway?

Identity, Mental Health, and Rural Place

> I was born and [have] lived in Gospel Hill all my life and look at me. I am a mess. I don't have any identity. I don't belong here or anywhere. This is not my home. Whites [who are the majority here] tell me I don't belong here. [And] Black folks don't let themselves think about themselves as Black. What are we? Colorless? So how do you learn how to be in this world? I think we [Blacks] are all depressed. [And] the Whites are all scared because they can't have their perfect little world because we [Blacks] are here. And more [Blacks] are coming from Philadelphia. Even if only 3 or 4 more come that's enough to make White folks go crazy. If they [Blacks] keep coming, maybe someday Whites won't have an identity either (Samuel, a 30-year-old African American male resident of a rural ghetto).

As we consider Samuel's comments, it is not surprising that the rural transformations we discussed and, particularly, the rise of rural ghettos have brought about changes in rural identity, too. By rural identity we are referring to the range of meanings given to the self that are rooted in residents' actions and experiences in agrarian and small-town locales. Such environments, which include the physical landscape and social relations found therein, serve as "external anchors" of our habits, motives, routines, and, hence, identities (Graumann 1974:397). Place, in this social-psychological sense, is shorthand for the resources – physical objects, social others, cultural rules, and scripts, etc. – for self-making that are contained within some bounded geographic location (see Burton and Lawson Clark 2005).

More specifically, identities are linguistic labels, indexes of the self (Singer 1980; Schwalbe and Mason-Schrock 1996) that individuals simultaneously claim and have imputed to them based on items, such as residence, group membership, shared social experience, and place identification. Identities signify both the self that we know and the self that we enact in everyday life. With this in mind, a rural identity can be both personal and social in nature. As a personal identity, rural has traditionally been seen as indicative of individual qualities and capabilities, such as hard-working, family-oriented, or self-sufficient, individual-level traits that are typically associated with countryside locations and nonurban milieu (see Naples 1994). Rural can also serve as a social identity, indicating membership in some geographically bounded and like-minded community of others who share values, beliefs, and a sense of belonging based on their residence and experiences in specific environments – e.g., a local township; agrarian settings marked by low-population densities, unspoiled natural space, and strong family ties (see Cobb 1992; Cuba 1984; Fitchen 1991; MacTavish and Salamon 2001; Naples 1994).

Identities are likewise relational in nature, often defined in contrast to other points of social reference based on differences in a person's residential location, age, kinship, social class, and so on. Hence, we find rural residents who identify themselves and others by way of familiar oppositional dichotomies, such as "town" vs. "country;" kin vs. non-kin; "old-timers" vs. "newcomers;" or Southerners vs. Northerners. Identities, too, are interactional realities that must be continually negotiated and realized based on individuals' social resources, their situated actions, and the immediate kinds of social arrangements within which they find themselves (e.g., types of cultural capital, forms of racialized or classed environments, etc.). Regardless of type, all identities serve to ground actors as meaningful and recognizable entities in their social worlds, whether as discrete individuals (e.g., Phyllis or Elijah) or members of some category or group (a Sanderson, Black, farmer). In each of these ways identities give substance to the self, linking it to the surrounding social order.

When local environments undergo substantial change, the ecology of the self – the set of relations with people and objects upon which the self is built – is likewise altered (see Erikson 1976; Garrett-Peters 2009; Hormuth 1990). In often reinforcing ways, structural changes taking place in rural areas, such as job losses, a move from family-sustaining production jobs to low-wage service work, demographic shifts in population, and the rise of rural ghettos have had consequences for identities and the structure of social relations around gender, race, and class that inform these (see Davis 1993, 2000; MacTavish 2007; Naples 1994; Salamon and Tornatore 1994; Tickamyer and Henderson 2003). With this movement has come the uncertainty and anxiety that many long-time rural residents experience as they adapt to the loss of place and the usual social arrangements which helped to give their lives a sense of stability and coherence (see Antonovsky 1979, 1987). Identity pressures and shifts within changing rural environments are not, however, limited to established residents. Such change can be experienced by urbanites and suburbanites seeking new lives in rural areas (see Hoey 2005, 2006; Salamon 2003), as well as in-migrating poorer populations searching for work or low-cost housing (see Salamon and Tornatore 1994). What is ultimately at stake for those involved are the self-conceptions and psychic costs and rewards that arise in the course of claiming, protecting, and/or rejecting various identities in these changing environments (see Schwalbe 2005).

Identity Challenges in the Context of Developing Rural Ghettos

A particular area of rural life where these changes can be seen is in the recent development of rural ghettos. We argue that rural change in the form of newly ghettoized sections of the community presents challenges to the identities and well-being of local residents in two main ways: via *stigmatization* and *a changing local landscape*. For both poor ghetto residents and established locals alarmed at the downward community spiral that areas of concentrated poor populations represent, emerging ghettos can stain rural residents' identities. Along with shrinking local economies, the allure of cheap local housing, and an influx of poor populations from outside the local area, comes an increasingly visible reminder of unwanted community change for many local residents. Rarely do rural residents foresee or fully comprehend the changes taking place, but their impacts are felt nonetheless: changes in the color and fabric of the community, fractured social relations, and damaged identities that are staked on features of the local environment that are no longer there.

Stigmatization and Spoiled Identities

Probably the most salient and identity-relevant feature of rural ghettos is that of stigma, where ghetto neighborhoods and populations are discredited as bad, inferior, or undesirable places and persons, respectively. In this sense, ghetto constitutes a "spoiled" identity (Goffman 1963) for both the physical space of the ghetto and those people living there. As concentrated areas of poverty, crime, and racial and class segregation become increasingly visible in rural communities, these ghettos come to signify moral and social inferiority (see Fitchen 1991; MacTavish 2007) for both the residents within and the rural community as a whole. Though we may find contemporary rural communities that are – or are at least *perceived* to be – relatively egalitarian in structure (see Fitchen 1991), beneath that image are always community residents classified into various groups or categories, identified based on markers of sex, race, residential location, and time in the local community. In rural communities where ghettos have developed, these distinctions and divisions often become amplified, where, for instance, long-time residents attempt to shore up their cherished identities as locals or rural folk by derogating newcomers, "othering" them (Schwalbe et al. 2000) as "ghetto" or categorizing them as outsiders, and hence, *illegitimate* residents (see Fitchen 1991:256; Naples 1994). Another familiar response in local residents' reactions to these undesirable developments is to scapegoat ghetto residents, blaming the newly visible poor or unwanted newcomers as responsible for negative community changes (see Naples 1994; Salamon and Tornatore 1994).

This stigmatization also has felt consequences for a range of ghetto residents. Most apparent are the poor and unemployed underclass of ghetto neighborhood residents, the most vilified being those on public assistance or engaged in criminal activities. Many ghetto residents, constrained by a real lack of work opportunities and increasingly marginalized by the larger local community, are unable and often unwilling to integrate into – and identity with – the larger, more upstanding portion of the rural community. But contrary to the stereotypical image of ghettos as entirely homogeneous neighborhoods populated by a poor underclass, ghetto neighborhoods can be heterogeneous places, comprised by working and professional classes, people who more often share beliefs, proclivities, and class location with those in the larger, traditional community (see Anderson 1990; Pattillo 2003). And, in places where a ghetto identity is conflated with race or ethnicity, nonghetto community residents can be rendered guilty by association (e.g., "decent," working-class Blacks who are lumped in as ghetto residents by local Whites).

A Changing Local Landscape

A second challenge to identity in the context of emerging rural ghettos is felt by established rural residents as they see and experience the local rural landscape change in unwanted and unsettling ways. Two features in particular that underlie a stable rural identity, *routine social relations* and *a sense of community*, are threatened for long-time residents who come to see the burgeoning rural ghetto and its residents as indicative of, and responsible for, unwanted changes (see Erikson 1976; Fitchen 1991; Greider et al. 1991).

Routine, recurring social relations between members of a community are both a feature of traditional rural life and one foundation upon which stable identities are built. Acting in established and expected ways, according to the recognized statuses (e.g., as female, a parent, etc.), role behaviors, and cultural scripts defined within a given social world, provides a basis for self-regulation and smooth social relations between actors in a community. In taking a growing "ghettoization" of the local rural community as an unwanted development, local residents often experience a loss of trust in their social relationships, particularly those relations with ghetto residents (cf. Erikson 1976; Lewis and Weigert 1985). For those who stake their identities on these usual social arrangements, changes in the nature of social relations can be unsettling, as taken-for-granted and valued aspects of their local environments are altered in uncontrollable and often unforeseen ways. As poor segments of the population reach a critical mass, social inequalities become more visible, and physical sections of the local community become unsightly, the developing rural ghetto disrupts the flow of "normal" life for many rural and small-town residents who have subscribed to particular definitions of rural (places and people) that no longer seem to apply (cf. Fitchen 1991:255–257).

Along with these same changes in social relations, local residents' sense of community, their sense of shared identity as members of a cohesive and familiar rural collectivity, can be challenged. Whether actual or a public fiction, the perception of solidarity among local rural residents provides a sense of commonality and a shared identity (see Fitchen 1991; Greider et al. 1991; Naples 1994). From the perspective of established rural residents, ghettoization processes introduce instability and uncertainty into their lives in a movement away from a preferred and sometimes idealized kind of local community. Similar to the predictable kind of reality that routine social relations provide, the sense of stability and coherence (cf. Antonovsky 1979, 1987) that comes with being part of, and identifying with, a local community of others is also at risk under these changing conditions. As undesirable groups of people come in, or formerly valued parts of the community disappear or become an eyesore, the local rural environment changes in unwanted ways, and local residents can come to sense that "things are falling apart." Valued rural identities and the sense of well-being that can come with such identifiers are casualties of these changes.

Discussion and Conclusion

In this essay, we explored the links between rural ghettos, morality, identity, and mental health. This volume provided us with a forum to take our ideas on this topic out for an intellectual walk and we seized the opportunity. As we indicated, the dialogue that we shared here represents our initial attempts to connect ideas that are relevant in our work as we develop an understanding of how recent changes in the landscape of rural America are affecting the mental health of the poor who reside within them. We are currently analyzing data on these themes from the *Family Life Project*, specifically the rural Pennsylvania site. That examination has revealed patterns that are very much in line with those identified by demographers including the restructuring of rural economies (Brown et al. 2003; Lichter and Brown in press), women supplanting men as the primary household breadwinners (Nelson 2005; Smith 2008), a rise in the number of urban racial/ethnic minority migrants to small towns and rural communities (Hamilton et al. 2008; Lawson Clark 2008), and a redistribution in the spatial concentration of rural poverty (Lichter et al. 2008).

We have also seen the trends in social relations around race that ethnographers such as Fitchen (1991), Naples (1994), and others have described (Duncan 1999; Salamon 2003; Sherman 2009). These relations have prodded us to look closely at the ways in which moral behaviors and beliefs are staged in these environments and used as a weapon by privileged Whites against poor minorities and poor Whites in their communities. It also has driven us to consider the role of place identity in the process and how it is perhaps more fragile and tenuous in rural contexts than most would guess. In all of this, observing how peoples' mental health and well-being appear to be "rattled" by changing moralities and identities is a cause for concern. To be sure, the implications of these dynamics will likely increase mental health disparities in rural environments although we can be sure who will most be affected – the poor, or those rural residents who, in the new rural order, are disquieted by the presence of a *certain type* of poor person.

We used the rural ghetto frame to contextualize our discussion because it directs attention to the mechanisms and processes that are involved in studying these very complex issues in ways that are more useful and satisfying than a lens that focuses only on concentrated poverty. The ghetto framework guided us to look at issues like stigma and social differentiation and how they are played out in light of the presence of a rural ghetto in larger rural ecologies. Most importantly, these concepts were theoretically aligned with our interest in morality, identity, and mental health in a changing rural America.

Although, at this point, we see our conceptual approach in this chapter as a work in progress, our hope is that it inspires readers to think about these issues relative to health outcomes in a serious way. There is a precedence for this kind of work as demonstrated by its ethnographic pioneers (see Fitchen 1991; Naples 1994), demographers (Lichter et al. 2008), and geographers (Aiken 1990). Furthermore, with the dramatic changes that are occurring in rural environments, it is our responsibility as social, behavioral, and biomedical scientists to explore these issues with due diligence and to do so in ways that test different perspectives and provide new insights on populations of rural Americans who have been sorely neglected in past and current research.

Acknowledgment Support for this research was provided by the National Institute of Child Health and Human Development (PO1-HD-39667), the National Science Foundation (SES-07-03968), and the National Institute on Drug Abuse.

References

Aiken, Charles S. 1987. "Race as a Factor in Municipal Underbounding." *Annals of the Association of American Geographers* 77:564–579.

Aiken, Charles S. 1990. "A New Type of Black Ghetto in the Plantation South." *Annals of the Association of American Geographers* 80:223–246.

Aiken, Charles. 1998. *The Cotton Plantation South Since the Civil War (Creating the North American Landscape)*. Baltimore: Johns Hopkins University Press.

Anderson, Elijah. 1990. *Streetwise: Race, Class, and Change in an Urban Community*. Chicago: University of Chicago Press.

Anderson, Elijah. 1999. *Code of the Streets: Decenty, Violence and the Moral Life of the Inner City*. New York: W.W. Norton & Company.

Antonovsky, Aaron. 1979. *Health, Stress, and Coping*. San Francisco: Jossey-Bass.

Antonovsky, Aaron. 1987. *Unraveling the Mystery of Health: How People Manage Stress and Stay Well*. San Francisco: Jossey-Bass.

Bageant, Joe. 2007. *Deer Hunting with Jesus: Dispatches from America's Class War*. New York: Crown Publishers.

Bourgois, Philippe. 1996. *In Search of Respect: Selling Crack in El Barrio*. New York: Cambridge University Press.

Brown, David L., Louis Swanson and Alan Barton (eds). 2003. *Challenges in Rural American in the 21st Century*. University Park: Penn State Press.

Burton, Linda M. and Sherri Lawson Clark. 2005. "Homeplace and Housing in the Lives of Low-Income Urban African American Families." pp. 166–188 in *Emerging Issues in African American Family Life*, edited by Vonnie C. McLoyd, Kenneth Dodge, and Nancy Hill. New York: Guilford Press.

Bushy, Angeline 1997. "Mental Health and Substance Abuse: Challenges in Providing Services to Rural Clients." *Bringing Excellence to Substance Abuse Services in Rural and Frontier*

America. Technical Assistance Publication (TAP) Series 20, DHHS Publication no (SMA) 97-3134. http://treatment.org/taps20/bushy.html.
Cobb, James. 1992. *The Most Southern Place on Earth: The Mississippi Delta and the Roots of Regional Identity*. New York: Oxford University Press.
Conger, Rand and Glen H. Elder Jr. 1994. *Families in Troubled Times: Adapting to Change in Rural America*. Hawthorne, NY: Aldine de Gruyter.
Cromartie, John B. and Linda L. Swanson. 1996. "Census Tracts More Precisely Define Rural Populations and Areas." *Rural Development Perspectives* 11(3):31–39.
Cromartie, John B. and Calvin L. Beale. 1996. "Increasing Black-White Separation in the Plantation South, 1970–90." *Economic Research Services*, USDA downloaded from downloaded on July 11, 2008 from: http://www.ers.usda.gov/publications/aer731/aer731e.pdf.
Cuba, Lee J. 1984. "Reorientations of Self: Residential Identification in Anchorage, Alaska." pp. 219–237 in *Studies in Symbolic Interaction* (Vol. 5), edited by N. Denzin. Greenwich, CT: JAI Press.
Davidson, Osha G. 1990. *Broken Heartland: The Rise of America's Rural Ghetto*. New York: The Free Press.
Davis, Dona L. 1993. "When Men Become 'Women': Gender Antagonism and the Changing Geography of Work in Newfoundland." *Sex Roles* 29:457–475.
Davis, Dona L. 2000. "Gendered Cultures of Conflict and Discontent: Living 'The Crisis' in a Newfoundland Community." *Women Studies International Forum* 23:343–353.
Dill, Bonnie Thornton. 1999. *Poverty in the Rural U.S.: Implications for Children, Families, and Communities*. Literature review prepared for the Annie E. Casey Foundation.
Dill, Bonnie Thornton and Bruce B. Williams. 1992. "Race, Gender, and Poverty in the Rural South." pp. 97–110 in *Rural Poverty in America*, edited by C. M. Duncan. New York: Auburn House.
Duncan, Cynthia M. 1999. *Worlds Apart: Why Poverty Persists in Rural America*. New Haven, CT: Yale University Press.
Duncan, C. M. and N. Lamborghini. 1994. "Poverty and Social Context in Remote Rural Communities." *Rural Sociology* 59:437–461.
Duneier, Mitchell. 1999. *Sidewalk*. New York: Farrar, Straus and Giroux.
Eason, John. 2010. *It's Like the City, Only Quieter: Making the Rural Ghetto*. Unpublished Paper. Tempe, AZ: Arizona State University.
Erikson, Kai T. 1976. *Everything in Its Path: Destruction of Community in the Buffalo Creek Flood*. New York: Simon & Schuster.
Falk, William 2004. *Rooted in Place: Family and Belonging in a Southern Black Community*. New Brunswick, NJ: Rutgers University Press.
Fitchen, Janet M. 1991. *Endangered Spaces, Enduring Places: Change, Identity, and Survival in Rural America*. Boulder, CO: Westview Press.
Fitchen, Janet M. 1994. "Residential Mobility Among the Rural Poor." *Rural Sociology* 59:416–434.
Flora, Cornelia Butler, Jan L. Flora with Susan Fey. 2004. *Rural Communities: Legacy and Change*. Boulder, CO: Westview Press.
Foulkes, Matt and K. Bruce Newbold. 2008. "Poverty Catchments: Migration, Residential Mobility, and Population Turnover in Impoverished Rural Illinois Communities." *Rural Sociology* 73(3):440–462.
Gans, Herbert J. 1972. "The Positive Functions of Poverty." *American Journal of Sociology* 78:275–289.
Garrett-Peters, Raymond. 2009. "'If I Don't Have to Work Anymore, Who Am I?': Job-Loss and Collaborative Self-Concept Repair." *Journal of Contemporary Ethnography* 38:547–583.
Gessert, Charles E. 2003. "Rurality and Suicide." *American Journal of Public Health* 93(5):698.
Goffman, Erving 1959. *The Presentation of Self in Everyday Life*. New York: Doubleday.
Goffman, Erving. 1963. *Stigma: Notes on the Management of Spoiled Identity*. Englewood Cliffs, NJ: Prentice-Hall.

Graumann, Carl F. 1974. "Psychology and the World of Things." *Journal of Phenomenological Psychology* 4:389–404.

Greenhouse, Carol J. 1986. *Praying for Justice: Faith, Order, and Community in an American Town.* Ithaca, NY: Cornell University Press.

Greider, Thomas, Richard S. Krannich, and E. Helen Berry. 1991. "Local Identity, Solidarity and Trust in Changing Rural Communities." *Sociological Focus* 24:263–282.

Hamilton, Lawrence C., Leslie R. Hamilton, Cynthia M. Duncan, and Chris R. Colocousis. 2008. *Place Matters: Challenges and Opportunities in Four Rural Americas*. Carsey Institute Reports on Rural America, Vol. 1(4). Durham, NH.

Harvey, David. 1993. *Potter Addition: Poverty and Kinship in a Heartland Community*. New York: Aldine de Gruyter.

Hirsch, Arnold. 1998. *Making the Second Ghetto: Race and Housing in Chicago 1940–1960.* Chicago: University of Chicago Press.

Hirschl, Thomas A. and Mark R. Rank. 1991. "The Effect of Population Density on Welfare Participation." *Social Forces* 70:225–235.

Hoey, Brian A. 2005. "From Pi to Pie: Moral Narratives of Noneconomic Migration and Starting Over in the Postindustrial Midwest." *Journal of Contemporary Ethnography* 34:586–624.

Hoey, Brian A. 2006. "Grey Suit or Brown Carhartt: Narrative Transition, Relocation: An Reorientation in the Lives of Corporate Refugees." *Journal of Anthropological Research* 62:347–372.

Hormuth, Stefan E. 1990. *The Ecology of the Self: Relocation and Self-Concept Change.* Cambridge: Cambridge University Press.

Jackall, Robert. 1988. *Moral Mazes: The World of Corporate Managers*. New York: Oxford University Press.

Johnson, Kenneth. 2003. "Unpredictable Directions of Rural Population Growth and Migration." In *Challenges in Rural American in the 21st Century*, edited by Brown, David L., Louis Swanson and Alan Barton. University Park, PA: Penn State Press.

Knapp, Tim. 1995. "Rust in the Wheatbelt: The Social Impacts of Industrial Decline in a Rural Kansas Community." *Sociological Inquiry* 65(1):47–66.

Lamont, Michele and Marcel Fournier (eds). 1992. *Cultivating Differences: Symbolic Boundaries and the Making of Inequality.* Chicago: University of Chicago Press.

Lawson Clark, Sherri. 2008. *Migration for Housing: Urban Families in Rural Living*. The Center for Rural Pennsylvania Report.

Lewis, David J. and Andrew Weigert. 1985. "Trust as Social Reality." *Social Forces* 63:967–985.

Lichter, Daniel T. and David L. Brown (in press). "Rural America in an Urbanizing Society: Changing Spatial and Social Boundaries." *Annual Review of Sociology.*

Lichter, Daniel T. and Kenneth M. Johnson. 2007. "The Changing Spatial Concentration of America's Rural Poor Population." *Rural Sociology* 72(3):29.

Lichter, Daniel T., Dominico Parisi, Steven M. Grice, and Michael Taquino. 2007a. "Municipal Underbounding: Annexation and Racial Exclusion in Small Southern Towns." *Rural Sociology* 72(1):47–68.

Lichter, Daniel T., Dominico Parisi, Steven M. Grice, and Michacl Taquino. 2007b. "National Estimates of Racial Segregation in Rural and Small-Town America." *Demography* 44(3):563–581.

Lichter, Daniel T., Dominico Parisi, Michael Taquino, and Bo Beaulieu. 2008. "Race and the Micro-Scale Spatial Concentration of Poverty." *Cambridge Journal of Regions, Economy and Society* 1:51–67.

MacTavish, Katherine. 2007. "The *Wrong Side of the Tracks*: Social Inequality and Mobile Home Park Residence." *Community Development* 38:74–91.

MacTavish, Katherine and Sonya Salamon. 2001. "Mobile Home Park on the Prairie: A New Rural Community Form." *Rural Sociology* 66:487–506.

MacTavish, Katherine, Michelle Eley, and Sonya Salamon. 2006. "Housing Vulnerability Among Rural Trailer-Park Households." *Georgetown Journal on Poverty Law and Policy* 13:95–117.

Massey, Douglas S. and Nancy A. Denton. 1993. *American Apartheid: Segregation and the Making of the Underclass*. Cambridge, MA: Harvard University Press.
McGranahan, David A. 1994. "Rural America in the Global Economy: Socioeconomic Trends." *Journal of Research in Rural Education* 10:139–148.
Moore, Robert M. 2001. *The Hidden America: Social Problems in Rural America for the Twenty-First Century*. London: Associated University Presses, Inc.
Naples, Nancy A. 1994. "Contradictions in Agrarian Ideology: Restructuring Gender, Race Ethnicity, and Class." *Rural Sociology* 59:110–135.
Nelson, Margaret K. and Joan Smith. 1999. *Working Hard and Making Do: Surviving in Small Town America*. Berkeley, CA: University of California Press.
Nelson, Margaret K. 2005. *The Social Economy of Single Motherhood*. New York: Routledge.
Pattillo, Mary. 2003. "Extending the Boundaries and Definition of the Ghetto." *Ethnic and Racial Studies* 26:1046–1057.
Reding, Nick. 2009. *Methland: The Death and Life of an American Small Town*. New York: Bloomsbury.
Salamon, Sonya. 2003. *Newcomers to Old Towns: Suburbanization of the Heartland*. Chicago: University of Chicago Press.
Salamon, Sonya and Jane B. Tornatore. 1994. "Territory Contested Through Property in a Mid-Western Post-Agricultural Community." *Rural Sociology* 59:636–654.
Sampson, Robert J. and Jeffrey Morenoff. 2006. "Durable Inequality: Spatial Dynamics, Social Processes, and the Persistence of Poverty in Chicago Neighborhoods." pp. 176–203 in *Poverty Traps*, edited by Samuel Bowles, Steve Durlauf, and Karla Hoff. Princeton, NJ: Princeton University Press.
Scaramella, Laura V. and Angela W. Keyes. 2001. "The Social Contextual Approach and Rural Adolescent Substance Use: Implications for Prevention in Rural Settings." *Clinical Child and Family Psychology Review* 4(3):231–251.
Schafft, Kai. 2006. "Poverty, Residential Mobility, and Student Transiency Within a Rural New York School District." *Rural Sociology* 71(2):212–231.
Schwalbe, Michael. 2005. "Identity Stakes, Manhood Acts, and the Dynamics of Accountability." *Studies in Symbolic Interaction* 28:65–81.
Schwalbe, Michael L. and Douglas Mason-Schrock. 1996. "Identity Work as Group Process." pp. 113–147 in *Advances in Group Processes*, edited by B. Markovsky, B. J. Lovaglia, and R. Simon. Greenwich, CT: JAI Press.
Schwalbe, Michael, Sandra Godwin, Daphne Holden, Douglas Schrock, Shealy Thompson, and Michele Wolkomir. 2000. "Generic Social Processes in the Reproduction of Inequality: An Interactionist Analysis." *Social Forces* 79:419–452.
Sherman, Jennifer. 2006. "Coping with Rural Poverty: Economic Survival and Moral Capital in Rural America." *Social Forces* 85:891–913.
Sherman, Jennifer. 2009. *Those Who Work, Those Who Don't: Poverty, Morality, and Family in Rural America*. Minneapolis, MN: University of Minnesota Press.
Singer, Milton. 1980. "Signs of the Self: An Exploration in Semiotic Anthropology." *American Anthropologist* 82:485–507.
Singh, Gopal K. and Mohammad Siahpush 2002. "Increasing Rural-Urban Gradients of U.S. Suicide Mortality, 1970–1997." *American Journal of Public Health* 92(7):1161–1167.
Small, Mario. 2007. "Is There Such a Thing as 'the Ghetto'?" *City* 11(3):413–421.
Smith, Kristin. 2008. *Working Hard for the Money: Trends in Womens' Employment: 1970–2007*. A Carsey Institute Report on Rural America.
Snyder, Anastasia R. and Diane K. McLaughlin. 2004. "Female-Headed Families and Poverty in Rural America." *Rural Sociology* 69(1):127–149.
Stack, Carol. 1996. *A Call to Home*. New York: Basic Books.
Tickamyer, Ann R. 1992. "Rural Labor Markets and the Working Poor." pp. 41–62 in *Rural Poverty in America*, edited by C. M. Duncan. Westport, CT: Auburn House.
Tickamyer, Ann R. and Cynthia M. Duncan. 1990. "Poverty and Opportunity Structure in Rural America." *Annual Review of Sociology* 16:67–86.

Tickamyer, Ann R. and Debra A. Henderson. 2003. "Rural Women: New Roles for the New Century?" pp. 109–117 in *Challenges for Rural America in the Twenty-First Century*, edited by D. Brown and L. E. Swanson. University Park, PA: The Pennsylvania State University Press.

Twiss, Pamela C. and Thomas R. Mueller. 2004. *Exploring Public Housing Use in Rural Pennsylvania*. Center for Rural Pennsylvania Report.

Van Gundy, Karen. 2006. *Substance Abuse in Rural and Small Town America*. Carsey Institute Report. A Carsey Institute Report on Rural America.

Venkatesh, Sudhir. 2009. *Off the Books: The Underground Economy of the Urban Poor*. Cambridge, MA: Harvard University Press.

Wacquant, Loïc. 2001. "Deadly Symbiosis: When Ghetto and Prison Meet and Mesh." *Punishment and Society* 3(1):95–134. Also in Garland, David. 2001. *Mass Imprisonment: Social Causes and Consequences*. London: Sage Publications.

Wacquant, Loic. 2002. "From Slavery to Mass Incarceration: Rethinking the 'Race Question' in the US." *The New Left Review* 13(Feb):41–60.

Wahl, Ana-Maria Gonzalez and Steven Gunkel. 2007. "From Old South to New South? Black-White Residential Segregation in Micropolitan Areas." *Sociological Spectrum* 27(5):507–535.

Weber, Burce, Leif Jensen, Mathleen Miller, Jane Mosley, and Monica Fisher 2005. "A Critical Review of Rural Poverty Literature: Is There Truly a Rural Effect?" *International Regional Science Review* 28:441–464.

Wilson, William J. 1987. *The Truly Disadvantaged.* Chicago: University of Chicago Press.

Wirth, Louis. 1956[1928]. *The Ghetto*. Chicago: University of Chicago Press.

Chapter 7
The Case of the Missing Mountain: Migration and the Power of Place

Lisa Sun-Hee Park and David Naguib Pellow

Introduction

A most amazing thing happened while conducting interviews for a research project on immigration and environmental politics in Aspen, Colorado. Mountains disappeared. These massive monuments that comprise the Rocky Mountains, which define much of the landscape, character, and history of the American West, ceased to exist.

In 2000, we entered this premier vacation spot to investigate the recent passage of an anti-immigration resolution by the city council of Aspen, Colorado, a town that sits more than 600 miles from the US–Mexico border. The resolution called on the federal government to implement greater restrictions on immigration in order to preserve the economic, cultural, and ecological integrity of the nation and this premier city. Aspen is an exclusive resort town with an international reputation for high-end service and a stunning landscape of pristine mountains, all configured to welcome wealthy skiers in the winter and wealthy hikers in the summer. And, like many communities, towns, and cities in the USA, Aspen depends upon cheap immigrant labor to fuel its local service economy. Ironically, what we found upon entering the field site was an invisibility, or disappearance, of immigrants as people, in direct relation to their hypervisibility as necessary workers.

We observed two different places called Aspen. The dominant, commercial Aspen was an idyllic, postindustrial refuge with stretch Range Rover limousines, toy poodles with diamond encrusted collars, world-class ski slopes, and film celebrities who live part of the year in multimillion dollar single-family homes. In this place, there are no ugly social problems like poverty, racism, and labor exploitation. Here, immigrants are ski instructors who are young and athletic with sport "charming" accents from Austria, Australia, or Nordic nations whose architecture is replicated in numerous "chalets" in town. The other Aspen is a place where foreign-born

L.S.-H. Park (✉)
Department of Sociology, University of Minnesota, Minneapolis, MN, USA
e-mail: lspark@umn.edu

L.M. Burton et al. (eds.), *Communities, Neighborhoods, and Health*,
Social Disparities in Health and Health Care 1, DOI 10.1007/978-1-4419-7482-2_7,

workers from Latin America drive 60–140 miles daily to work in low-status jobs for low wages with few benefits. Many of these workers live in deplorable housing conditions, including cars, campers, and even caves.

In the glossy, commercial version of Aspen, these immigrants do not exist. However, if you look in the back of any restaurant, hotel, or residential home, immigrants cook and clean kitchens and bathrooms, mow lawns, and pour concrete over outdoor heated driveways. Like so many communities, immigrants are made invisible in multiple ways. For example, the lack of affordable housing forces many to live "down valley" in trailer parks that are hidden along the highway and away from the commercial center. The increasing presence of federal Immigration and Customs Enforcement (ICE) in targeted sweeps at Wal-Mart (one of the only affordable stores in the area) and the building of a new immigrant detention center (i.e., jail) in a neighboring town also works to keep immigrants in hiding. But, perhaps the most persistent and commonplace acts of enforcing immigrant invisibility are the everyday indignities experienced at work, school, and home that remind them of their marginality as people despite, or in direct contradiction to their centrality within both the local and global economies.

When we interviewed Latino immigrants in Aspen and across the larger Roaring Fork Valley about their living and working experiences, we heard about a very different place. At the end of an hour-long interview, we asked what s/he thought about the natural beauty of Aspen's mountains. This question consistently brought what was a fairly smooth conversation to an abrupt stop. In almost every case, one of two things happened. Some just broke out in laughter, dismissed the question, and asked if the interview was over. Others gave us a blank look and asked, "Mountain? What mountain?" In their cognitive geography, the massive Rocky Mountains of Aspen disappeared. People didn't "enjoy" the mountains; one simply worked on them.

However, in our lengthy conversations, it was clear that Aspen did not disappear with its mountains. Rather, Aspen existed as a different place with an alternative set of meanings. In both literal and figurative ways, immigrants "made" Aspen in accordance with their own experiences – one that apparently has nothing to do with skiing down a mountain or taking in a show at the Aspen Music Festival. This kind of place-making is fundamental to "self-making." Philosopher Jeff Malpas (1999:15) argues that place is not a mere by-product of humans; it is a necessity for being: "being and place are inextricably bound together in a way that does not allow one to be seen merely as an effect of the other; rather being merges only in and through place." Meaning, a localized sense of place is necessary in defining personal identity and social belonging, particularly within a context that works so hard to make them disappear. It appears that this self-making is not derived purely from the transnational memories of "home" immigrants hold onto, but also requires a more immediate, material construction of place that makes their presence real and helps them to survive, if not thrive, in their new community.

This chapter investigates the power of place through the lens of transnational migration. We begin by arguing that within the growing political economy of globalization, the power and significance of place, and particularly of borders, have intensified. We then discuss the ways in which immigrants construct another Aspen in contrast to efforts to "displace" them. Here, we briefly outline two of the more familiar strategies used by Aspenites and introduce a more novel approach (environmentalism) that has strong potential for widespread future adaptations. Following the creative direction of Thomas Gieryn (2000), our revisit to this research site using a "place-sensitive" lens provides new insights into the power of place and place-making in immigrant adaptation and alienation.

Migration, Globalization, and the Increasing Significance of Borders

As Saskia Sassen (1990) argues, transnational labor migration is an integral part of the global movement of capital, goods, and services (Sassen 1990). And despite efforts to limit the flow of migration, the establishment of global political, military, and economic linkages continues to foster large-scale emigration to particular nations, including the USA. In this way, migration patterns are not haphazard. Large-scale emigration is directly tied to foreign investment in export production. For instance, US trade with Mexico grew by a factor of eight from 1986 to 2004 (Sassen 2006). Despite this embedded connection between the movement of capital and the movement of people, national immigration policy remains almost entirely fixated on border control. This is a pivotal flaw in many countries. Sassen writes, "Yet with all these differences immigration policy and the attendant operational apparatus in all these countries reveal a fundamental convergence regarding immigration. The sovereignty of the state and border control, whether land borders or airports, lie at the heart of the regulatory effort" (Sassen 1999:150). The popular preoccupation with the literal US–Mexico border has been an easy scapegoat for multiple national anxieties, particularly with regard to the economy and terrorism. It provides big political gains while in reality doing little toward national "security" or economic stability (Massey 2003). Instead, we have witnessed continuous disintegration of civil rights and the social safety net for both citizens and noncitizens in the name of border control and national security.

Borders are demarcations of power. Whether of literal physical place or figurative abstract assumptions, borders are socially constructed entities. Geographer David Sibley (1997) explains that these social boundaries can provide both security and comfort as well as provoke risk and fear, depending upon where you stand and with what resources. Subsequently, the ability to cross such boundaries – or, to move from a familiar space to an alien space under the control of someone else – can be an anxious experience.[1] Borders are also liminal spaces. As such, they are

[1]In some circumstances it can be fatal, as graphically illustrated by the 400+ deaths of Latin American women working in Maquila factories in Juarez.

messy spaces in which the contradictions and confusion of boundary maintenance are exposed. Legal scholar Robert Chang (1996) astutely observes, "The Border is everywhere" and yet can be rendered invisible. "It is through this invisibility that the border gains much of its power" (Chang 1996). Chang notes that because national borders are imperfect, supplementary mechanisms for exclusion are deployed.

The border took on even greater symbolic and cultural importance for US national identity during the 1990s. Certainly, anxiety regarding national security helped solidify the southern borderlands as a tangible front in the frequently intangible "global war on terror." At the same time, the rapidly growing immigrant population began to settle in nontraditional destination states. Work opportunities in the Southeast, Midwest, and Rocky Mountain states attracted immigrants away from the usual coastal cities. The foreign-born population more than doubled in many of these new destinations between 1990 and 2000 (Urban Institute 2002). According to the Urban Institute, "The dispersal of our newest arrivals to regions that historically have attracted relatively few immigrants means that the integration issues previously confined to only a handful of states – issues such as access to language classes, health care, welfare benefits, and jobs – are now central concerns for most states" (Urban Institute 2002:1). In fits and starts, immigration has topped the agenda in many towns across the nation, from Aspen, Colorado to Durham, North Carolina to Nashville, Tennessee.[2] Similar to what Alex Kotlowitz found in his analysis of Carpentersville, a small town in Illinois with 37,000 residents, immigration politics is experienced in a very personal way with a strong tendency to turn nasty. Carpentersville is described as a town "without a center." Longtime residents report a growing sense of alienation and isolation within a global economy that dramatically changed the racial demographics from 17% Latino in 1990 to 40% a decade later (Kotlowitz 2007). And, while Kitty Calavita, Ruth Milkman, and other scholars repeatedly note the historical fact that wage levels fell and income inequality grew as a result of deindustrialization, capital flight, economic restructuring, and the dismantling of labor unions in the 1970s and 1980s (all of which occurred *before* the current influx of immigrants into middle America), immigrants remain easy targets during these unsettling times (Calavita 2008). The US–Mexico border, then, is seen as necessary for regaining a sense of stability, particularly perhaps for those communities further away from the borderlands who see their lives in the "heartland" changing in ways that no longer center their experience (Kotlowitz 2007).

The underlying role of these border-making enforcement measures is what Nicholas DeGenova (2005) calls "deportability" (or, from a place-sensitive perspective, "displacement"). He writes, "The US nation-state's enforcement of immigration law and policing along the US–Mexico border, notably, have long sustained the operation of a revolving-door policy – simultaneously implicated in *im*portation as

[2]For discussion of Aspen, CO, see Park and Pellow (forthcoming) The Slums of Aspen. For Carpentersville, IL, see Alex Kotlowitz (2007). For Nashville, TN, see Pat Harris (2009).

much as (in fact, far more than) deportation"(DeGenova 2005:8) The border and its programs create its own legitimacy through the production of migrant "illegality" or criminality. At the same time, illegality and the possibility of deportation facilitates continued displacement, which serves to preserve immigrant labor's vulnerable status.

Power and Place, Aspen Style

Public Emplacement

Given the heavy presence of the increasingly militarized border, immigrants in Aspen and the larger Roaring Fork Valley have devised multiple methods of emplacement. One method directly and publicly addressed a border-making facility: an INS detention center. With the organizational assistance of key local, nonprofit agencies, immigrants participated in a public march, a town hall forum, and petition drives in protest. Their efforts culminated in early November 1999 with hundreds of people descending on the town of Carbondale, the proposed site for the facility, for several hours of marching and speeches at a rally. Participants carried signs with messages such as "Permite vivir en paz" (Let us live in peace); "Respeto a los derechos humanos" (Respect human rights); "There goes the neighborhood"; "We want the Latinos to stay, the INS should go" (Stiny 1999); "Deport the INS"; and "Aliens = people" (Craig 1999). Each of these placards attests to the view that immigrants are whole human beings, beyond a disembodied labor force. In an unusual turn of events, Latino immigrants, in conjunction with Anglo allies, collectively established a public presence in an effort to legitimize their place within this locality. In doing this, the INS facility – itself a criminalizing social force – was rendered illegitimate, or "deportable." And, in fact, it was "deported" (at least to the neighboring town of Glenwood Springs).

The successful "displacement" of the facility out of Carbondale required a multipronged approach. In addition to public actions like the rally, Latinos Unidos, Stepstone Center, and the Roaring Fork Legal Services, the main nonprofit organizations leading this effort, articulated three different place-based arguments. First, they framed their concern as one of a jail being located in a quiet neighborhood and how that would be hazardous because of the risk to the public associated with criminals being held there. Of course that framing explicitly accepted the INS' own labeling of immigrants as criminals. Another frame was that the danger this public building posed to the community constituted a "taking" of property owners' rights under the US Constitution – a classic conservative western populist argument. And still a third frame was built on a more critical social justice perspective that argued against the broader ripple effects of such a facility's presence – that it would instill fear, terror, and lend itself to racial profiling of Latinos, whether documented or not. Felicia Trevor, former director of the Stepstone Center and a resident of Carbondale, filed an appeal of the building permit issued for the facility. Her letter read, "One of the primary uses of this facility would be as a detention point for dangerous criminals, and the building would become a staging point for detaining and transporting these criminals… This will present a danger to many Carbondale residents, both in the kinds of persons that will be processed, as well as the danger of this office becoming a target from those outside." The letter also stated,

> There is a highly populated residential neighborhood surrounding the site, and property owners in this area have not been provided adequate notice that this 'public building' would include a secure facility designed to harbor federal criminals. Permitting occupation of the site by the QRT [Quick Response Team] is an unjustified taking of these property owners' rights to quiet enjoyment of their homes in safety, and a violation of the residents' constitutional rights.
>
> Daniels (1999)

Trevor and Roaring Fork Legal Services director Kathy Goudy appeared before the town board to express their concern that the presence of the INS facility would lead to more harassment of Latinos, causing many to leave the area. Activists deliberately combined these three seemingly contradictory frames to gain the widest possible support for opposition efforts directed at the facility. While contradictory, these frames are continuous in their place-based logic. Each exploits people's vulnerability to social change or disruptions to their sense of place. At issue is their sense of themselves – their identity and belonging that is so tied to the identity of their town. For Carbondale, a small town that lives and struggles under the shadows of Aspen's blinding glitter, even an outcome that is clearly pro-immigrant was achieved through arguments that adhere to normative constructions of "good" and "bad" immigrants. This has significant long-term limitations as illustrated by the fact that an INS facility was built in the region, just not in Carbondale. These place-based arguments, however, helped define a distinct political identity and boundary. In January 2000, the Carbondale Zoning Board of Adjustment voted to deny the INS its building permit (Daniels 2000). But to their credit, Latinos Unidos and Stepstone acknowledged these larger limitations and took proactive steps to propose new directions for the INS. In a letter to an area newspaper, they stated "We also believe the INS should restructure their present immigration procedures to include greater emphasis and resources on processing of immigration documents and the creation of temporary work visas, and to lessen the focus on the detention of undocumented workers" (Stroud 2000).

Everyday Emplacement

A second method of emplacement Latino immigrant residents utilized is of a more everyday variety in which they formulate a sense of stability despite the regular harassment of local police, federal immigration enforcement presence, and some very vocal white native-born residents. In addition to working long hours, immigrants develop a collective sense of community by volunteering at local charities, going to church, taking night classes at the community college, participating at local primary schools, and, of course, caring for each other within and across families. Carla is one example. She told us: "I have been working in Snowmass at the hotel. I'm a housekeeper, for two years. I work five days there, and on my extra day, I clean houses. I get up at six I finish at seven [pm]. And every other Friday I volunteer at the Aspen thrift shop." Federico, a longtime resident of the Valley, leads a full life that integrates different opportunities in the area. He and his family have been able to enjoy an existence that is beyond the labor of survival. Federico proudly told us:

> I'm a carpenter. I also work in Aspen. I remodel houses, very big houses. I work eight hours a day, 7-3. Tuesday and Thursday evenings, I go to the Colorado Mountain College in Carbondale for classes. I also help my kids with homework, to help them with their Spanish because they speak more English than Spanish and we want our kids to maintain both languages. Two of my youngest sons dance for the city of Aspen ballet. We go to church on Saturdays – the Spanish masses – because it's very important for us to maintain our religion, pass it on to our children. Another routine is that I referee soccer.

Carla and Federico are the lucky ones. Having lived in the USA for a number of years, they have established a sense of place. However, many others still struggle to do so. Lupe is one example:

> It's been twelve years since I arrived in the US. I am from Honduras. I heard stories from people who used to come here for work. Financially, they were paid more here than other places. But when I arrived here, it was a different issue. I came here and I was having trouble finding a place to live, finding a job. For the reason of being undocumented, it's been difficult. They don't pay what they said sometimes. Instead, they would pay you how much they want to pay. I've been in Glenwood Springs for five years now. We have to do a lot of work and we don't get paid very well.

The increasing militarization of the border has made life increasingly difficult and consequently, the necessity of emplacement is greater than ever. Like many tourist towns, the nature and availability of work can change dramatically with the change in season. Juanita, a staff member at Catholic Charities, explained, "In winter it's very difficult to pay the bills and rent because a lot of people get laid off. In the winter it is only the people who work in the hotels or restaurants in Aspen that have work. Other than that, a lot of people are laid off. That's the worst part of the year." This flexibility of labor demand facilitated a transnational response in which migrants crossed the US–Mexico border multiple times each year in search of work. Julio's story is one illustration of this practice. He lives half the year in Mexico and the other half in a trailer park in the Roaring Fork Valley with his daughter, who is an adult. The trailer park manager knows he is undocumented and will not allow him to live there even though his daughter is a resident. Julio said,

> I have to go in, sneaking in. The manager is always watching. But if the manager finds out that I'm there with my daughter, he will just tell her to move out of the park. I have to park like a mile away and just walk home, sneaking, you know. So that's why we don't even go out, we don't even enjoy the garden, we have to be in the house. My wife doesn't work, so she's in the house 24 hours a day. Even though we have good salaries out here, with the rent and things they have to pay, you don't get to enjoy, you don't get any extra time or money to go bowling, to do fun stuff with your family. We don't get to have fun stuff like most people do.

In effect, Julio finds himself under house arrest and immobile unless he is laboring for someone else. With increasing border security (this includes beyond the literal border), migrants like Julio are finding border crossing more difficult and dangerous. According to an Associated Press report published in 2004, border crossings by undocumented persons claimed one life every day (Pritchard 2004). And, once inside the country proper, transportation routes can also be fraught with danger. In February 2000, two vans transporting undocumented persons slid off an icy highway and into a snow bank in Wolf Creek Pass, Colorado. No one was hurt in that accident, but a month earlier (January 2000), fifteen people were injured and three killed in a similar accident near Walsenburg, Colorado. An INS supervisor in Alamosa, Colorado told reporters that these "smuggle vans… remind me of slave ships… They jam people into them just like the holds of slave ships. They are being exploited" (Hunter 2000). Once migrants reach their destinations, they are often working the most unrewarding, lowest paid, and high-risk jobs available, even if they arrive here legally through the federal H2-A visa program (Yeoman 2001). The job-related death rate in Colorado for a Mexican worker is four times greater than the average US-born worker (Pritchard 2004).

Seasonality also has specific gendered effects. Evita Salinas, a temporary labor contractor in the area said as follows:

> Most of the guys here are doing construction labor – about 80% of them. It all depends on the season. During the summer time you can have like 60% working construction and the other 40% are landscaping. During the winter it's very tough and there's not a lot to do, so many people are getting out and working in hotels and restaurants. There is a little bit of construction. And snow shoveling. For women, during winter time there is the hotel. You can do piece rate and you do as many units as you can – they pay you per unit – or you can work on shifts at hotels. That's tough for women because there's not a lot, just cleaning and landscaping. Or on the golf course the girls are doing some restaurant work. And it's tough because most of the girls in this town have kids. There is no real childcare here. There is a lot of childcare for gringos, but you need to pay a lot of money and you cannot afford it. So what we do is to have one friend take care of ten kids, but it's awful, it's tough. It's like a system. Somebody will take care of the babies and they will get maybe $10 per baby, but its very difficult. That's why I don't have babies [laughter].

As with many tourist economies, services like affordable childcare for the manual workforce are nonexistent. The available choices for the care of children of immigrants are extremely limited. We interviewed Gustavo, a grandfather in his late 1960s, who, once again, crossed the treacherous Sonoran desert. He did so at the request of his daughter who asked him to come to the States in order to care for his ill young grandson. Like many immigrants, Gustavo had worked for much of his adult life in the USA sending his paychecks to his family in Mexico with the intent of building a house in Mexico and retiring there. After many years of hard labor, Gustavo achieved his goal only to find that his grown children needed his help while they struggled in Colorado. Now, he spends his days inside a trailer home that he shares with his daughter's family of four, looking after a grandchild with special needs who requires round-the-clock care, while his daughter and son-in-law work as janitors in Aspen. His deeply lined face, marked with years of labor in construction sites and agricultural fields, showed little emotion as he cracked a polite smile and said with a shrug, "Of course I'm here. My grandson needs me. Who else is going to take care of him?"

Given that health care is often a struggle for native-born US citizens, 47 million of whom currently have little or no coverage (Appleby 2006), we found significant inconsistencies in the cost and quality of health care for migrants in Aspen and the Roaring Fork Valley. For low-income immigrants, whether they receive health care and how much it costs seems to be completely at the whim of clinic administrators, sheer luck, or divine intervention.

We spoke to one young couple – Josefa and Tomas – who had arrived from Mexico just a few months prior to our visit. Tomas had a chronic health condition related to a perforated liver, and Josefa was 7 months pregnant. She told us:

> We are worried about the health care because everything here's pretty expensive. We tried to sign up for some services and couldn't get them here. They told us that we have to pay 400 dollars up front, and it's a cost between 7 and 8 thousand dollars to have the baby in the hospital.

Like everything else in this exclusive mountain resort, the cost of living is exorbitant, including health care.[3] Given that labor and delivery are covered under emergency health care and therefore available for everyone – including undocumented immigrants – we asked if the clinic and hospitals Josefa visited had signed her up for public health insurance.[4] She said, "I already went for one office visit and had an ultrasound and it was 800 dollars. And I haven't been able to pay, and now I have another appointment on the 29th, but if I don't bring 400 dollars they won't see me." Already in her third trimester, Josefa had only had one prenatal care visit and did not expect to go back to the hospital until the labor.[5] Another interviewee experienced similar treatment. She said, "I paid six thousand dollars for my birth. I gave four hundred the first visit, eight hundred the next, and now I'm making payments." However, in an earlier focus group, we spoke with another Latina who had just given birth a few weeks ago at the same clinic that Josefa visited. She was determined to be an indigent case and was not charged for her delivery.

Other immigrants and advocates we spoke with related similar inconsistencies. Juanita, a staff member at Catholic Charities in Glenwood Springs, told us, "There's

---

[3]For a more detailed analysis of the politics of immigrant health care, see Lisa Sun-Hee Park's *Bearing the Burden* (forthcoming NYU Press).

[4]Emergency Medicaid, for which undocumented immigrants qualify, covers labor and delivery. Also, Colorado is one of 12 states that provide prenatal care coverage for "qualified" immigrants who have resided in the USA for less than 5 years (see Kaiser Family Foundation & Center on Budget and Policy Priorities. 2004. *Covering New Americans: A Review of Federal and State Policies Related to Immigrants' Eligibility and access to Publicly Funded Health Insurance*. Menlo Park, California. November).

[5]Prenatal care for undocumented pregnant immigrants can be serviced through presumptive eligibility programs in many states. Presumptive eligibility allows uninsured pregnant women to obtain immediate prenatal care while their Medicaid eligibility is processed (National Latina Institute for Reproductive Health. 2005. *Prenatal Care Access among Immigrant Latinas*. New York. December).

a clinic in Rifle, but we've been receiving a lot of complaints that they are being really racist – the people who work up there – they don't tell clients that there's a low-income service up there. So even people from Rifle are coming up here for services." Jasmine, another immigrant Valley resident, stated, "Health care is a huge issue. We don't have health care. I had to pay $600 for $100 worth of insurance. It's really bad here. There are programs to help Latinos for health care but I don't know which ones they are. There is Medicaid, but in order to qualify, you have to make *no* money. We don't get health insurance through the job."

The lack of such basic and relatively cheap reproductive care illustrates the "vagabond" nature of late capitalism. Cindy Katz (2001) writes as follows:

> Globalized capitalism has changed the face of social reproduction worldwide over the past three decades, enabling intensification of capital accumulation and exacerbating differences in wealth and poverty. The demise of the social contract as a result of neoliberalism, privatization, and the fraying of the welfare state is a crucial aspect of this shift.
>
> Katz (2001)

Here, Katz places the irresponsibility on capitalist production that extracts the profitable benefits of migrant labor but does not pay minimal costs. She adds, "A vagabond, as is well known, moves from place to place without a fixed home. However, vagabondage insinuates a little dissolution – an unsettled, irresponsible, and disreputable life, which indeed can be said of the globalization of capitalist production." Capitalism apparently has no place, no loyalties to specificity or the everyday material realities of workers. Instead, it moves across transnational borders in ways that not only delink social reproduction from production but also use the borders themselves to make migrants invisible.

The immigrants we spoke with counter this disembodiment in an everyday context by finding ways to develop friendships and build meaningful community connections. For example, José Cordova stated,

> I go to church, you know? And usually we have mass and a little youth group. And I'm involved in that, in helping teenagers. On weekends, we have retreats and stuff like that. And we've become friends with the youth and we go sometimes to camping or we play football, soccer and stuff like that. Even just sitting around and talking about different topics, that's what we do usually.

Others find or make time to relax after work, in ways that would be familiar to most people. Javier said, "After work sometimes we have a beer and play soccer, here in Carbondale. Behind the middle school there's a basketball court and we organize there to play soccer in the field." Josefa is also involved in a church group and works hard to carve out a place for the Latino community. She explains, "We can't do skiing and other things that are expensive sports that the Aspen people do. We do baseball, though. The whole Latino community reads *La Mision* – that's our paper. And we also listen to radio." These actions are reminiscent of what bell hooks calls "homeplace" in the lives of African Americans: "Black women resisted by making homes where all black people could strive to be subjects, not objects, where we could be affirmed in our minds and hearts despite poverty, hardship, and deprivation, where we could restore to ourselves the dignity denied us on the outline in the public world (hooks 1990)."

Questioning Environmental Privilege

A third method of emplacement is in response to a more novel form of migrant displacement. On December 13, 1999, the City Council of Aspen unanimously passed a resolution petitioning the US Congress and the President to enact legislation that would stabilize the nation's population. The language of the resolution suggests that this goal could be achieved by enforcing existing laws regulating undocumented immigration and reducing authorized immigration. City Council member Terry Paulson, who is also a longtime immigration critic and self-avowed environmentalist, led this effort. He received support and guidance from nationally prominent immigration control organizations such as the Carrying Capacity Network and the Center for Immigration Studies, who reportedly told him, "other communities haven't had the courage to do so… Because many current immigrants are members of minority groups in the US, attempts to limit immigration may be seen as racist."

Paulson wasted no time in calling for an expansion of the resolution beyond the city of Aspen. He announced his intention to engage a statewide campaign to "promote overpopulation awareness" and declared, "If we address population and do something about it everything else will fall in line." Aspen, located in Pitkin County, Colorado, then successfully persuaded the county to follow the city's lead and in March of 2000, the County commissioners voiced unanimous approval for a "population stabilization" resolution. The Aspen city council document combines classic nativist language around immigration with ideas that many persons of a liberal or left political persuasion would embrace. For example, the document includes the following seemingly progressive statements regarding environmental and labor conditions:

> The people of the United States and the City of Aspen, Colorado envision a country with… material and energy efficiency, a sustainable future, a healthy environment, clean air and water, ample open space, wilderness, abundant wildlife and social and civic cohesion in which the dignity of human life is enhanced and protected.

The goal for Aspen is to be a "city beautiful," a beacon of sustainability and social responsibility. Unfortunately, underpinning this goal is nativist ideology. Aspen Councilman Terry Paulson sponsored the resolution with the following opening statement:

> Fellow Council Members. This resolution we will be considering for adoption tonight could be the most important consideration we will ever make as representatives of our constituents and their children. … "We have agitated, confused and deluded ourselves with the illusion that we are being overwhelmed by many, many problems – when in fact we have primarily only one. But it is the one that terrifies us the most, and we handle that terror by chattering endlessly about everything else. Denying... and minimizing population growth in the 1990s is a *hate crime against future generations*, and it must end."[6] Please, join me…, by passing this resolution as written, and thereby insuring a sustainable future for America and her children.

---

[6]Here, Paulson cites Jonette Christian from Mainers for Immigration Reform, who gave a presentation at the Aspen Institute in October 1999.

Following this logic, immigration becomes the major cause of our ecological crisis. Similar initiatives have been proposed in numerous states and cities across the West and Southwest and in other nations under the banner of "green" policy making. However, the city of Aspen experienced a momentary embarrassment when it was reported that its resolution was featured on American Patrol's website – a California-based organization that the Southern Poverty Law Center characterizes as a "hate group."

In response to this and other reports of concern about the resolution, the Aspen City Council took great pains to stress that the initiative "was not racially motivated." The countywide resolution, passed 4 months later, contained the following statement: "Immigration is the leading cause of population growth in the Unites States. Population is the leading cause of environmental degradation." Thus, by implication, immigration must be the leading cause of ecological degradation. Like the Aspen resolution, the county's resolution underscores the longstanding link between nativism and environmentalism in the USA and elsewhere.

As Aspen Council member Tom McCabe cautioned, "The planet's a finite resource…We can't indefinitely welcome people and expect to maintain our quality of life." And that is precisely the point: Aspenites and others in similarly privileged places across the USA want to protect *their* "quality of life," which includes resources and wealth derived from the ecosystems that only they have access to and from the hard work of others.

The innocent claim that environmentalists in the Roaring Fork Valley only want to "preserve our way of life" is belied by the fact that such a lifestyle requires the domination of the environment and of certain groups of people (e.g., people of color, immigrants, and workers who make such privileges possible for the wealthy and mostly white elite). It also underscores an enduring belief that there are essential differences between people of different ethnic, racial, and national backgrounds. Aspen and the surrounding Roaring Fork Valley of Colorado is just one of many sites on the planet built as a refuge from undesirable people and where nature can be manipulated for the convenience and enjoyment of a handful of elites. Moreover, in the case of the nativist environmentalists of Aspen, these environmentally privileged communities are claiming victim status. A Roaring Fork Valley area progressive activist and educator told us: "Environmental racism is when people of color are dumped on. But here, especially in Aspen, we have rich white folks who are saying *we're* getting dumped on! So it's like the idea has been totally turned around and upside down." In other words, Aspenites are essentially crying "reverse environmental racism" because they view immigrants not only as a cause of environmental harm, but as a kind of social contamination, a form of pollution. This strongly parallels much of the discourse on population control within the US environmental movement historically.

Geographer David Sibley argues bluntly that Western society is based on exclusion. The flipside of exclusion is inclusion, so every act that repels others sends a message of belonging to those who are "like us" (Sibley 1997). As Sibley writes "The human landscape can be read as a landscape of exclusion… Because power is expressed in the monopolization of space and the relegation of weaker groups in society to less desirable environments." He suggests that we take a closer look at the "curious practices" of the "majority" "who consider themselves to be normal or mainstream" in order to uncover "the oddness of the ordinary" (Sibley 1997). Herein lies the third method of emplacement: questioning environmental privilege.

Immigrant residents of the Valley may not always be visible and public with their politics, but this does not mean they do not have strong feelings about the way they are treated. We asked local resident, worker, and activist José Cordova what he thought about the claim that immigrants harm local ecosystems. He stated, "I think that's a misperception because I've been working with construction companies and the mess that they do with that stuff! There's no ecological preservation. They just throw away everything. I don't think it's the Latinos affecting the environment." He reframed the social problem as one of privilege:

> My position is that that the concept of overpopulation is not that accurate. That's one of the arguments of groups to justify policies, to say there is poverty because of overpopulation. But if we go into details about wealth and the lands that are available, we see that maybe we may all fit in the world. I don't think the problem is overpopulation; the problem is redistribution of the wealth and the redistribution of knowledge.

With an advanced degree in environmental sciences from a university in Central America, Cordova offered a critique of the general orientation of environmental policy in this nation. He contends that the focus is never on the point of production, but rather on what to do *after* we've produced or consumed goods. Like the population–environment debate, the postproduction and postconsumer recycling fixation of US environmental policy and environmental movements benefits powerful institutions that remain unchallenged (Gould et al. 1996; Szasz 1994):

> I understand all these programs of recycling, reuse, rethinking. It's OK, it's nice. But that's not the problem. The problem is from the beginning – how you produce those goods. You can produce something and make something new out of this, but the problem is that they are producing it in the first place, so the problem is conceptual and ideological. The forest and all the resources will suffer because you have not changed the approach to nature. …So we produce more and we are working in this [consumer] phase of the production cycle, so they say we can recycle and reuse, but the problem is the same. And from that perspective you cannot say or argue that the foreigners or immigrants are the cause of the environmental problems. The companies are drilling for oil right now, it's right here, these companies need natural gas and money, so it's not the foreigners. It's how you use nature.

Finally, Cordova issues a criticism of the USA in its lack of commitment to global environmental agreements, implying that the immigration-environment debate not only benefits corporate polluters but also the federal government, which does not take seriously its environmental responsibilities within and beyond its national borders.

> The US has not signed the Kyoto Protocol [on global warming] and all those agreements that are well accepted all over Europe, and other countries have accepted it. I understand that they say that it's not economically sound to change all the production systems. But all these other countries are doing it. Germany has changed legislation to change the way the companies work.

Cordova's analysis and assessment of US environmental politics coincides with what progressive scholars, policy makers, business leaders, and activists here and in other nations have been arguing for years (Agyeman et al. 2003; Gould et al. 2008; Pellow 2007).

His appraisal of the population–environment debate speaks directly to the overarching quest for environmental privilege in the Roaring Fork Valley and elsewhere. Environmental privilege is not just about maintaining exclusive access to ecological amenities (mountains, rivers, lakes, beaches, parks, trails, etc.); it is also about maintaining access and belonging to the broader reality of social place, of which both ecological and nonecological amenities are a part.

Another resident offered her views on the subject:

> The problem is when the Hispanic community are getting businesses and they're interacting more with the organizations, and they're getting more involved with the important issues in this valley. That is when it pops up as a problem. That is my experience. More than, "I don't like you because you're Mexican."

In other words, structural or institutional racism, not just interpersonal racism, is at the core of the struggle for white environmental privilege and is deployed strategically as immigrants form more permanent, material claims to place. Environmental privilege is ultimately an exertion of power that employs nativism and its racist logic to demarcate where particular people belong. Carlos Loya works as a laborer throughout the Valley and has had plenty of experience with racism. Sometimes when native-born whites yell epithets at him he responds in one of two ways. He might tell Anglos, "My ancestors were here in Aspen long before you got here. This land used to be our land." Or he poses a question: "You call me wetback because I crossed a river, so what can I call you? You crossed an ocean." Loya stated, "Without knowing it, they are making us tough and giving us patience and strength when they do this. We have a strong shell" (Aguilera 2004).

Loya's response to nativists is a quintessential example of this method of emplacement. He questions environmental privilege by evoking a new narrative of national origins. He asks, what demarcates belonging? Who got here first? And, if my migration makes me inferior, what does your migration across the Atlantic mean? How are you not an immigrant? Loya exerts his power by "flipping the script" and questioning their taken-for-granted entitlement of place.

Scholars working in the field of environmental justice studies have, for more than three decades, presented evidence that poor, working class, indigenous, and people of color communities face greater threats from pollution and industrial hazards than other groups. While these studies reveal the hardships and crimes associated with environmental inequality and environmental racism, fewer studies consider the flipside of that reality. Environmental privilege results from the exercise of economic, political, and cultural power that some groups enjoy, which enables them near exclusive access to coveted environmental amenities such as forests, parks, mountains, rivers, coastal property, open lands, and elite neighborhoods. Questioning environmental privilege identifies the wealthy Aspenites as the social problem, not the immigrants.

Place-Making in a Global World

Within the context of globalization, the ability to freely choose whether to stay in one place or to traverse multiple borders of nation-states appears to be increasingly limited to elites. The heightened militarization of national borders in conjunction with neoliberal trade policies imposes immobility on some while coercing migration on others. What appear consistent in this scenario are the persistent significance of place and the importance of place-making as an empowering act. Citing the importance of Doreen Massey's work on the multiple spatial scales in which people develop a "global sense of place," feminist geographer Linda McDowell (1999) argues, "Places are made through power relations which construct the rules which define boundaries." These boundaries are socially and spatially constructed to include some and exclude others. What emplacement methods employed by immigrants living in Aspen tells us is that place-making is a necessary part of their lives, in both ordinary (everyday) and extraordinary (public) ways. They use both local and global strategies to produce this sense of place (Isabel 2006; McLafferty and Chakrabarti 2009). And, while their experience of Aspen may not match the power behind the glittery, goliath rendition of Aspen splayed across glossy magazine covers, it is real and it is theirs. Evidently, a sense of place is a requisite for a sense of self, particularly for transnational migrants.

References

Aguilera, Elizabeth. 2004. "A Wealth of Diversity in a Valley of Riches." *The Denver Post*. July 20.

Agyeman, Julian, Robert Bullard, and Bob Evans, editors. 2003. *Just Sustainabilities: Development in an Unequal World*. Cambridge, MA: The MIT Press.

Appleby, J. 2006. "Ranks of Uninsured Americans Grow." *USA Today*. August 29.

Calavita, Kitty. 2008. "Deflecting the Immigration Debate: Globalization, Immigrant Agency, "Strange Bedfellows and Beyond"." *Contemporary Sociology* 37(4):302–305.

Chang, Robert S. 1996. "A Meditation on Borders," pp: 244–253. In *Immigrants Out! The New Nativism and the Anti-immigrant Impulse in the United States*. Edited by Juan F. Perea. New York, NY: New York University Press.

Craig, Bill. 1999. "Protesters Decry Possible INS move." *Glenwood Post*. November 6.

Daniels, Donna. 1999. "Appeal Filed Against INS Office." *Glenwood Independent*. December 2.

Daniels, Donna. 2000. "INS Loses in C'dale, Renews Search for Office." *Glenwood Independent*. January 28.

DeGenova, Nicholas. 2005. *Working the Boundaries: Race, Space, and "Illegality" In Mexican Chicago*. Durham, NC: Duke University Press.

Dyck, Isabel. 2006. "Traveling Tales and Migratory Meanings: South Asian Migrant Women Talk of Place, Health and Healing." *Social and Cultural Geography* 7(1):593–617.

Gieryn, Thomas F. 2000. "A Space for Place in Sociology." *Annual Review of Sociology* 26:463–493.

Gould, Kenneth, Allan Schnaiberg, and Adam Weinberg. 1996. *Local Environmental Struggles: Citizen Activism in the Treadmill of Production*. New York, NY: Cambridge University Press.

Gould, Kenneth, David N. Pellow, and Allan Schnaiberg. 2008. *The Treadmill of Production: Injustice and Unsustainability in the Global Economy*. Boulder, CO: Paradigm Publishers.

Harris, Pat. 2009. "City of Nashville rejects English-only law." *Reuters*. January 22.
hooks, bell. 1990. "Homeplace: A Site of Resistance," pp: 41–49. In *Yearning: Race, Gender and Cultural Politics*. Edited by hooks, bell. Boston, MA: South End Press.
Hunter, Mark. 2000. "'Slave Ships' Keep INS Busy as Flood of Smugglers Surges." *Denver Post*, February 24.
Katz, Cindy. 2001. "Vagabond capitalism and the Necessity of Social Reproduction." *Antipode* 33(4):710–727.
Kotlowitz, Alex. 2007. "All Immigration Politics is Local (and Complicated, Nasty and Personal)." *The New York Times Magazine*. August 5, Section 6.
Malpas, Jeff. E. 1999. *Place and Experience: A Philosophical Topography*. Cambridge: Cambridge University Press.
Massey, Douglas. 2003. *Beyond Smoke and Mirrors: Mexican Immigration in an Era of Economic Integration*. New York, NY: Russell Sage Foundation.
McDowell, Linda. 1999. *Gender, Identity, and Place: Understanding Feminist Geographies*. Minnesota, Minnesota University Press.
McLafferty, Sara and Ranjana Chakrabarti. 2009. "Locating Diversity: Race, Nativity and Place in Health Disparities Research." *GeoJournal* 74:107–113.
Pellow, David N. 2007. *Resisting Global Toxics: Transnational Movements for Environmental Justice*. Cambridge, MA: The MIT Press.
Pritchard, Justin. 2004. "US Mexican Worker Deaths Rising Sharply." *Aspen Daily* News/ Associated Press.
Sassen, Saskia. 1990. *Mobility of Labor and Capital*. Cambridge, MA: Cambridge University Press.
Sassen, Saskia. 1999. *Guests and Aliens*. New York: The New Press.
Sassen, Saskia. 2006. "The Bits of a New Immigration Reality: A Bad Fit with Current Policy." http://borderbattles.ssrc.org/Sassen/printable.html. Accessed on April 26, 2010.
Sibley, David. 1997. *Geographies of Exclusion: Society and Difference in the West*. London: Routledge.
Stiny, Andrew. 1999. "Carbondale March Protests INS." *Aspen Daily News*. November 6.
Stroud, John. 2000. "Zoning Board Denies INS Permit for Carbondale Site." *Glenwood Post*. Friday, January 28.
Szasz, Andrew. 1994. *EcoPopulism: Toxic Waste and the Movement for Environmental Justice*. Minneapolis: University of Minnesota Press.
Urban Institute. 2002. "The Dispersal of Immigrants in the 1990s. Facts and Perspectives: Immigrant Families and Workers", Brief No.2. Washington, DC: Urban Institute.
Yeoman, Barry. 2001. "Silence in the Fields." *Mother Jones*. January/February 2001.

Chapter 8
Moving Beyond Geography: Health Practices and Outcomes Across Time and Place

Karen Albright, Grace Chung, Allison De Marco, and Joan Yoo

Places cannot be divorced from the people and things that act on them (Cummins et al. 2007; Macintyre et al. 2002). Beyond this accepted statement, there is considerable debate on how place affects health, which effects matter, and how they should be measured. Macintyre and colleagues (2002) identify five features of place that may affect health: its physical characteristics (e.g., the climate, water, and air quality shared by all residents), the availability of healthy environments within it (e.g., decent housing, secure and nonhazardous employment, safe play areas for children), its publicly or privately provided support services (e.g., education, transportation, policing, and health and welfare services), its sociocultural features (e.g., political, economic, ethnic, religious history, norms and values, degree of community integration, crime level, incivilities, and networks of community support), and the reputation of the area (i.e., how a place is perceived, which may influence the self-esteem and morale of residents and, thus, may affect efforts to improve infrastructure). Dimensions of place are not universally experienced, but they have differential impacts based on the social location of communities and individuals within them. The lack of local health services, for example, may be more detrimental to less mobile residents than to people who are able to travel longer distances for service. High local poverty is typically associated with a greater likelihood of poor health compared to residents of more affluent places (Cohen et al. 2000; Malmström et al. 1999; Pampalon et al. 2007).

This chapter adds to this literature by focusing on the place effects on health that may persist or change over time and distance. We are explicitly concerned with the interaction of place and health in communities of immigrants, who bring historical, individual, social, political, and cultural experiences from their place of origin to a new setting. The transnational movements of people add a layer of complexity to discussions of place and community. When seen in this context, place is an even

K. Albright (✉)
Department of Community and Behavioral Health, Colorado School of Public Health, University of Colorado Denver, Anschutz Medical Campus, Denver, CO, USA
e-mail: karen.albright@ucdenver.edu

L.M. Burton et al. (eds.), *Communities, Neighborhoods, and Health*,
Social Disparities in Health and Health Care 1, DOI 10.1007/978-1-4419-7482-2_8,

more dynamic construct than as a single, static geographic location. We examine how place of origin affects health beyond its original geographic boundaries and how such effects may change over time. Examining the interaction between immigrants' places of origin and their host societies allows deeper insight into *how* place effects work.

Immigrants often create fluid and multiple identities grounded in both the society of origin and the host society (Glick Schiller et al. 1996). Several broad types of migrant incorporation are identified: assimilation, exclusion, integration, and multiculturalism (Tambiah 2000). Immigrants may consciously attempt to preserve their collective identity and ties to a geographic location by maintaining explicit and implicit ties with the homeland and resisting full acceptance by the host society or assimilation into the new culture. At the same time, they may also actively work to develop identity and community in their new society.

Groups may immigrate for many reasons. They may seek employment in more prosperous countries, experience dislocation due to civil wars or natural disasters, such as floods, earthquakes, and drought, or seek escape from pogroms of ethnic cleansing and genocide (Tambiah 2000). Individuals' connections to their countries of origin following their departure may be cultural and/or economic. They may reinforce relationships with the community of origin by making remittances, seeking investment capital, returning to marry homeland members, sponsoring new migrants, returning to build or refurbish old family seats, sponsoring/financing local festivals, making pilgrimages, or inviting cultural groups and holy people to the new country (Tambiah 2000). The Chinese Man clan, which migrated across Europe and North America and is now in the fifth generation, no longer speaks Chinese yet still perceives itself as different from Chinese neighbors in the host communities where they have settled and goes to great lengths to maintain a sense of connection with their place of origin through close contact with fellow Man members.

We examine the state of knowledge of the persistent effects of place on health practices and outcomes among three distinct immigrant communities. We seek to describe how shared identities, a shared culture, and/or a shared experience with a particular place of origin may impact health outcomes and practices, and how those outcomes and practices may change over time. We first examine health practices among Chinese living in England. These practices reflect an integration of both Chinese and Western approaches to health care while also revealing the importance of sustaining Chinese identity and ties with place of origin across generations. We then turn to the study of health outcomes across time and place by examining notable health phenomena among two groups of immigrants to the USA. In the first case, we describe the town of Roseto, Pennsylvania, which was settled and populated by immigrants from Roseto Val Forte, Italy, in the late-1800s. For several decades in the mid-twentieth century, Rosetans had the lowest mortality rate from heart disease in the USA. In the second case, we examine the "epidemiological paradox" (Markides and Coreil 1986), which refers to the finding that Hispanics, particularly immigrants from Mexico, have better mortality rates and birth outcomes in the USA than do their White and African-American counterparts, despite the fact that many have low socioeconomic status and lack access to adequate medical care.

Both the "Roseto effect" and Hispanic "epidemiological paradox" have been the focus of much interest in medical and social scientific circles in recent decades and, as we discuss below, suggest the centrality of the social aspects of community in place effects on health.

Health Practices Across Time and Place: The Chinese in England

Chinese immigration has existed since at least 202 BCE, when the Chinese journeyed to establish political and military alliances, settling along the Silk Road (Ma 2003). Chinese immigrants are now found in almost every country on earth (Djao 2003). Pushed by repeated foreign invasion, domestic rebellions, regional armed conflicts, drought, and natural disasters and pulled by high demand for laborers abroad, Chinese immigrants left to live a life not possible in China (Ma 2003). Many hoped for major improvements in the political and social conditions in their homeland that would allow them to return and were motivated to maintain a keen interest in China, teach their children the language and culture, sustain economic and social ties, and visit often (Ma 2003).

Indeed, for many Chinese immigrants, the connection to their homeland is a constant presence (Wai-sum 2008). However, the degree of assimilation with the indigenous population has varied considerably due in part to the difficulties in navigating the complex realities associated with membership in two cultures (Skeldon 2003). In Thailand and Cambodia, for example, the assimilation of Chinese immigrants has been virtually complete, but in other areas an intermediate culture developed that was neither indigenous nor Chinese. In still other areas, Chinese immigrants have encountered high barriers to assimilation. For example, in orthodox Islamic societies, such as Aceh in Indonesia, Chinese immigrants must convert to the host culture to gain access to marriage partners, high social status, and economic opportunities. Not coincidentally, the differences in the openness of these societies help determine the persistence of health beliefs and practices. In the following section, we focus specifically on the health beliefs and practices of Chinese immigrants to England because the research examining the use of traditional and Western medicine over multiple generations facilitates our examination of place effects over time. We highlight how shared beliefs and culture from the place of origin, as well as experiences within the host country, influence health beliefs and practices.

Health Practices of Chinese Immigrants in England

The first Chinese migration to England occurred in the 1960s, originating from Hong Kong. These first immigrants, who now make up the elderly generation of the immigrant Chinese in England, typically speak little or no English and remain confined to their ethnic enclaves (Gervais and Jovchelovitch 1998). The next generation, consisting of both newcomers and the children of the first wave of immigrants, is largely comprised of two groups: a bilingual and highly educated professional group and a socially isolated working class group with low English proficiency. The first group is well integrated and either British-born or from cosmopolitan Hong Kong, Malaysia, Singapore, and China, while the working class group consists of newcomers who originate mainly from rural areas in China, Vietnam, and Hong Kong.

Many Chinese immigrants to England have embraced both their place of origin and their place of settlement by integrating Chinese and Western approaches to health care (Gervais and Jovchelovitch 1998). Traditional Chinese medicine is based on herbal and diet therapy and is used to correct underlying states of imbalance for both emotional and physical maladies (Kleinman et al. 2006). Restoration of energetic balance in all aspects of one's bodily and social domains is the fundamental approach to cure illness. Such an explanatory model of health and illness, along with the cultural concept of shame and Confucian principles of conduct and loyalty, forms the basis of how health conditions are explained and health-related decisions are made by the Chinese (Tabora and Flaskerud 1996). Although the Western model of medicine is the dominant paradigm within the English health care system and it differs from the Chinese approach in fundamental ways, the Chinese English have integrated the two by continuing to value and practice Chinese medicine (Gervais and Jovchelovitch 1998; Green et al. 2006; Jovchelovitch and Gervais 1999). According to Jovchelovitch and Gervais (1999), the Chinese orientation to health and illness serves as an anchor on which to appropriate Western knowledge of medicine. In this way, an integrated repertoire of health beliefs and practices has been constructed, wherein Chinese and Western knowledge coexist. Indeed, Green et al. (2006) report an overwhelming trend toward the complementary use of both Chinese and Western medicine among Chinese immigrants. Other studies have suggested that place of origin effects are enduring among the Chinese English such that traditional Chinese concepts of health and illness have been sustained over generations and permeate the core of health orientations shared and practiced by the Chinese English to this day (Kleinman 1975; Unschuld 1987; Gervais and Jovchelovitch 1998).

Traditional Chinese health beliefs and practices are sustained over time in England primarily through three key mechanisms: (1) engaging in Chinese dietary management through family-oriented practices of food preparation and consumption, (2) the use of Chinese social networks to access both Chinese and Western treatment in England and their place of origin, and (3) claiming Chinese-ness in non-Chinese society (Gervais and Jovchelovitch 1998; Green et al. 2006; Jovchelovitch and Gervais 1999). Chinese immigrants share the belief that health principles are enacted, passed down, and reproduced through key cultural practices such as food preparation and consumption and the Chinese language (Jovchelovitch and Gervais 1999). Every food item and cooking method is denoted as having either hot or cold or neutral properties that affect flow of energy, thus used in accordance with a bodily condition to maintain balance and harmony. These practices take place mainly within the family and, therefore, the Chinese way of thinking and talking about health and illness is perpetuated through kinship relations across generations. Green and colleagues (2006) found that regardless of when they immigrated to England, all the women whom they interviewed engaged in the Chinese practice of dietary management to maintain bodily balance and harmony, although not all sought out a Chinese medicine specialist for medical treatment. As these women's everyday health habits are grounded in the Chinese tradition, a discrepancy appears almost inevitable between the understandings and health perceptions of Chinese English women and that of Western practitioners, serving as a barrier to seeking Western health care. As these studies suggest, maintenance of Chinese health beliefs is a remarkable commonality among the Chinese English, regardless of the number of years of residence in England. Despite the fact that some are dismissive of Chinese medicine in theory, most seem to take a complementary approach to medical treatment.

Chinese social networks serve as an additional mechanism through which Chinese immigrants continue traditional practices from the place of origin. Recommendations by friends and relatives are helpful sources for locating practitioners back in China. In Green et al.'s (2006) study, more than half of the women reported seeking treatment from "home." Even though there are Chinese healers in England, medical visits to mainland China or Hong Kong are not uncommon because home-based practitioners are perceived as more trustworthy and experienced compared to England-based practitioners. These recommendations allow women with limited English skills (and, thus, more limited access to Western health care) to receive needed care.

Claiming one's Chinese-ness in non-Chinese society appears to further facilitate the persistence of the original place effect among the Chinese English. Although the way in which Chinese cultural assumptions about health and health practices are appropriated and perceived varies by generation, it is regarded as a symbolic act of affirming ties to their place of origin. A higher level of acculturation is associated with a greater use of Western medicine, but not to decreased use of Chinese medicine for similar problems (Tabora and Flaskerud 1996; Wade et al. 2007). Further, increased acculturation is associated with use of more mainstream complementary and alternative medicine, whereas less acculturation is associated with the use of Chinese herbs and acupuncture (Wade et al. 2007). Among members of the older, less acculturated generation, the integration of Chinese and Western practices occurs without much tension or negotiation with their Chinese identity (Jovchelovitch and Gervais 1999). Among the Chinese English, the sense of being Chinese is grounded in the traditional Chinese way of thinking about health and illness, which values embracing all existing resources. Thus, adoption of available Western health practices is a natural course of action and is seen as being pragmatic rather than contradictory to the Chinese tradition. In contrast, the younger, more acculturated generation has experienced psychological stress from the clash between the different health practices and beliefs considered normative by each culture. Although they maintain the Chinese health beliefs transmitted through familial rituals, it is a struggle to negotiate and make health-related choices in a way that both reaffirms their Chinese roots and establishes their acculturated identity in England. For the British-born generation, their understanding of the Chinese way is not entirely their own, since it has been established indirectly through their parents. However, their Chinese appearance prevents them from fully identifying with the British. In this context, embracing the Chinese health tradition serves as an important mechanism through which to maintain and claim cultural ties to their place of origin when they lack a sense of belonging to either culture. Overall, research indicates that the health beliefs the first Chinese immigrants brought with them to England decades ago continue to endure as they are upheld, practiced, and integrated with the practices of Western culture.

Health Outcomes Across Time and Place: The Roseto Effect

The small town of Roseto, Pennsylvania, illuminates another way place can affect health. Settled in the late nineteenth century by immigrants primarily from Roseto Val Forte, Italy, Roseto became known in medical circles in the early 1960s for its markedly low rates of coronary disease. Indeed, Rosetans' incidence of and mortality rate from myocardial infarction (i.e., heart attack) were less than half that of the rest of the nation and, perhaps even more notably, less than half that of four neighboring towns: Bangor, Nazareth, Stroudsburg, and East Stroudsburg (Wolf et al. 1974). Each of these towns was larger than Roseto (i.e., in the 1960 census, Bangor had a population of 5,766, Nazareth 6,209, Stroudsburg 6,070, and East Stroudsburg 7,674, compared to Roseto's 1,630) and had different ethnic and social histories (e.g., Nazareth had been settled by Moravians, a Southern German religious group, and continued to be largely populated with ethnic Germans, while Bangor's mix of Welsh, Scotch-Irish, German, Italian, and other immigrants created a high degree of ethnic and social heterogeneity). However, each of these towns shared with Roseto the physical trappings of geographic location that often dominate the discussions of place, particularly their proximity to the Appalachian Ridge "slate belt" that provided the industry that would support them throughout the late-nineteenth and twentieth centuries (Wolf and Bruhn 1993).

In an effort to explain these rather surprising findings, scientists studying Roseto first turned to the most obvious explanation: that Rosetans' remarkably resilient hearts were due to their particular health behaviors, their good genes, and/or the quality of health care they received. However, none of these factors could entirely explain Rosetans' uniquely low prevalence of heart disease. Though differences in coronary heart disease have often been attributed to differences in diet and other behavioral risk factors (Lasker et al. 1994), Rosetans did not engage in particularly healthy habits. Indeed, their lifestyles theoretically should have led to a much higher incidence of heart failure. Their fat intake, obesity levels, cigarette smoking, and serum cholesterol concentration did not differ significantly from those of their eastern Pennsylvania neighbors (Wolf et al. 1974). The men, in particular, led unhealthy lifestyles: not only did the vast majority engage in dangerous, backbreaking work every day in the nearby slate quarries but they also smoked freely, drank copiously, and ate meals centered on animal protein fried in lard (Bruhn and Wolf 1979; Wolf and Bruhn 1993).

Nor could heredity provide a satisfying explanation. Although most Roseto residents in the mid-twentieth century were descended from the same handful of immigrants who had arrived in America in 1882 and settled in "New Italy" (Roseto's original name) five years later, not all descendents of those immigrants experienced healthy hearts as the Rosetans did. Indeed, descendants who moved elsewhere in eastern Pennsylvania, or to nearby New Jersey or New York, experienced heart disease and failure at the national rate (Bruhn and Wolf 1979; Wolf and Bruhn 1993). Death from myocardial infarction was also experienced by young Italians who were born in Roseto but lived most of their lives in other communities (Wolf and Bruhn 1993). Further, Roseto was served by the same water supply, physicians, and hospital facilities as was the immediately adjacent Bangor, where rates of myocardial infarction approximated the national average (Egolf et al. 1992; Stout et al. 1964).

Scientists' inability to explain Rosetans' low incidence of myocardial infarction by the usual dietary, genetic, and/or service utilization factors ultimately led them to the conclusion that something in the structure of the community itself was affecting heart health (Lasker et al. 1994; Wolf et al. 1974). Specifically, they found that the discrepancy in the prevalence of and mortality from myocardial infarction in Roseto could be attributed directly to its culture and social cohesion (Egolf et al. 1992; Bruhn et al. 1966). Rosetans enjoyed a stable social structure that emphasized family and community cohesion. The town had high levels of ethnic and social homogeneity, including predominantly intra-ethnic and local marriages. It was also characterized by a strong commitment to religion, an absence of ostentation even among the wealthy, and nearly exclusive patronage of local businesses (Egolf et al. 1992). In what would become known as "the Roseto effect," these elements of social cohesion – and the "social milieu" (Wolf et al. 1974:106) that they created and enabled – together acted as protective factors against heart attacks and, thus, were significantly related to Rosetans' longevity (Wolf et al. 1974; Wolf and Bruhn 1993).

The finding that strong social bonds were the determining factor in Rosetans' longevity is aligned with other research in the medical and social scientific literatures indicating that a number of social and community level factors are associated with physical and mental health. For example, Kawachi et al. (1999) find that lower levels of social trust are associated with higher rates of most major causes of death, while higher levels of social trust are associated with positive assessments of health and well-being. But although Roseto has been widely cited for highlighting the relationship between social cohesion and health (Gladwell 2008; Lynch 1979), parsing out what is known about both the origins of and the changes in this community also helps to shed light on how place effects on health may work over time. This, in turn, furthers the task of trying to understand the *how*, *what*, and *why* in the broader relationship between place and health.

The story of Roseto offers us two vantage points from which to examine how place may affect health. First, the migration from Roseto Val Forte, Italy to what became Roseto, Pennsylvania provides information on how factors pertaining to health may be transplanted into new environments. Second, the changes in Rosetans' mortality rates over time-as the original community members aged, died out, and were replaced by third-generation Italian-Americans who preferred to abandon the old ways for more modern, individualistic lifestyles-suggest that both place effects on health and place itself are best understood as fluid, rather than static, concepts.

Changes Across Place: From Italy to Pennsylvania

Compared to the volumes that have been written about Roseto, Pennsylvania, few specifics are known about health behaviors and practices in Roseto Val Forte, Italy. However, scholars have argued that the Italian tradition of strong social ties and family coresidence (Kunitz 1990) were among the cultural practices carried over with the migration to America. Indeed, Lasker et al. (1994) have suggested that some of the differences between Roseto and Bangor may be rooted in the traditions each brought to the USA from different parts of Europe. "In contrast to countries in North, West, and Eastern Europe, households in Southern Europe [e.g., Italy] were much more likely to be large, multi-generational, and to contain multiple families" (Lasker et al. 1994:61).

Not surprisingly, the Italian customs and norms that encouraged and enabled social cohesion were especially strong when the majority of Roseto residents were either foreign-born immigrants or their children. The number of first-generation Rosetans remained quite high for a long period of time; indeed, compared to Bangor, Roseto had more than twice as high a percentage of foreign-born residents until 1970 (Lasker et al. 1994). The old customs and community solidarity were maintained through a variety of social mechanisms, including high levels of activity in local organizations and marriage with other Italians (and, often, with other Rosetans). However, these numbers declined over time: in 1925–1934, 93% of all marriages were between two Italians or those of Italian descent, while by 1975–1984, only 22% were so (Lasker et al. 1994).

Changes Within Place: From the First Generation to the Third

For much of the twentieth century, Roseto was a relatively homogeneous, endogamous, and locally active community, dominated by foreign-born residents who were primarily working class. In the mid-1960s, the community began to change. The ethos of the first and second generation of immigrants began to be replaced by American-born generations, who abandoned the old community ways in favor of behavior that reflected the more materialistic, less cohesive, and less family-driven American culture (Bruhn and Wolf 1979). These younger Rosetans were not isolated by the social discrimination against Italians that had initially forced their elders to become self-sufficient. Because this generation attended college in unprecedented numbers, they were familiar with the outside world in a way that their parents had never been (Lasker et al. 1994). Highly educated and hungry for upward mobility, the younger generations valued the old world values of family and community solidarity less than they did acculturation. Interethnic marriages became much more common, local church attendance began to decline, people joined more exclusive country clubs or moved into the suburbs, and the formerly tight cohesive social structure became noticeably looser (Wolf et al. 1974).

It was at this precise cultural moment when Rosetans' relative immunity against early death from myocardial infarction was lost. Myocardial infarction increased significantly in 1965–1974, as did higher mortality rates, particularly in younger Rosetan men and older women. Although by the following decade (1975–1984) the sharp rise in heart disease leveled off to approximate the national average, the loss of Rosetans' special status as coronary outliers seems to illustrate well the argument, put forth by Cassel and colleagues (1960), that though populations are adaptable to new circumstances, they are most vulnerable in times of rapid change, and it is during these times that their health prospects suffer most (Cassel et al. 1960).

Health Outcomes Across Time and Place: The Mexican "Epidemiological Paradox"

Mexicans are the largest immigrant population in the USA, comprising 32% of all foreign-born residents and 66% of Hispanic immigrants in 2007 (Passel and Cohn 2009). These immigrants have been found to be at a disadvantage when compared to their US-born counterparts. For example, Mexican immigrants are more likely to live in poverty, more likely to work in low-wage industries, and less likely to have health insurance than their US-born counterparts. (Crowley et al. 2006; Rutledge and McLaughlin 2008). Previous health inequality research examining the relationship between socioeconomic status and health has found that low socioeconomic status (SES) is associated with poor health for the vast majority of health indicators including mortality and morbidity (Lynch and Kaplan 2000). Moreover, racial and ethnic minority groups have worse health outcomes when compared to non-Hispanic Whites (Budrys 2003).

However, the combined effects of race/ethnicity and SES on minority groups' health have been found to be more complex. Numerous studies suggest that Hispanics as a whole have similar or better health outcomes (e.g., mortality, life expectancy, birth outcomes) than non-Hispanic Whites in the USA (Carter-Pokras et al. 2008; Franzini et al. 2001; Sorlie et al. 1993) despite the low socioeconomic profile of Hispanics as a group. These findings are somewhat surprising when the health of African-Americans, whose socioeconomic profile as a group is comparable to that of Hispanics, has consistently been found to be worse than their non-Hispanic White counterparts (Budrys 2003). The term "epidemiological paradox" has been used to describe the finding that Hispanics as a group demonstrate better-than-expected health and mortality outcomes despite their low socioeconomic profile (Markides and Coreil 1986). Foreign-born Hispanics, in particular, exhibit better health and mortality than their US-born counterparts (Carter-Pokras et al. 2008; Sorlie et al. 1993), a fact that some argue largely accounts for the "epidemiological paradox" (Hummer et al. 1999). In the following section, we examine the importance of place of origin and its long-term effects on Mexican immigrants' health.

The term "epidemiological paradox" was adopted by Markides and Coreil (1986) to summarize previous research suggesting that Mexican Americans (as identified by Spanish surnames) have similar or even better mortality rates in Texas than their White counterparts. Since then, numerous studies have documented the better-than-expected mortality rates of US-born and foreign-born Mexicans using various datasets, including the National Longitudinal Mortality Study and the National Health Interview Survey linked with the National Death Index (Hummer et al. 1999; Sorlie et al. 1993). Despite the low rates of prenatal and medical care, infant mortality rates among infants of Mexican immigrant mothers were found to be substantially lower than infants of other race and ethnic groups (Hummer et al. 2007). Similar birth outcomes are reported for infants of other Hispanic immigrant women, except for infants of Puerto Rican mothers (Hummer et al. 2007). In addition, with the exception of the younger Mexican male population (aged 15–24), which has higher mortality rates than non-Hispanic Whites, mortality rates for Mexicans in other age ranges are similar to or better than those of non-Hispanic Whites (Sorlie et al. 1993). Other studies have found that Mexican Americans have favorable mortality rates compared to other Hispanics (Hummer et al. 2000; Sorlie et al. 1993). Researchers hypothesize that these positive health findings may be explained by the large percentage of foreign-born individuals among Mexican Americans. Interestingly, when mortality rates were compared between US-born and foreign-born Mexicans, studies found that foreign-born Mexicans have lower mortality rates and higher life expectancies than their US-born counterparts (Cho et al. 2004; Cunningham et al. 2008; Sorlie et al. 1993). Similarly, when Hummer and colleagues (1999) examined the association between race/ethnicity, nativity, and health, their findings suggest that differences in mortality between various race/ethnic groups are partly influenced by the proportion of foreign-born individuals in each race/ethnic group. In other words, race/ethnic groups with a greater proportion of foreign-born individuals exhibit lower mortality rates than race/ethnic groups with greater proportions of US-born individuals. However, duration in the US is not significantly associated with mortality rates (Hummer et al. 1999), although it has been found to be significantly associated with healthy behaviors (Carter-Pokras et al. 2008).

Several hypotheses have been presented in an attempt to explain the "epidemiological paradox." The first hypothesis is the cultural or social buffering hypothesis. This hypothesis proposes that social networks, stronger family ties, traditional health practices, and strong ethnic identity may buffer the negative effects of low SES, discrimination, and other health risks. Specifically, studies have found that Mexican immigrants are less likely to smoke, drink alcohol, and have better dietary intakes including higher average intake of protein, vitamins, folic acid, and calcium (Carter-Pokras et al. 2008; Franzini et al. 2001; Guendelman and Abrams 1994). These cultural buffers have been found to have a significant protective effect on birth outcomes, including infant mortality rates (Kelaher and Jessop 2002).

Nonetheless, these protective cultural effects diminish as foreign-born Mexicans become more acculturated. Indeed, there is growing evidence that positive health behaviors among foreign-born Mexicans decrease as their length of residence in the US increases (Lara et al. 2005). Studies have found that those who have been living in the US longer are more likely to smoke, drink, and have poor eating habits than their more recently arrived counterparts (Black and Markides 1993; Himmelgreen et al. 2001).

Residential characteristics in the USA are also associated with the persistence of these protective cultural factors and their potential health benefits. For example, the prevalence of asthma is lower in neighborhoods where there are higher proportions of foreign-born Hispanics, mostly Mexicans (70.4%; Cagney et al. 2007). When the impact of nativity, neighborhood characteristics, and low birth weight were examined, Johnson and Marchi (2009) found that Spanish-speaking Mexican mothers living in immigrant-oriented Hispanic neighborhoods were less likely to have babies with low birth weight than their English-speaking counterparts. According to the segmented assimilation theory, immigrants who reside in neighborhoods with a greater proportion of other immigrants have better sociocultural resources, which allow them to maintain their traditional health practices (Finch et al. 2007). One study reports that living in neighborhoods with higher proportions of Mexican immigrants improves the birth outcomes of second generation US-born Mexicans, and suggests that the sociocultural resources that allow Mexicans to maintain traditional health behaviors and practices may be a strategy for maintaining the "epidemiological paradox" of Mexican Americans (Peak and Weeks 2002).

However, further investigation is needed to fully explain the "epidemiological paradox" among Mexican immigrants. Researchers have suggested that the paradox, particularly the superior health of foreign-born Mexicans, may be driven by the selective nature of migration (Franzini et al. 2001). The healthy migrant hypothesis suggests that individuals who are both physically and psychologically healthier than those in the country of origin are selected for migration (Carter-Pokras et al. 2008; Franzini et al. 2001). Not only is there self-selection involved in the migration process but immigration laws in the USA have also been used to screen and permit entry to individuals who are in good health (Carter-Pokras et al. 2008). The healthy migrant hypothesis posits that as a result, immigrants are generally healthier than both their counterparts from the country of origin and the country to which they have migrated. However, this hypothesis has not been supported by empirical research yet (Abraido-Lanza et al. 1999).

Similarly, others have hypothesized that the "epidemiological paradox" can be explained by return migration among immigrants who become ill (Carter-Pokras et al. 2008). Individuals who migrate to the USA are identified in various health data, from which vital statistics and other US health statistics are derived. However, it is not currently possible to identify those who return to their countries of origin, nor the reason(s) for their return. As a result, these individuals are more likely to remain in the population count but are not likely to be identified in the death count after their death, which may underestimate the mortality rates of the foreign-born population (Carter-Pokras et al. 2008). Palloni and Arias (2004) have found some evidence that the return migration effect does partially explain the "epidemiological paradox" found in the mortality rates for older foreign-born Mexicans.

Discussion: What Can We Deduce About Place Effects Across Time and Geography?

In this chapter, we focused primarily on the sociocultural features of place that influence health (e.g., political, economic, ethnic, religious history, norms and values, degree of community integration, and networks of community support) as described by Macintyre and colleagues (2002). Where you live matters for health, although perhaps not as much as who you are (Pickett and Pearl 2001). The new places where immigrants settle make a difference to their health. However, the characteristics that are brought from the homeland and culture of origin also matter – significantly. Place effects are transmitted from the place of origin to the host country as individuals migrate from one place to another. These effects are maintained for a certain period in the hostland, manifested in both practices (e.g., traditional medicine among Chinese migrants, social practices among the Roseto, and healthy behaviors among Mexican immigrants) and outcomes (e.g., unusually good heart health among the Roseto community and low mortality rates and good birth outcomes among Mexican transplants in the USA).

In each case presented in this chapter, new immigrants settled in places inhabited by other immigrants from their home culture. These enclaves helped immigrants to maintain their traditional practices by lessening exposure to conditions in these new places. However, these place effects changed over time as duration in the host country increased, new generations were born, and the immigrants and/or their offspring became more assimilated into the dominant culture. Assimilation into the host culture led to the abandonment of original practices among the Roseto and the Mexican Americans, including reduced social cohesion and changes in diet and lifestyle. In the case of the Chinese English, assimilation led to the merging of old and new practices (i.e., the integration of traditional and Western medicine), as well as a renewed interest in native culture for later generations. In the case of the Pennsylvania Rosetans, strong ties to their place of origin loosened as generations born in the USA embraced the more materialistic, less cohesive, and less family-driven American culture (Bruhn and Wolf 1979). As discrimination against Italians dissipated, descendents of the original immigrants became less socially isolated and more ensconced in the dominant culture, attending college, marrying outside the community, and assimilating to a much greater extent than their parents had (Lasker et al. 1994). Among the Mexican immigrants characterized by the "epidemiological paradox," acculturation led them away from the healthy practices that had provided them with an edge, although considerable debate remains regarding exactly how this advantage operates.

In these examples, place effects over space and time can be enduring, such as among the Chinese, or more transitory, as seen in the Roseto and Mexican cases. The question is why this happens. It may be a function of the culture that immigrants encounter within their hostlands. In the introduction, we briefly mentioned the variation in the experiences of Chinese immigrants who have settled in different countries. In some host countries, they have been better able to maintain their unique culture, whereas in others, such as Islamic Indonesia, immigrants are more inclined to abandon their traditional practices to gain access to valuable opportunities (Skeldon 2003). In England, the existence of the Chinese community helps Chinese immigrants build ethnic social networks, through which they are able to gain access to, and connect with, health resources in their place of origin. In a Western society such as England, with a medical paradigm that contrasts that of the Chinese, it may be important for Chinese immigrants to create their own space both physically, by forming an ethnic enclave where they can exchange resources and share many features of being Chinese (e.g., skin color, food, cultural practices, etc.), and symbolically, where they can enact Chinese-ness by sustaining traditional health beliefs and practices. Does such a physical space function as a platform facilitating immigrants' identification with their ethnic roots by maintaining health beliefs and practices from their place of origin over time? It seems that both physical and symbolic spaces reinforce each other, sustaining the original place effects on health beliefs and practices over generations. Empirical testing of this premise in future research will be useful for a better understanding of why and how place effects endure among immigrants in some places but not others.

Similar trends were also found in the case of the "epidemiological paradox" of Mexican Americans. Based on the segmented assimilation hypothesis, studies have reported that Mexican mothers who live in unacculturated neighborhoods or ethnic enclaves are more likely to maintain traditional health practices and to achieve better birth outcomes (Finch et al. 2007; Peak and Weeks 2002). This suggests that maintaining a physical space in the host country may help immigrants, whether from Mexico or Italy, sustain original place effects on health beliefs, practices, and outcomes over generations. However, the mechanisms for understanding the lasting effects of place of origin on health may not be that simple. Johnson and Marchi (2009) suggest that benefits of living in ethnic enclaves may occur only when there is consonance between the individual and neighborhood residents on language, cultural orientations, migration histories, and socioeconomic backgrounds. They also highlight the fact that Mexican-American mothers who experience cultural dissonance between themselves and their neighbors may be at greater risk for poor birth outcomes (Johnson and Marchi 2009). While preserving a unique physical space (e.g., ethnic enclave) in the host country seems to help immigrants maintain health benefits brought from their country of origin, the process(es) through which these health benefits last or evolve over time is still unclear. Further investigation is needed to fully understand the mechanisms between the effects of place in host countries and place of origin on health practices and outcomes.

Place effects may also depend upon a match between the practice and the new environment. For example, Chinese tradition values all available resources, which may help to explain why the Chinese English have come to maintain both traditional and Western practices, whereas in the USA, harmful health behaviors (e.g., consumption of convenience products that are cheap and easily available) have moved Mexican immigrants away from their traditional healthier behaviors (Black and Markides 1993; Himmelgreen et al. 2001), thus negatively affecting health outcomes. Further, whereas younger generations of Rosetans and Mexican Americans increasingly adopted the mores of their host society, the younger generations of Chinese English experienced a renewed interest in their identities as Chinese and actively sought to restore those ties and practices (Jovchelovitch and Gervais 1999).

Acknowledgments We are grateful to the editors for facilitating this thoughtful volume and inviting us to be a part of it. We also thank the National Cancer Institute for sponsoring the conference on place, health, and equity, and the presenters and attendees for stimulating our thoughts and furthering our research. Finally, we are indebted to Belinda Tucker, Andrew Fuligni, David Takeuchi, Cheryl Boyce, and the Family Research Consortium IV for providing an excellent postdoctoral training experience.

References

Abraido-Lanza, Ana, Bruce Dohrenwend, Daisy Ng-Mak, and J. Blake Turner. 1999. "The Latino Mortality Paradox: A Test of the "Salmon Bias" and Healthy Migrant Hypotheses." *American Journal of Public Health* 89: 1543–1548.

Black, Sandra and Kyriakos Markides. 1993. "Acculturation and Alcohol Consumption in Puerto Rican, Cuban-American, and Mexican-American Women in the United States." *American Journal of Public Health* 83: 890–893.

Bruhn, John G., Betty Chandler, M. Clinton Miller, and Stewart Wolf. 1966. "Social Aspects of Coronary Heart Disease in Two Adjacent Ethnically Different Communities." *American Journal of Public Health* 56: 1493–1506.

Bruhn, John G. and Stewart Wolf. 1979. *The Roseto Story: An Anatomy of Health*. Norman: University of Oklahoma Press.

Budrys, Grace. 2003. *Unequal Health: How Inequality Contributes to Health or Illness*. Lanham, MD: Rowman & Littlefield Publishers Inc.

Cagney, Kathleen, Christopher Browning, and Danielle Wallace. 2007. "The Latino Paradox in Neighborhood Context: The Case of Asthma and Other Respiratory Conditions." *American Journal of Public Health* 97: 919–925.

Carter-Pokras, Olivia, Ruth Zambrana, Gillermina Yankelvich, Maria Estrada, Carlos Castillo-Salgado, and Alexander Ortega. 2008. "Health Status of Mexican-Origin Persons: Do Proxy Measures of Acculturation Advance our Understanding of Health Disparities?" *Journal of Immigrant Minority Health* 10: 475–488.

Cassel, John, Ralph Patrick, and David Jenkins. 1960. "Epidemiological Analysis of the Health Implication of Cultural Change: A Conceptual Model." *Annals of the New York Academy of Sciences* 84: 938–949.

Cho, Youngtae, W. Parker Frisbie, Robert Hummer, and Richard Rogers. 2004. "Nativity, Duration of Residence, and the Health of Hispanic Adults in the United States." *International Migration Review* 38: 184–211.

Cohen, Deborah, Suzanne Spear, Richard Scribner, Patty Kissinger, Karen Mason, and John Wildgen. 2000. "Broken Windows' and the Risk of Gonorrhea." *American Journal of Public Health* 90: 230–236.

Crowley, Martha, Daniel T. Lichter, and Zhenchao Qian. 2006. "Beyond Gateway Cities: Economic Restructuring and Changing Poverty Among Mexican Immigrants." *Family Relations* 55: 345–360.

Cummins, Steven, Sarah Curtis, Ana V. Diez-Roux, and Sally Macintyre. 2007. "Understanding and Representing 'Place' in Health Research: A Relational Approach." *Social Science and Medicine* 65:1825–1838.

Cunningham, Solveig, Julia Ruben, and Venkat Narayan. 2008. "Health of Foreign-Born People in the United States: A Review." *Health and Place* 14: 623–635.

Djao, Wei. 2003. *Being Chinese: Voices from the Diaspora.* Tucson, AZ: The University of Arizona Press.

Egolf, Brenda, Judith Lasker, Stewart Wolf, and Louise Potvin. 1992. "The Roseto Effect: A 50-Year Comparison of Mortality Rates." *American Journal of Public Health* 82: 1089–1092.

Finch, Brian Karl, Nelson Lim, William Perez, D. Phuong Do. 2007. "Toward a Population Health Model of Segmented Assimilation: The Case of Low Birth Weight in Los Angeles." *Sociological Perspectives* 50: 445–468.

Franzini, Luisa, John Ribble, and Arlene Keddle. 2001. "Understanding the Hispanic Paradox." *Ethnicity and Disease* 11: 496–518.

Gervais, Marie-Claude and Jovchelovitch, Sandra. 1998. "Health and Identity: The Case of the Chinese Community in England." *Social Science Information* 37: 709–729.

Gladwell, Malcolm. 2008. *Outliers: The Story of Success.* New York: Little, Brown, & Co.

Glick Schiller, Nina, Linda Basch, and Cristina Blanc-Szanton. 1996. "Transnationalism: A New Analytic Framework for Understanding Migration." Pp. 1–24 in *Toward a Transnational Perspective on Migration*, edited by N. Glick Schiller, L. Basch, and C. Blanc-Szanton. New York: New York Academy of Sciences.

Green, Gill, Bradby, Hannah, Chan, Anita, and Lee, Maggie. 2006. "We are Not Completely Westernised": Dual Medical Systems and Pathways to Health Care among Chinese Migrant Women in England." *Social Science & Medicine* 62: 1498–1509.

Guendelman, Sylvia and Barbara Abrams. 1994. "Dietary, Alcohol, and Tobacco Intake among Mexican-American Women of Childbearing Age: Results from HANES Data." *American Journal of Health Promotion* 8: 363–372.

Himmelgreen, David, Rafael Perez-Escamilla, Yukuei Peng, Dinorah Martinez and Alva Wright. 2001. "Length of Time in US, Acculturation Status, and Overweight and Obesity Among Latinos in Two Urban Settings." *American Journal of Physical Anthropology (Supplement)* 12: 81

Hummer, Robert, Richard G. Rogers, Sarit H. Amir, Douglas Forbes, Douglas, and W. Parker Frisbie. 2000. "Adult Mortality Differentials among Hispanic Subgroups and Non-Hispanic White." *Social Science Quarterly* 81: 459–476.

Hummer, Robert, Daniel A. Powers, Starling G. Pullum, Ginger L. Gossman, and W. Parker Frisbie. 2007. "Paradox Found (Again): Infant Mortality among the Mexican-Origin Population in the United States." *Demography* 44: 441–457.

Hummer, Robert, Richard Roger, Charles Nam, and Felicia LeClere. 1999. "Race/Ethnicity, Nativity, and U.S. Adult Mortality." *Social Science Quarterly* 80: 136–153.

Johnson, Michelle and Kristen Marchi. 2009. "Segmented Assimilation Theory and Perinatal Health Disparities Among Women of Mexican Descent." *Social Science and Medicine* 69: 101–109.

Jovchelovitch, Sandra and Gervais, Marie-Claude.1999. "Social Representations of Health and Illness: The Case of the Chinese Community in England." *Journal of Community & Applied Social Psychology* 9: 247–260.

Kawachi, Ichiro, Bruce P. Kennedy, and Roberta Glass. 1999. "Social Capital and Self-Rated Health: A Contextual Analysis." *American Journal of Public Health* 89: 1187–1193.

Kelaher, Margaret and Dorothy Jessop. 2002. "Differences in Low-Birthweight Among Documented and Undocumented Foreign-Born and US-Born Latinas." *Social Science and Medicine* 55: 2171–2175.

Kleinman, Arthur. 1975. Medicine in Chinese Cultures. Bethesda, MD: Fogarty International Center, NIH

Kleinman, Arthur, Leon Eisenberg, and Byron Good. 2006. "Culture, Illness, and Care: Clinical Lessons from Anthropologic and Cross-Cultural Research." *Focus 4*(1): 140–149.

Kunitz, S. J. 1990. "Social Support and Mortality in Post-transition Populations." In *Disease in Populations in Transition: Anthropological and Epidemiological Perspectives*, edited by A. C. Swedlund and G. J. Armelagos. New York: Bergin & Garvey.

Lara, Marielena, Cristina Gamboa, M. Iya Kahramanian, Leo Morales and David E. Hayes Bautista. 2005. "Acculturation and Latino Health in the United States: A Review of the Literature and its Sociopolitical Context." *Annual Review of Public Health* 26:367–397.

Lasker, Judith, Brenda Egolf, and Stewart Wolf. 1994. "Community, Social Change and Mortality." *Social Science & Medicine* 39: 53–62.

Lynch, James J. 1979. *The Broken Heart: The Medical Consequences of Loneliness.* New York, NY: Basic Books.

Lynch, John and George Kaplan. 2000. "Socioeconomic Position." pp. 13–35 in *Social Epidemiology*, edited by Lisa F. Berkman and Ichiro Kawachi. New York: Oxford University Press.

Ma, Laurence J. C. 2003. "Space, Place, and Transnationalism in the Chinese Diaspora." pp. 1–50 in *The Chinese Diaspora: Space, Place, Mobility, and Identity,* edited by L. J. C. Ma and Carolyn Cartier. Lanham, MD: Rowman & Littlefield Publishers, Inc.

Macintyre, Sally, Anne Ellaway, and Steven Cummins. 2002. "Place Effects on Health; How Can We Conceptualize and Measure Them?" *Social Science and Medicine* 55:125–139.

Malmström, Marianne, Jan Sundquist, and Sven-Erik Johansson. 1999. "Neighborhood Environment and Self-Reported Health Status: A Multilevel Analysis." *American Journal of Public Health* 89: 1181–1186.

Markides, Kyriakos and Jeannine Coreil. 1986. "The Health of Hispanics in the Southwestern United States: An Epidemiologic Paradox." *Public Health Reports* 101: 253–265.

Palloni, Alberto and Elizabeth Arias. 2004. "Paradox Lost: Explaining the Hispanic Adult Mortality Advantage." *Demography* 41: 385–415.

Pampalon, Robert, Denis Hamel, Maria De Koninck, and Marie-Jeanne Disant. 2007. "Perception of Place and Health: Differences Between Neighbourhoods in the Quebec City Region." *Social Science and Medicine* 65: 95–111.

Passel, Jeffrey and D'Vera Cohn, 2009. *Mexican Immigrants: How Many Come? How Many Leave?* Washington, DC: Pew Hispanic Center, July 2009.

Peak, Christopher and John Weeks. 2002. "Does Community Context Influence Reproductive Outcomes of Mexican Origin Women in San Diego, California?" *Journal of Immigrant Health* 4: 125–136.

Pickett, Kate and Michelle Pearl. 2001. "Multilevel Analyses of Neighborhood Socio-Economic Context and Health Outcomes: A Critical Review." *Journal of Epidemiology and Community Health* 55: 111–122.

Rutledge, Matthew and Catherine McLaughlin. 2008. "Hispanics and Health Insurance Coverage: The Rising Disparity." *Medical Care* 46: 1086–1092.

Skeldon, Ronald. 2003. "The Chinese Diaspora or the Migration of Chinese Peoples?" pp. 51–68 in *The Chinese Diaspora: Space, Place, Mobility, and Identity,* edited by L. J. C. Ma and Carolyn Cartier. Lanham, MD: Rowman & Littlefield Publishers, Inc.

Sorlie, Paul, Eric Backlund, Norman Johnson, and Eugene Rogot. 1993. "Mortality by Hispanic Status in the United States." *JAMA* 270: 2464–2468.

Stout, Clarke, Jerry Morrow, Edward N. Brandt, and Stewart Wolf. 1964. "Study of an Italian-American Community in PA: Unusually Low Incidence of Death from Myocardial Infarction." *JAMA* 188: 845–849.

Tabora, Betty L. and Jacquelyn H. Flaskerud. 1996. "Mental Health Beliefs, Practices, and Knowledge of Chinese American Immigrant Women." *Issues in Mental Health Nursing* 18: 173–189.

Tambiah, Stanley J. 2000. "Transnational Movements, Diaspora, and Multiple Modernities: Transnational Movements of People and Their Implications." *Daedulus* 129: 163–194.

Unschuld, Paul U. 1987. "Traditional Chinese Medicine: Some Historical and Epistemological Reflections." *Social Science and Medicine* 24: 1023–1029.

Wade, Christine, Maria T. Chao, and Fredi Kronenberg. 2007. "Medical Pluralism of Chinese Women Living in the United States." *Journal of Immigrant and Minority Health* 9: 255–267.

Wai-sum, Amy L. 2008. "Look Who's Talking: Migrating Narratives and Identity Construction." pp. 206–223 in *At Home in the Chinese Diaspora: Memories, Identities, and Belongings,* edited by E. K. Khun and A. P. Davidson. New York: Palgrave Macmillan.

Wolf, Stewart and John G. Bruhn. 1993. *The Power of Clan: The Influence of Human Relationships on Heart Disease.* New Brunswick, NJ: Transaction Publishers.

Wolf, Stewart, Kay Linda Grace, John G. Bruhn, and Clarke Stout. 1974. "Roseto Revisited: Further Data on the Incidence of Myocardial Infarction in Roseto and Neighboring Pennsylvania Communities." *Transactions of the American Clinical and Climatological Association* 85: 100–108.

Chapter 9
Sacred Place: An Interdisciplinary Approach for the Social Science

Jennifer Abe

...Every encounter of the sacred is rooted in a place, a socio-spatial context that is rich in myth and symbol.

(Belden Lane 1994, p. 19)

Last spring, I experienced an Easter Vigil for the first time. I was then visiting the *L'Abbaye de Senanc*, a monastery built in the thirteenth century, nestled in fields of lavender outside the hillside town of Gorda in southern France. We, a small band of pilgrims and tourists, gathered in the middle of the night in a covered stone courtyard, shivering in air so cold that each exhalation created tiny clouds. In the interior of the fireplace, large enough for a tall person to stand, lay several sheaves of dried lavender. A procession of monks, robed in rough cloth held and knotted with thick rope, filed into that silent space, then dimly lit by the thin candles we cradled in our hands. One of the garbed men threw a lighted branch into the dried bundle of fragrant herbs. With an astonishing roar, the Easter flame flared and rose up steeply, casting long, strange shadows against the ancient limestone. The haunting song of the monks who dwelled in that place reverberated in the air, their ageless sound echoing in the stillness. I felt a sense of timelessness, even of the eternal. I sensed the presence of all those who had stood there in the same place, keeping watch on that same night for the past several hundred years, who had listened to these chants echoing against the walls, and who had also smelled the pungent lavender in the cold air. In that space, that sacred place, I felt a strong sense of connection to those countless unknown others, my sense of time and history suddenly punctured and porous. So, the Easter Vigil began.

What makes a place sacred? How is it that some places hold such profound meaning that they feel critical to us as human beings in helping to locate ourselves as persons and as communities? An ancient stone monastery in a distant land

J. Abe (✉)
Department of Psychology, Loyola Marymount University, 1 LMU Drive Suite 4700, Los Angeles, CA 90045, USA
e-mail: jsabe@lmu.edu

L.M. Burton et al. (eds.), *Communities, Neighborhoods, and Health*, Social Disparities in Health and Health Care 1, DOI 10.1007/978-1-4419-7482-2_9,

mediated a strong connection for me with individuals long gone from this world. How did a sense of kinship arise with those who spoke a different tongue, with whom I shared only a faintly similar tradition? Sacred places mediate human experiences of the transcendent. To be sure, these are not the only places in which such experiences occur, but such places, long experienced as holy or "set apart," often contain and encourage the potential for such a connection.

Little research has been conducted on the notion of sacred place in the social sciences, although interest in the related constructs of spirituality and religiousness is evident in research that has burgeoned dramatically over the past several decades (Weaver et al. 2006). Spirituality and religiousness have been linked, both directly and indirectly, to a variety of health outcomes (Rasic et al. 2009; Franch 2008; Blumenthal et al. 2007; WHOQOL SRPB Group 2006; Szaflarski et al. 2006 Powell et al. 2003; Koenig and Cohen 2002; Pargament 1997, George et al. 2002; Miller and Thoresen 2003). Evidence suggests that some "hard" indicators of religion, such as church attendance, are strongly associated with mortality rates; across studies, regular churchgoers appear to outlive those who do not attend church, even after controlling for a range of other factors (Musick et al. 2004; Oman et al. 2002; Hummer et al. 1999; Koenig et al. 1999). Empirical findings related to less behavioral indicators of religion, including spirituality, religious beliefs, values, and attitudes, have had more mixed associations with health and well-being (WHOQOL SRPB Group 2006; Powell et al. 2003). In an international study of 5,087 individuals in 18 countries, however, findings indicated a positive association between spirituality, religion, and personal beliefs, and overall quality of life, with the strongest correlations for psychological and social domains (WHOQOL SRPB Group 2006).

Despite the renewed interest in this area, there is little attempt to examine spirituality and religiousness as contextualized in the places they are experienced and practiced. Current measures are oriented almost exclusively towards self-reported, decontextualized, individual behaviors and attitudes. How might an examination of sacred places contribute to an understanding of the ways in which places, when experienced as sacred, may mediate well-being? What are the communal practices, rituals, symbols, values, and beliefs embedded in sacred places that contribute to an individual's experience of the divine or transcendent? Such questions have the potential to help unpack the relationship between individual experiences of sacred place and their collective meanings (i.e., their social, spiritual, religious, political, historical, geographical significance). In addition, these questions can help illumine the role of specific "place-making" activities in these places, activities that not only help sustain their sacred meaning to persons and communities over time but that may also represent beneficial health-related practices in themselves.

Research on place in the social sciences has demonstrated that place and place-related constructs such as *sense of place* (Relph 1976), *place identity* (Proshansky et al. 1983), and *place attachment* (Low and Altman 1992), for example, contribute to differences in human health and well-being (Fullilove 1996; Jackson et al. 2008; Frumkin 2003; Macintyre et al. 2002; Bolam et al. 2006; Stain et al. 2008). Consequently, an examination of sacred place may also help address an important gap in the literature on place and health. The primary aim of this chapter is to develop a model of sacred place and sacred place-making for the social sciences, one that is grounded in a rich interdisciplinary understanding of place and can help frame future research on the intersections between place, spirituality, and health. In doing so, this research may contribute to both literatures on (a) spirituality and religiousness, by contextualizing beliefs and practices in sacred places, as well as (b) place and health, by identifying sacred places as potentially important sites for promoting human health and well-being.

The chapter has four parts. First, the notion of "sacred place" is reviewed in an interdisciplinary context, with particular attention given to recent theological understandings of sacred place. Second, a conceptualization of sacred place for social science research is developed, drawing on the contributions of three divergent theoretical understandings of place that cross disciplinary boundaries (essentialist, social constructivist, and person–place frameworks). Third, the notion of "sacred place-making" is introduced and applied to the experience of sacred place in two different contexts (wilderness experiences and everyday life). Finally, concluding observations about sacred place and sacred place-making that may contribute to future research in this area are provided.

Theological Understandings of Sacred Place: An Interdisciplinary Approach

The notion of "place" has long held the attention of philosophers engaged with the idea of human *dwelling* in the universe (Heidegger 1972; Weil 1952; Bachelard 1969). Because we are embodied beings, we are physically in the world "somewhere." (Heidegger 1972). Whereas traditional geography has often regarded place as simply a "portion of space occupied by a thing or human being" (Billinge 1986), humanistic geography has treated human experience as central to the study of place (Paasi 1991; Relph 1976; Tuan 1974). These divergent perspectives mirror competing notions of place in ancient Greece: Aristotle viewed place as *topos*, an inert container to be filled with human experience, whereas the Platonic notion of place as *chora* implied the active capacity of a place to "resonate to the immediacies of human experience" with its own energy and power (Lane 2001). Scholarly inquiry has also resulted in place being "unbounded" from geography altogether, both as a term reflecting social hierarchy, power, and position (Stowkowski 2002), as well as a frame for understanding the "spatiality of experience," and one's life as a never-ending spiritual search (i.e., Gregory of Nyssa).

Nowhere are the spiritual underpinnings of the meaning of place more evident than in work that examines the universal human yearning for "home" or the feeling of being at home in the world. "To be rooted," claims Weil (1952), "is perhaps the most important and least recognized need of the human soul." Bachelard (1969), in *The Poetics of Space*, describes "home" as "…our first universe, a real cosmos in every sense of the word" (p. 4). But, "home" is more than simply where we originate. "All really inhabited space bears the essence of the notion of home" (Bachelard 1969, p. 5). Sheldrake (2001), a theologian, identifies some of the multiple meaning of "home": it represents a place in which we feel grounded as we move through life, a sense of belonging as part of a community, a yearning to be in relationship with nature, and an experience of *life itself as sacred* (italics in the original, p. 10).

In his book *Landscapes of the Sacred*, Belden Lane (2001), a historian of religion in American life, describes sacred place as "…a construction of the imagination that affirms the independence of the holy" (p. 19) and proposes four "axioms" for understanding the character of sacred places. His first axiom, *sacred place is not chosen, it chooses,* shows the manner in which sacred place is held in the imagination: these places seemingly take hold of us, and not the other way around, underscoring the mystery and power of such places. This idea is illustrated in the experience of Jack Turner who described his experience as a young man, dazed but uninjured following a plane crash in Utah, when he first encountered the "Harvest Site" pictographs in the "Maze" area of the Canyonlands National Park:

> Then, in the last light of day, I was startled by a line of dark torsos and a strange hand on a wall just above the canyon floor. I froze, rigid with fear. My usual mental categories of alive and not-alive became permeable. The painted figures stared at me, transmuted from mere stone as if by magic, and I stared back in terror…After a few seconds, my body intervened with my mind, pulling it away from a gaze that engulfed me. The torsos became "just" pictures. My mind discovered a comfortable category for the original perception and the confusion passed. But strangely, seeing them as representations did not reduce the emotion I felt….I could not override the feeling that the figures were looking at me, and that I was seeing what I wasn't supposed to see.
>
> (Turner 1996, p. 8)

Turner recounts how he returned to the same spot 31 years later and how the experience could not be recaptured, no matter how he tried: "The pictographs were still wonderful, but now they were just things we were visiting. I had become a tourist to my own experience…I tried sitting with them alone in the dark, but they neither gazed at nor engulfed me now" (p. 11).

Places also become recognized as sacred because of what happens within them. Lane (2001) suggests that *sacred place is ordinary place, ritually made extraordinary* (p. 19). In a Hindu home, one such area, the *pooja* room, is considered the most important sacred home space, where household deities reside, sacred objects are kept, and daily rituals are performed (Mazumdar and Mazumdar 1999). It is one of several domestic spaces that serve to underscore the importance of Hindu women's roles in sustaining religious practices and in caring for sacred spatial domains in the Hindu household. Such places are "set apart" and experienced as unique from other places even if they are physically not so distinguishable from other places.

The recognition and awareness of a place as sacred also require a state of attention and consciousness that enables a person to "see" it. Lane suggests in his third axiom that *sacred places can be tread upon without being entered.* When one's perceptual frame is tuned in, it is possible to respond to and experience a place as sacred; conversely, one can be *in* a place and not be *present* in it at all. In his book, *Wisdom Sits in Places*, anthropologist Keith Basso (1996) recounts the shift in his perceptions of the Arizona desert as he traveled through the landscape and learned many of the place-names from his Western Apache companions. His landmark study illumined the vast difference between moving through a landscape known mostly as dots on a map and moving through a landscape known at a deeper level – through the collective memory, history, stories, identity, and moral lessons contained in its place-names. As a result of this process, Basso observed, "...for me, riveted and moved, the country takes on a different cast, a density of meaning – and with it a formidable strength – it did not have before" (p. 28).

Finally, Lane suggests that *the impulse of sacred place is both centripetal and centrifugal, local and universal*, which he describes as both "a pulling in and a pushing out from a center, a tendency alternately between localization and universalization" (p. 32). The centripetal impulse is reflected in the yearning to be rooted, to belong, and to identify the divine in the particulars of the local. The centrifugal impulse represents the restless quest, the journey to move away from what is known. Heidegger's notion of "dwelling" encompasses both of these impulses, rootedness and belonging, as well as movement and journey. The notion of *pilgrimage* expresses this duality; in the journey toward encountering sacred places, pilgrims become more firmly rooted in their religious traditions. *Pilgrimage* as a religious requirement for Islam, for instance, allows pilgrims to visit places associated with the Prophet and to experience them with all their senses, in the physical reality of these places, in ways that "...engage the believer in the sacred geography and history of the place" (Mazumdar and Mazumdar 2004, p. 393).

Lane's four axioms provide a flexible structure for capturing the complexity, richness, mystery, and power of sacred place. They point to how the exploration of sacred place may not only renew our appreciation for the continuing resonance and power of place in influencing our personal and collective identity but also how a greater understanding of sacred place may help in examining the potential "sacred character" of our lives (Pargament 2008).

Conceptualizing Sacred Place for the Social Sciences

Edward Relph (1976) described sacred places as those enabling individuals to experience "existential insideness" or "the unselfconscious and authentic experience of place as central to existence" (p. 142). What are the qualities that characterize experiences of the sacred? "Sacred qualities" include the notion of (a) *transcendence* ("the perception that there is an extraordinary dimension to our lives, something that goes beyond our immediate selves, our everyday experience, and our usual understanding"), (b) *boundlessness* ("the perception of endless space and time"), and (c) *ultimacy* ("the perception of an essential and ultimate truth that underlies the foundation of experience") (Pargament 2008, p. 24).

How are these "sacred qualities" related to an understanding of spirituality? Moberg (2002) views spirituality as "...the essence of the religious life, a transcendent quality that cuts across and infuses all of the core dimensions of religiosity" (p. 48). In the social sciences, spirituality has been variously described as "a search for the sacred" (Pargament 1999) or as a search for transcendent or ultimate meaning (Astrow et al. 2001), among many other definitions. *Spirituality* is closely related to *religion*, which primarily reflects an institutional, social phenomenon, whereas spirituality "…is usually understood at the level of the individual within specific contexts" (Miller and Thoresen 2003, p. 28; Thoresen 1998). Another term, *religiousness*, reflects the conceptualization of religion at the individual level, emphasizing an individual's identification with institutional practices, values, and beliefs that are rooted in a formal religious tradition. Whereas religious individuals are often highly spiritual, many spiritually oriented individuals do not identify with any specific religious tradition, leading to a consensus that spirituality reflects a broader concept than religiousness (Miller and Thoresen 2003; Hill and Pargament 2003).

When religion, religious beliefs, or ideas are connected to the attachment people feel to places, such feelings are identified as "religious place attachment" (Mazumdar 2005). Mazumdar and Mazumdar (1999, 2005) have demonstrated in a number of important studies the importance of considering religion in research on place and place attachment, with close attention to the role of religion in defining places as sacred. The present chapter on sacred place does not attempt to provide a comparative analysis of place across religious traditions, nor is it oriented towards detailed descriptions of specific rituals and religious practices (see the Mazumdars' body of work for this kind of careful analysis). Instead, this chapter conceptualizes sacred place broadly as it relates to spirituality, both as it is central to religious traditions and experienced apart from specific religious traditions. From this perspective, sacred places are defined in terms of how they *point to the transcendent*, whether or not they are explicitly grounded in religious traditions, with physical features (natural and/or built) and/or geography that have been richly imbued with symbol and meaning through rituals and ceremonies over time. This conceptualization of sacred place draws from the contributions of three divergent approaches (essentialist, social constructivist, and person–place frameworks) to the study of place. These approaches are not set "against" each other as competing perspectives on sacred place; rather, the specific ways in which each approach can deepen our understanding of sacred place are lifted out and emphasized.

Sacred Place: Contributions from Essentialist Approaches

Classic formulations of sacred place begin with Mircea Eliade's work, *The Sacred and the Profane* (1959), and his view of particular geographical locations as representing earthly points of intersection (or *axis mundi*) between different "cosmic regions" in which "passage from one cosmic region to another is made possible (from heaven to earth and vice versa; from earth to the underworld)." *Stupas*, Buddhist temples rounded and built with sharp towers that appear to pierce the earth's skin at precisely identified geographical locations, for instance, represent architectural forms designed around the concept of *axis mundi*.

This approach contributes to an understanding of sacred place through its focus on defining places in the world as either "sacred" or "profane." To identify a place as sacred was to also implicitly name the area outside its boundaries as profane. Mt. Kailash, in western Tibet, for instance, links heaven and the earth and is sacred to the Hindus because it is believed to be "the abode of Lord Shiva" (Ruback et al. 2008, p. 175). For the Navajo, the first humans came into being at The Place of Emergence, located in Southwestern Colorado, another sacred place. In addition, specific rivers (e.g., the Ganges and the Jordan), mountains (e.g., Mt. Sinai, Mt. Fuji, "Tahoma" or Mt. Ranier), and even entire cities (for example, Jerusalem, Mecca, and Benares) have been "set apart" in our collective imagination from other places as particular sites of holiness, long considered sacred by many cultures (Mazumdar and Mazumdar 1993; Lane 2001).

From a slightly different approach, in ancient Rome, it was considered necessary to understand the *genius loci*, or spirits of the place, to become truly known of a particular geographic location (Walter 1988). Thus, from this perspective, to define a place as sacred was to acknowledge the spirit of the place as sacred. The notion of *genius loci* "...symbolized the place's generative energy, and it pictured a specific, personal, spiritual presence who animated and protected a place...on the deepest level, [it represented] the energy, definition, unifying principle, and continuity of place" (Walter 1988, p. 150). Similarly, a common thread in diverse Native American conceptions of spirituality includes viewing the natural world as infused with spirit, with all "relations" (i.e., animals, plans, minerals, earth, sky, people) experienced as interdependent and interconnected with each other (Garrett and Wilbur 1999; Voss et al. 1999). From these perspectives, the land itself as well as all its inhabitants is alive to each other.

The concepts of *axis mundi* and *genius loci* represent *essentialist* views of place, in that the sacred character of the setting is endemic to the place itself. A limitation of this approach is that it can greatly narrow the view of sacred place because what falls outside the boundaries of "sacred" may be considered "profane" by default, creating an automatic opposition and tension between sacred space and everyday life (Sheldrake 2007). Yet, the major contribution of this approach is its imaginative, even mythic reach, linking human experience to the divine, as mediated through place. This approach may also illuminate how the natural world is often encountered and experienced in a deeply spiritual manner.

Sacred Place: Social Constructivist Contributions

Many scholars have critiqued the study of place as perhaps too narrowly focused on its tangible, physical features, questioning the assumptions underlying traditional concepts of place (Stowkowski 2002). Instead, they argue that places should be conceived of as rich "texts" representing a diverse set of socially, historically, culturally, politically, and religiously contested meanings and symbols (Stowkowski 2002; Manzo 2003; Zerubavel 1996). Jerusalem, claimed as a sacred city by three major world religions, is probably the most visible example of the contested, multiple identities of a place long regarded as sacred. This perspective contributes to our understanding of sacred place by illuminating its socially constructed elements, the complex, multiple layers of meaning that accrue over time through the social interaction and activities of individuals and groups around a place.

A "relational" view of place emphasizes human "constellations of connections" so that places are viewed as "nodes in networks" characterized by long or short "reaches" and with differing levels of complexity (Cummins et al. 2007). Because relationships and networks are highlighted, this perspective also enables an examination of how power relationships, and the use of language, and symbols affect the creation, naming, meaning, and use of places (Stowkowski 2002; Stokols and Shumaker 1981).

From a social constructivist perspective, places become "inscribed as sacred through the cultural production of the groups which claim them" (Nelson 2006). Day (2008) completed an ethnographic study of two churches, housed in urban buildings whose original purpose was secular, and describes the process by which these buildings were reconstructed as sacred. These unassuming buildings on a busy street, Germantown Avenue, in Philadelphia, Pennsylvania, became experienced as *holy ground* in their urban setting, blurring traditional boundaries between sacred and profane. In her study, she examined how the physical form and space of the buildings expressed and shaped the religious identity of the congregations that housed them, and how the "sweat equity" invested by members of each congregation to renovate these spaces served to make them sacred. That is, these places become sacred through the work of "sacralization," a form of place-making (Relph 1976; Basso 1996). The Mennonite congregation transformed "…the dark attic-like space into a sun-drenched worship space, elegant in its utter simplicity" (Day 2008, p. 430). The neighboring Pentacostal congregation, in contrast, not only renovated their space quite differently but also carried out an ongoing set of cleansing rituals to sacralize their new space, literally room by room (Day 2008).

A major contribution of this perspective is the dynamic, unbounded nature of this view of place in its emphasis on relationships and networks, in a way that is not constrained by geography (Cummins et al. 2007; Relph 2008). As such, the complex, rich network of social, cultural, political, historical narratives and realities grounding these places, as well as their often-contested nature, is highlighted. A limitation of this approach is that the place itself – its physically and geographically constituted reality – often gets relegated to the background and may even be rendered invisible compared with the study of social networks, relationships, and power, as it relates to an understanding of the significance of place. Yet, the social constructivist framework also provides a powerful lens for us to better understand how persons work on places to "inscribe them as sacred."

Sacred Place: Person–Place Relationships as Reciprocal and Mutually Constitutive

In contrast to an *essentialist* perspective, in which place is emphasized more than persons, as well as a *social constructivist* view, in which persons are emphasized more than places, in a *person–place* approach, the influence is more reciprocal and even perhaps mutually constitutive. "We are not only *in* places but *of* them" observes Edward Casey (1996, 1997), in describing a long philosophical tradition of examining how being "emplaced" and "embodied" is foundational to a phenomenological understanding of experience. "The primacy of perception," from the phenomenological perspective, is also "the primacy of the lived body" (Casey 1996), such that place and body are mutually constitutive and are further seen as "inter-animated." This perspective contributes to our understanding of sacred place in reminding us that experiences of the sacred are grounded in the "lived body" in particular places, experienced through our senses: *This* is what the light looks like in *this* place, *this* is the manner of vegetation and animal life, *this* is the line of the horizon, *these* are the scents, the taste of the air (Riegner 1993; Casey 1996).

The "mutually constitutive" view of the relationship between places and persons draws greater attention to the way places "work" on people so that the direction of influence is not simply from persons to places but also the other way around, from places to persons. Places "gather" the animals, plants, stories, myths, culture, history, geography, language, and people in a place and "keep" this configuration in a way that holds it together with the form of the place (mountain, mesa, gully) (Casey 1996). When a person is in such a gathered place, the place can "release memories" that belong as much to the place as to the individual (Casey 1996).

Sacred places may also be "intensely gathered" with physical features, whether of the natural world or a built environment, that are imbued with symbols, radiant in their spiritual and religious significance, as well as historical, cultural, political, and social narratives. Basso's (1996) account of the Western Apache relationship to the Arizona desert landscape underscores how places speak to communities; "For Indian men and women, the past lies embedded in features of the earth – in canyons and lakes mountains and arroyos, rocks and vacant fields – which together endow their lands with multiple forms of significance that reach into their lives and shape the ways they think" (p. 34). Landscapes embody meaning precisely because their specific characteristics hold individual and collective identities, with the power to convey spiritual and moral truths for communities (Basso 1996; Gone 2008).

Sacred Place-Making: Sacralization and Sacrilization Processes

The work of creating places, places that feel genuine, authentic, and significant to us, requires the work of *place-making*. Place-making involves all the conscious and unconscious ways in which we invest places with meaning through our ongoing activities and rituals, contributing to them in ways that express the dreams, passions, needs, and values of those in them in harmony with the physical features of the environment surrounding them (Relph 1976; Basso 1996). Further, the notion of place-making as a process illustrates how geographic setting or physical space may shift from being experienced as *topos*, or "only" geography, to *chora*, vibrant "authentic" place. In addressing this "total and unified experience of place," Relph (1976) notes that "the end result is places which fit their context and are in accord with the intentions of those who created them, yet have a distinct and profound identity" (p. 68). Thus, place-making may be viewed as the primary means through which places imprint themselves on people, their identity, and sense of self, as well as the way in which people shape places, both physically as well as imaginatively. Of place-making, Basso (1996) observes, "what people make of their places is closely connected to what they make of themselves … We are, in a sense, the place-worlds we imagine" (p. 7).

What does place-making mean with respect to sacred place? Burton-Christie (2009) describes how "place-making" may be viewed as a contemplative spiritual practice. Using the work of the great landscape photographer, Robert Adams, he lifts out the imaginative element of place-making, noting the delicate and complex nature of this contemplative work that weaves together the "verities" of place, including not only the physical geography of the place but also our personal experience or story evoked in the place ("autobiography"), as well as what the place "stands for" in the broader collective imagination ("metaphor"). *Geography, autobiography, and metaphor*, these three elements help account for the process, yes, even spiritual practice by which whole "place-worlds" come into being.

In *sacred place-making*, these elements are further woven together in the imagination to create authentic, meaningful places through the reciprocal processes of *sacralization*, which refers to the myriad of socially constituted ways in which people create and sustain sacred places (emphasizing the influence of persons upon places), and *sacrilization*, which refers to the avenues whereby [sacred] places work on persons so that they are "sensitized to the spiritual" (emphasizing the influence of places upon persons) (Heintzman 2002; Chandler et al. 1992). Rituals, symbols, artifacts, icons, texts, stories, memories – all have potent meaning in contributing to the rich social and cultural significance in *sacred place-making* to reflect and represent not only the core values and beliefs of the community, but also the meanings, physical features, and geography of the sacred place itself.

Sacrilization, the ways in which places "work" on individuals to orient them to the sacred, to the spiritual, and *sacralization* or the place-making activities, rituals, and processes that enable a place to be "inscribed" as sacred may potentially contribute to high levels of *place identity* (Proshansky et al. 1983) and *place attachment* (Low and Altman 1992), as well as to a strong *sense of place* (Relph 1976) among individuals. Research on *place identity* indicates that aspects of the self develop as a result of one's relation to the environment (Proshansky et al. 1983). This notion views place as not just a means for satisfying human needs (see Stokols and Shumaker 1981, for the notion of *place dependence*), but also views place as essential to one's very sense of self, resulting in a strong sense of *place attachment* (Williams et al. 1992). These place-based constructs emphasize affective experiences or impacts within an individual that are elicited by place and that may be associated with health outcomes (Fullilove 1996; Bolam et al. 2006; Frumkin 2003; Stain et al. 2008). Through sacred place-making processes, individuals open themselves to the power and mystery of sacred places (sacrilization) as well as invest sacred places with personal meaning and memory through their time and activity (sacralization). What remains to be seen, perhaps, is how individuals may also contribute to their own well-being through these sacred place-making processes.

For instance, one way in which experiences of sacred place may foster well-being is through a sense of *leisure*, defined in terms of "…a mental and spiritual attitude…a condition of the soul…a receptive attitude of mind, a contemplative attitude" (Pieper 1963, pp. 40, 41), which involves the "interplay of time, activity, motivation, and setting" (Heintzman 2002, p. 154). A sense of leisure may be fostered in the company of others as well as be experienced alone and may occur in culturally or institutionally defined sacred places as well as in places that are not explicitly named as sacred. Two examples of sacred place and place-making processes are presented below, with a focus on places (i.e., wilderness experiences and everyday living) that are not necessarily explicitly identified as sacred.

Sacred Place-Making: Wilderness Experiences

> I remember the night, and almost the very spot on the hilltop, where my soul opened out, as it were, into the Infinite, and there was a rushing together of the two worlds, the inner and the outer. It was deep calling unto deep, – the deep that my own struggle had opened up within being answered by the unfathomable deep without, reaching beyond the stars... (p. 68).
>
> An anonymous account in "Varieties of Religious Experience"

In *The Varieties of Religious Experience*, William James (1902) offers several accounts of individuals who have undergone profound spiritual experiences in the natural world. Contact with the natural world has long been regarded as having spiritual benefits (Heintzman 2002; Stringer and McAvoy 1992; Frederickson and Anderson 1999). While health-related implications and outcomes are a major focus of the present chapter, this work also underscores the need to differentiate between a focus on the natural world as significant – even perhaps sacred – for its own sake, and a focus on the natural world for its salutatory effects on human health and well-being (Stokols 1990). Nonetheless, there are at least three ways in which wilderness experiences may facilitate spiritual well-being: (1) as a *restorative environment*, (2) through the experience of *leisure*, and (3) through *solitude* that promotes deep reflection.

First, research has examined characteristics of the natural world that facilitate spiritual development (Williams et al. 1992). Kaplan (1995), for example, describes wilderness as a "restorative environment" that (1) provides individuals with a sense of "getting away," (2) represents a "whole other world" that is rich, coherent, and can fully engage the mind (an environment characterized by "extent"), (3) fits an individual's inclinations and purposes ("compatibility"), and (4) facilitates and encourages opportunities for reflection (high levels of "soft" fascination). Second, wilderness places may promote spiritual well-being (see Heintzman 2002, 2008; Chandler et al. 1992) through the experience of leisure: (1) through "grounding" experiences that allow individuals who are in a state of "spiritual emergency" to "work through" these matters by connecting them to the physical world and (2) through experiences of "sacrilization" resulting from contact with the physical world.

Finally, wilderness experiences may foster well-being through the experience of *solitude*, especially as it may foster contemplation and reflection (Frederickson and Anderson 1999; Heintzman 2002, 2008). Research suggests that solitude may have a positive effect on mood state, provide opportunities for individuation as well as creative thinking (Larson et al. 1982; Suedfeld 1982). Regarding the "healing" nature of solitude, Suedfeld (1982) observes, "There seem to be no loneliness; rather the individual feels a freedom from distraction, from the usual restrictions imposed by social norms and the need to maintain face, and the benefits of reducing external stimulation to the point where the still, small internal voices can be heard" (p. 61).

Sacred Place-Making: Everyday Living

Although experiences of the wilderness may be deeply spiritual, even transformative, it is not necessary to go to the wilderness, or anywhere for that matter, to have a spiritual experience. What can be overlooked in a discussion of sacred place is how ordinary experience in everyday settings also may be experienced as sacred. Andre Dubus (1998) gives an account of making sandwiches in his kitchen from his wheelchair that reflects this "sacramental" orientation towards everyday life:

> On Tuesdays when I make lunches for my girls, I focus on this: the sandwiches are sacraments….and each motion is a sacrament, this holding of plastic bags, of knives, of bread, of cutting board, this pushing of the chair this spreading of mustard on bread, this trimming of liverwurst, of ham. All sacraments, as putting the lunches into a zippered book bag is, and going down my six ramps to my car is. I drive on the highway, to the girls' town, to their school, and this is not simply a transition; it is my love moving by car from a place where my girls are not to a place where they are; even if I do not feel or acknowledge it, this is a sacrament. If I remember it, then I feel it too (pp. 89–90).

Such experiences are intensely personal, and such places are wholly specific to each individual. Nonetheless, everyday settings can be experienced as "more than" individual in their meaning, connecting individuals to a larger fabric of meaning through shared memories, relationships, and communal experiences of a place. Hester (1993) worked with the residents of the town of Manteo on the outer banks of North Carolina, for example, to identify the places in their village waterfront that were most important to them. As a community designer asked to redesign the area, Hester wanted to honor the residents' strong, but largely unconscious, passion for their town. He began with "behavior mapping," identifying the locations and activities that served to anchor the daily patterns of the townspeople. What was revealed through this activity was a "powerful cultural mosaic that illustrated not only how space related to the town's present social patterns but suggested how collective memory had been invested in certain parts of the landscape" (p. 273). The places that were identified as "sacred structures" by residents included such ordinary places as:

> "…the marshes surrounding the town, Jule's Park, a drugstore and soda fountain where local teens and the elderly were served freshly squeezed lemonade and chicken salad sandwiches, the post office, churches, the Christmas Shop, front porches, the town launch, a statue of Sir Walter Raleigh, the Duchess Restaurant where locals gathered for morning

> coffee and political discussions, the town hall, locally made unreadable street signs, the town cemetery, the Christmas tree in the gravel parking lot, park post lamps placed there in memory of loved ones, and two historic sites" (p. 276).

These were places that were essential to Manteo residents in fostering place identity, and a sense of place, in this town. "Place-based meanings tell us something about who we are and who we are not, how we have changed and into what we are changing" (Hull et al. 1994, p. 110). What was also revealed through Hester's work, however, was how residents were largely unaware of how important these ordinary places were to them. These "sacred structures" helped to knit them together as a community, connecting them not only to each other through daily rituals but also in a sense of a communal past, invoking a shared sense of identity and history.

Conclusion

The idea that sacred places may mediate an individual's experience of the transcendent may contribute to our understanding of the relationships between spirituality, place, and health. Several features of this relationship may be important in exploring sacred place as it may relate to health outcomes. *First, methodological approaches to examining sacred place should take seriously the embodied nature of experience.* Mazumdar and Mazumdar (1993, 2004) show how an examination of religion and place identity cannot be described apart from an abundance of religious rituals, symbols, artifacts, and activities that includes all the senses. This sensory richness may be an important aspect of the "soft" fascination referred to by Kaplan (1995) in his description of "restorative environments" as well.

Second, sacred place may perhaps be best understood as a social construct (Relph 1976; Mazumdar and Mazumdar 2004). While experiences of sacred place may be deeply personal and private, they are embedded within a larger frame of collective, social meaning. Zerubavel (1996) describes *social* memories as impersonal, not dependent on individual experience, but on the passing on of traditions, stories, myths, and collective memories as members of *mnemonic communities*. Individuals may have powerful experiences of these places, experiences that point to existential, transcendent meanings, but these meanings occur within the context of a richly layered complex of social, spiritual, religious, political, and cultural meanings. Indeed, the relationship between individual (private) experience and sacred place may even be considered *intersubjective* in nature (Good 2007; Relph 1976).

Third, it is important to examine how individuals experience sacred place, that is, the phenomenology of their experiences. A few empirical studies suggest that the affective dimensions of religious experience – specifically the experience of "spiritual emotions" as awe, gratitude, and connectedness to others – may be more salient when individuals perceive different aspects of their lives to be sacred (Haidt 2003; Emmons and McCullough 2003). Pargament (2008) has raised the intriguing notion that the experience of such positive spiritual emotions could be associated with positive health outcomes. Might the experience of sacred place be associated with the elicitation of such emotions? At the same time, Manzo (2005) underscores that place meanings are often ambiguous in nature and may be negative in valence (not just a positive experience), a point that may be particularly important in understanding sacred places as a much broader construct than that of "restorative environments" (Kaplan 1995) or "therapeutic landscapes" alone (Williams 1998; Gone 2008). Consequently, while sacred places may be experienced by some individuals as restorative or even therapeutic, the same places may also elicit grief, sadness, and reignite disturbing, traumatic experiences within other individuals. The range of responses to sacred place should be viewed as potentially highly variable.

Fourth, the experience of the transcendent may occur through solitude as well as strong experiences of community. Solitude provides time for reflection and contemplation, as well as the space for spiritual experience (Heintzman 2002). Heintzman (2002) hypothesizes that while solitude may provide the time and space for sacrilization and the development of spiritual well-being related to one's life purpose and meaning, social activities may provide the opportunity to develop spiritual well-being related to concern and connectedness with others (also see Stringer and McEvoy 1992; Frederickson and Anderson 1999; Suedfeld 1982).

In conclusion, the construct of sacred place and sacred place-making holds much potential for exploring the potential avenues through which sacred places may impact human well-being. Current research does not contextualize spirituality and/or religiousness in the places in which they are practiced and experienced so that an examination of sacred place can potentially enrich an understanding of the mechanisms by which spirituality and/or religiousness affect health and well-being. Furthermore, research on sacred place may also contribute to the literature investigating the effects of place on health by examining how experiences of the sacred, as experienced in particular places, may mediate health and well-being.

The intent of the current chapter has also been to expand the lens of research on place to *see* the sacred in places, whether it is searching out community beliefs about *genius loci* and *axis mundi* in the land, to uncover *sacred structures* in communities (Hester 1993), or to elicit reflection about experiences of the sacred in particular places among individuals. Exploring the processes of place-making within sacred places can help us better understand the reciprocal, even mutually constitutive nature of person–place relationships: how do people engage in *sacralization* to help create and sustain sacred places over time? What specific characteristics and experiences of sacred places foster and sensitize people to spiritual concerns, or *sacrilization*? The richness of the construct of sacred place as a bounded, geographic, physical reality as well as an unbounded, sacramental view of the world can contribute to the study of the relationship between place and health among different groups and communities of people in a way that is only beginning to be explored.

References

Astrow, A.B., Puchalski, C.M., & Sulmasy, D.P. 2001. Religion, spirituality, and health care. Social, ethical, and practical considerations. *American Journal of Medicine*, *110*, 283–287.

Bachelard, G. 1969. *The Poetics of Space*. Boston, MA: Beacon Press.

Basso, K. 1996. *Wisdom Sits in Places: Landscape and Language Among the Western Apache.* Albuquerque, NM: University of New Mexico Press.
Billinge, M.D. 1986. Place. In R.J. Johnston, D. Gregory, & D.M. Smith (Eds.). *The Dictionary of Human Geography*, p. 346. Oxford, UK: Basil Blackwell.
Blumenthal, J., Babyak, M., Ironson, G., Thoresen, C., Powell, L., Czajkowski, S., et al. 2007. Spirituality, religion, and clinical outcomes in patients recovering from an acute myocardial infarction. *Psychosomatic Medicine*, *69*(*6*), 501–508.
Bolam, B., Murphy, S., & Gleeson, K. 2006. Place-identity and geographical inequalities in health: a qualitative study. *Psychology and Health*, *21*(*3*), 399–420.
Burton-Christie, D. 2009. Place-making as contemplative practice. *The Anglican Theological Review*, *91*(*3*), 347–371.
Casey, E.S. 1996. How to get from space to place in a fairly short stretch of time: phenomenological prolegomena. In S. Feld & K.H. Basso (Eds.). *Senses of Place.* Santa Fe, NM: School of American Research Press.
Casey, E.S. 1997. *The Fate of Place: A Philosophical History*. Berkeley, CA: University of California Press.
Chandler, C.K., Holden, J.M., & Kolander, C.A. 1992. Counseling for spiritual wellness: theory and practice. *Journal of Counseling and Development*, *71*, 168–175.
Cummins, S., Curis, S., Diez-Roux, A.V., & Macintyre, S. 2007. Understanding and representing 'place' in health research: a relational approach. *Social Science & Medicine*, *65*, 1825–1838.
Day, K. 2008. The construction of sacred space in the urban ecology. *Crosscurrents*, *58*(*3*), 426–440.
Dubus, A. 1998. *Meditations from a Movable Chair.* New York, NY: Vintage.
Eliade, M. 1959. *The Sacred and the Profane: The Nature of Religion*. Chicago, IL: Harcourt Brace and World.
Emmons, R.A., & McCullough, M.E. 2003. Counting blessings versus burdens: experimental studies of gratitude and subjective well-being in daily life. *Journal of Personality and Social Psychology*, *84*, 377–389.
Franch, M. 2008. Spirituality, religion, and meaning. *Journal of Nervous and Mental Disease*, *196*(*8*), 643–646.
Frederickson, L.M., & Anderson, D.H. 1999. A qualitative exploration of the wilderness experience as a source of spiritual inspiration. *Journal of Environmental Psychology*, *19*, 21–39.
Frumkin, H. 2003. Healthy places: exploring the evidence. *American Journal of Public Health*, *93*(*9*), 1451–1456.
Fullilove, M. (1996). Psychiatric implications of displacement: Contributions from the psychology of place. *The American Journal of Psychiary*, *153*(*12*), 1516–1523.
Garrett, M.T., & Wilbur, M.P. 1999. Does the worm live in the ground? Reflections on Native American spirituality. *Journal of Multicultural Counseling and Development*, *27*(*4*), 193–206.
George, L.K., Ellison, C.G., & Larson, D.B. 2002. Explaining the relationships between religious involvement and health. *Psychological Inquiry*, *13*(*3*), 190–200.
Good, J.M.M. 2007. The affordances for social psychology of the ecological approach to social knowing. *Theory & Psychology*, *17*(2), 265–295.
Gone, J. 2008. "So I can be like a Whiteman": The cultural psychology of space and place in American Indian mental health. *Culture & Psychology*, *14*, 369–399.
Haidt, J. 2003. Elevation and the positive psychology of morality. In C.L.M. Keyes & J. Haidt (Eds.). *Flourishing: The Positive Person and the Life Well Lived* (pp. 275–289). Washington, DC: APA Press.
Heidegger, M. 1972. *On Being and Time*. New York, NY: Harper & Row.
Heintzman, P. 2002. A conceptual model of leisure and spiritual well-being. *Journal of Park and Recreation Administration*, *20*(*4*), 147–169.
Heintzman, P. 2008. Leisure-spiritual coping: a model for therapeutic recreation and leisure services. *Therapeutic Recreation Journal*, *42*(*1*), 56–73.
Hester, R. 1993. Sacred structures and everyday life: a return to Manteo, North Carolina. In D. Seamon (Ed.). *Dwelling, Seeing, and Designing* (pp. 271–297). New York, NY: State University of New York Press.

Hill, P., & Pargament, K. 2003. Advances in the conceptualization and measurement of religion and spirituality: implications for physical and mental health research. *American Psychologist, 58*, 64–74.
Hull, R.B., Lam, M., & Vigo, G. 1994. Place identity: symbols of self in the urban fabric. *Landscape and Urban Planning, 28*, 109–120.
Hummer, R.A., Rogers, R.G., Nam, C.B., & Ellison, C.G. 1999. Religious involvement and U.S. adult mortality. *Demography, 36*, 273–285.
Jackson, C.H., Richardson, S., & Best, N.G. 2008. Studying place effects on health by synthesizing individual and area-level outcomes. *Social Science & Medicine, 67(12)*, 1995–2006.
James, W. 1902. *2004 The Varieties of Religious Experience.* New York, NY: Barnes & Noble Classics.
Kaplan, S. 1995. The restorative benefits of nature: toward an integrative framework. *Journal of Environmental Psychology, 15*, 169–182.
Koenig, H.G., & Cohen, H.J. (Eds.). 2002. *The Link Between Religion and Health: Psychoneuroimmunology and the Faith Factor*. Oxford, England: Oxford University Press.
Koenig, H.G., Hays, J.C., Larson, D.B., George, L.K., Cohen, H.J., McCullough, M.E., et al. 1999. Does religious attendance prolong survival? A six-year follow-up study of 3,968 older adults. *Journals of Gerontology Series A Biological Sciences and Medical Sciences, 54A*, M370–M376.
Lane, B.C. 1994. Galesville and Sinai: the researcher as participant in the study of spirituality and sacred space. *Christian Spirituality Bulletin, 2(1)*, 19.
Lane, B.C. 2001. *Landscapes of the Sacred: Geography and Narrative in American Spirituality.* Baltimore, MD: The Johns Hopkins University Press.
Larson, R., Czikszentmihalyi, M., & Graef, R. 1982. Time alone in daily experience: lonelines or renewal? In L.A. Peplau & D. Perlman (Eds.). *Loneliness: A Sourcebook of Current Theory, Research and Therapy* (pp. 40–53). New York, NY: John Wiley & Sons.
Low, S.M., & Altman, I. 1992. Place attachment: a conceptual inquiry. In I. Altman & S.M. Low (Eds.). *Place Attachment* (pp. 1–12). New York, NY: Plenum Press.
Macintyre, S.A., Ellaway, A., & Cummins, S. 2002. Place effects on health: how can we conceptualise, operationalise and measure them? *Social Science & Medicine, 55(1)*, 125–139.
Manzo, L.C. 2003. Beyond house and haven: toward a revisioning of emotional relationships with places. *Journal of Environmental Psychology, 23*, 47–61.
Manzo, L.C. 2005. For better or worse: exploring multiple dimensions of place meaning. *Journal of Environmental Psychology, 25*, 67–86.
Mazumdar, S. 2005. Religious place attachment, squatting, and "qualitative" research: a commentary. *Journal of Environmental Psychology, 25*, 87–95.
Mazumdar, S., & Mazumdar, S. 1993. Sacred space and place attachment. *Journal of Environmental Psychology, 13*, 231–242.
Mazumdar, S., & Mazumdar, S. 1999. "Women's significant spaces": religion, space, and community. *Journal of Environmental Psychology, 19*, 159–170.
Mazumdar, S., & Mazumdar, S. 2004. Religion and place attachment: a study of sacred places. *Journal of Environmental Psychology, 24*, 385–397.
Miller, W., & Thoresen, C. 2003. Spirituality, religion, and health: an emerging research field. *American Psychologist, 58(1)*, 24–35.
Moberg, D. 2002. Assessing and measuring spirituality: confronting dilemmas of universal and particular evaluative criteria. *Journal of Adult Development, 9(1)*, 47–60.
Musick, M.A., House, J.S., & Williams, D.R. 2004. Attendance at religious services and mortality in a national sample. *Journal of Health and Social Behavior, 45*(2), 198–213.
Nelson, L.P. (Ed.) 2006. *American Sanctuary: Understanding Sacred Spaces.* Bloomington, IN: Indiana University Press.
Oman, D., Kurata, J.H., Strawbridge, W.J., & Cohen, R.D. 2002. Religious attendance and cause of death over 31 years. *International Journal of Psychiatry in Medicine, 32*, 69–89.
Paasi, A. 1991. Deconstructing regions: notes on the scales of spatial life. *Environment and Planning, 23*, 239–256.
Pargament, K. 1997. *The Psychology of Religion and Coping: Theory, Research, Practice.* New York, NY: Guilford.

Pargament, K. 1999. The psychology of religion *and* spirituality? Yes and no. *International Journal for the Psychology of Religion*, *9*, 3–16.
Pargament, K. 2008. The sacred character of community life. *American Journal of Community Psychology*, *4*, 22–34.
Pieper, J. 1963. *Leisure: The Basis of Culture*. New York, NY: The New American Library.
Powell, L.H., Shahabi, L., & Thoresen, C.E. 2003. Religion and spirituality: linkages to physical health. *American Psychologist*, *58(1)*, 36–52.
Proshansky, H.M., Fabian, A.K., & Kaminoff, R. 1983. Place identity: physical world and socialization of the self. *Journal of Environmental Psychology*, *3*, 57–83.
Rasic, D., Belik, S., Elias, B., Katz, L., Enns, M., & Sareen, J. 2009. Spirituality, religion and suicidal behavior in a nationally representative sample. *Journal of Affective Disorders*, *114*(*1*), 32–40.
Relph, E. 1976. *Place and Placelessness*. London, UK: Pion Limited.
Relph, E. 2008. Sense of place and emerging social and environmental challenges. In J. Eyles & A. Williams (Eds.). *Sense of Place, Health, and Quality of Life*. Burlington, VT: Ashgate.
Riegner, M. 1993. Toward a holistic understanding of place: reading a landscape through its flora and fauna. In D. Seamon (Ed.). *Dwelling, Seeing, and Designing: Toward a Phenomenological Ecology* (pp. 181–215). Albany, NY: State University of New York Press.
Ruback, R.B., Pandey, J., & Kohli, N. 2008. Evaluations of a sacred place: role and religious belief at the *Magh Mela*. *Journal of Environmental Psychology*, *28*, 174–184.
Sheldrake, P. 2001. *Spaces for the Sacred: Place, Memory, and Identity*. Baltimore, MD: The Johns Hopkins University Press.
Sheldrake, P. 2007. Placing the sacred: transcendence and the city. *Literature & Theology*, *21*(*3*), 243–258.
Stain, H.J., Kelly, B., Lewin, T.J., Higginbotham, N., Beard, J.R., & Hourihan, F. 2008. Social networks and mental health among a farming population. *Social Psychiatry and Psychiatric Epidemiology*, *43*, 843–849.
Stokols, D. 1990. Instrumental and spiritual views of people-environment relations. *American Psychologist*, *45*(*5*), 641–646.
Stokols, D., & Shumaker, S.A. 1981. People in places: a transactional view of settings. In J.H. Harvey (Ed.). *Cognition, Social Behavior, and the Environment* (pp. 441–488). Hillsdale, NJ: Erlbaum.
Stowkowski, P.A. 2002. Languages of place and discourses of power: constructing new senses of place. *Journal of Leisure Research*, *34*(*4*), 368–382.
Stringer, L.A. & McAvoy, L. H. (1992). The need for something different: Spirituality and wilderness adventure. *Journal of Experiential Education, 15(1)*, 13–20.
Suedfeld, P. 1982. Aloneness as a healing experience. In L.A. Peplau & D. Perlman (Eds.). *Loneliness: A Sourcebook of Current Theory, Research and Therapy* (pp. 54–65). New York, NY: John Wiley & Sons.
Szaflarski, M., Ritchey, P., Leonard, A., Mrus, J., Peterman, A., Ellison, C., et al. 2006. Modeling the effects of spirituality/religion on patients' perceptions of living with HIV/AIDS. *Journal of General Internal Medicine*, *21*(*5*), S28–S38.
Thoresen, C.E. 1998. Spirituality, health and science. In S. RothRoemer, S.R. Kurpius, & C. Carmin (Eds.). *The Merging Role of Counseling Psychology in Health Care* (pp. 409–431). New York, NY: Norton.
Tuan, Y. 1974. Topophilia: *A Study of Environmental Perception, Attitudes and Values*. Englewood Cliffs, NY: Prentice-Hall, Inc.
Turner, J. 1996. *The Abstract Wild*. Tucson, AZ: The University of Arizona Press.
Voss, R.W., Douville, V., Little Soldier, A., & Twiss, G. 1999. Tribal and Shamanic-based social work practice: a Lakota perspective. *Social Work*, *44*(*3*), 228–241.
Walter, E.V. 1988. *Placeways: A Theory of the Human Environment*. Chapel Hill, NC: University of North Carolina Press
Weaver, A., Pargament, K., Flannelly, K., & Oppenheimer, J. 2006. Trends in the scientific study of religion, spirituality, and health: 1965–2000. *Journal of Religion & Health*, *45*(*2*), 208–214.
Weil, S. 1952. *The Need for Roots*. New York, NY: Routledge Classics.

WHOQOL SRPB Group. 2006. A cross-cultural study of spirituality, religion, and personal beliefs as components of quality of life. *Social Science & Medicine*, *62*(*6*), 1486–1497.

Williams, A. 1998. Therapeutic landscapes in holistic medicine. *Social Science & Medicine*, *46*(*9*), 1193–1203.

Williams, D.R., Patterson, M.E., Roggenbuck, J.W., & Watson, A.E. 1992. Beyond the commodity metaphor: examining emotional and symbolic attachment to place. *Leisure Sciences*, *14*, 29–46.

Zerubavel, E. 1996. Social memories: steps to a sociology of the past. *Qualitative Sociology*, *19*(*3*), 283–299.

Chapter 10
Dis-placement and Dis-ease: Land, Place, and Health Among American Indians and Alaska Natives

Karina L. Walters, Ramona Beltran, David Huh, and Teresa Evans-Campbell

This land is mine
All the way to the old fence line
Every break of day
I'm working hard just to make it pay

This land is mine
Yeah I signed on the dotted line
Camp fires on the creek bank
Bank breathing down my neck

They won't take it away...
They won't take it away from me

--White Australian Farmer – "Father"

This land is me
Rock, water, animal, tree
They are my song
My being's here where I belong

This land owns me
From generations past to infinity
We're all but woman and man
You only fear what you don't understand

They won't take it away...
They won't take it away from me

--Indigenous Australian Tracker – "Albert"

"This Land is Mine/This Land is Me" from the film, *One Night the Moon* (2001)

Inspired by real events and the documentary *Black Tracker*, indigenous Australian Director Rachel Perkins' (Arrernte People) musical film *One Night the Moon* illustrates the complex and difficult relationships between aboriginal and settler communities of Australia as their respective worldviews and consequential actions determine the outcome of a life-and-death situation. The story revolves around a young farm girl (Emily) who wanders off one night into the Australian outback. In a pivotal scene, men are gathered on the White farm owner's property, ready to begin the search for the missing girl. An indigenous Australian Tracker, Albert, is there to assist but is ordered off the land by the White farmer and father of the lost girl who does not want "some darkie leading the search" – a decision that later

K.L. Walters (✉)
University of Washington, 4101 15th Avenue, NE, Seattle, WA 98105-6299, USA
e-mail: kw5@u.washington.edu

L.M. Burton et al. (eds.), *Communities, Neighborhoods, and Health*, Social Disparities in Health and Health Care 1, DOI 10.1007/978-1-4419-7482-2_10,

proves to be tragic. At the moment of ordering Albert off of his land, the father enters into song with the lyrics noted above, "This land is mine…," articulating his fierce and resolute stance of contracted ownership and therefore ultimate stewardship of the land. Forced out of the scene and away from the search, Albert joins the song with contrasting lyrics, "This land is me…," reflecting an entirely different relationship to the land, one which is intrinsic, relational, and without dominion. This is a key turning point in the film, where indigenous knowledge of land and place is rejected with devastating consequences for the young girl, her family, the community, and ultimately everyone involved. The story is clearly allegorical of the devastating consequences of colonization and racism; in this case, rejection of indigenous knowledge and practice proved to be fatal. Juxtaposing indigenous and Western European ways of relating to land, place, and time, its implications are consistent with contemporary social and environmental challenges. Global climate change and its resulting consequences are rapidly endangering indigenous communities worldwide. As market interests in land-based resources from water and mining interests to genetically engineered food crops continue to erode the landscape, the critical link between place and health becomes evident and the need for immediate intervention becomes imminent. Now, more than ever, the deeply situated land-based knowledge of indigenous peoples is pressing to be heard – not only to save the planet but to save all of our collective health and well-being.

Indigenous peoples (IP) throughout the world suffer devastatingly high rates of health disparities, many of which are linked to land loss and destruction, as well as general lack of access to healthy land environments (La Duke 1999). Globally, IP have disproportionately high rates of chronic and communicable diseases (Gracey and King 2009; King 2009) coupled with poor living conditions, inadequate housing, poor nutrition, and exposure to high environmental contaminants, leading to a disproportionate burden of chronic health deficits as well as high levels of morbidity and mortality (Gracey and King 2009; King 2009). The 2006 Indigenous World International Working Group on indigenous affairs states the following: "Indigenous peoples remain on the margins of society: they are poorer, less educated, die at a younger age, are much more likely to commit suicide, and are generally in worse health than the rest of the population" (Stidsen 2006: 10). This is particularly true for indigenous groups "whose original ways of life, environment, and livelihoods have been destroyed and often replaced with the worst of Western lifestyle – i.e., unemployment, poor housing, alcoholism, and drug use" (Stephens et al. 2005: 11). To date, research has just begun to incorporate a more holistic orientation to understanding health and wellness (Burghardt and Nagai-Jacobson 2002; Mark and Lyons 2010; Wilson 2003), with a focus on moving beyond "the absence of disease" model of wellness (King 2009; Krieger 2005) to defining and articulating the social, cultural, spiritual, mental, and more recently, environmental aspects (including geography and place) of well-being and health (Burgess et al. 2005; King 2009; Mark and Lyons 2010). In terms of IP, a more holistic or *wholistic* orientation is clearly consonant with cultural worldviews and traditional knowledge relevant to health and well-being

(Mark and Lyons 2010; Walters and Simoni 2002; Wilson 2003). In recent years, the interconnectedness of the mind, body, and spirit has gained acceptance, particularly in the fields of psychoneuroimmunology (Lyons and Chamberlain 2006), and epigenetics (Jasienska 2009; Krieger 2004, 2005; Olden and White 2005), as well as with particular psychophysiological health outcomes including cardiovascular (Kuzawa and Sweet 2009), inflammation disorders, and neuroendocrine and immune functions (Seeman et al. 2003). Although the relationships among land, wellness, and health are well articulated in Indigenous origin stories and tribally specific Original Instructions[1] (Deloria 1992, 1995; Pierotti and Wildcat 2000), only recently have these relationships been empirically examined in the health sciences (Burgess et al. 2005; Oneha 2001; Wilson 2003). The indigenous philosophical–spiritual orientation to land and ethical code of conduct is captured in this quote from a Ggudju elder (indigenous Australian):

> Our story is in the land.
> It is written in those sacred places.
> My children will look after those places,
> That's the law.
>
> Cited in Burgess et al. (2005: 118)

The land–health nexus is also captured by Anderson (1995); as cited in Burgess et al. (2005: 120), an aboriginal scholar who states

> Our identity as human being remains tied to our land, to our cultural practices, our systems of authority and control, our intellectual traditions, our concepts of spirituality, and to our systems of resource ownership and exchange. Destroy this relationship and you damage – sometimes irrevocably – individual human beings and their health.

IP Original Instructions were and are tied to the land and cosmos. Gregory Cajete, a Tewa scholar (2000: 186) notes

> Native people expressed a relationship to the natural world that could only be called 'ensoulment'...which for Native people represented the deepest level of psychological involvement with their land and which provided a kind of a map of the soul. The psychology and spiritual qualities of Indigenous peoples' behavior...were thoroughly 'in-formed' by the depth and power of their participation mystique with the Earth as a living soul. It was from this orientation that Indian people developed 'responsibilities' to the land and all living things, similar to those that they had to each other. In the Native mind, spirit and matter were not separate: They were one and the same.

[1]Original Instructions is a lingua franca term used by some Native scholars and community leaders to represent the tribal-specific spiritual and ethical codes of conduct and instructions handed down for millennia as to how the people should conduct themselves, honor their relationships, and fulfill their responsibilities and obligations to all of creation, ancestors, future generations, and spirit worlds.

Although classic social determinants of health, such as poor socioeconomic status, substandard housing, and poor access to appropriate health care all contribute to poor health among IP, these factors do not sufficiently explain the high rates of poor health and mental health, particularly with respect to post traumatic stress disorder (PTSD), anxiety, and depression among IP, specifically American Indians and Alaska Natives (Walters et al. 2002). As a result, indigenous scholars have turned their attention to examining how historical and societal determinants of health, particularly the role of place-based historically traumatic events (e.g., forced relocation and land loss), environmental microaggressions (discrimination distress based on land desecration), and disproportionate exposures to high rates of lifetime trauma, not only are hazards to contemporary IP health but may also persist for generations (Evans-Campbell and Walters 2006; Evans-Campbell 2008; Krieger et al. 2010).

After reviewing the literature on indigenous place and health, this chapter shares empirical findings related to land and place loss on physical and mental health outcomes among a national sample of gay, lesbian, bisexual, or transgender (hereafter collectively referred to as two-spirit) American Indian and Alaska Natives (hereafter referred to as AIAN or Native; The Honor Project, RO1MH65871). Two-spirit AIAN face additional health stressors associated with negotiating multiply oppressed statuses. Preliminary empirical evidence indicates that two-spirits experience elevated rates of antigay and anti-Native violence, including sexual and physical assault during childhood and adulthood (Balsam et al. 2004; Evans-Campbell 2008; Walters et al. 2002; Simoni et al. 2006), historical traumatic event exposure (Balsam et al. 2004), and microaggression distress (Chae and Walters 2009) – experiences typically associated with adverse physical and mental health outcomes, including self-rated poor health and high rates of pain (Chae and Walters 2009). Historical and contemporary traumas concurrent with socioeconomic vulnerabilities undercut the health of AIANs, especially among two-spirit populations (Fieland et al. 2007; Walters and Simoni 2002).

The major aim of this chapter is to stimulate work in the area of place and health, specifically examining how AIAN health outcomes can be contextualized and understood in light of historical losses and disruptions tied to place or land. In fact, the very definition of "indigenous" intimates a sacred thread or reciprocal tie to land, place, and identity (King 2009). Cajete (1999: 6) notes that the word "*indigenous*" "is derived from the Latin root *indu* or *endo*, which is related to the Greek word *endina,* which means 'entrails.' Indigenous literally means being so completely identified with a place that you reflect its entrails, its insides, its soul." Any disruption in indigenous land, place, or culture clearly has a potentially harmful effect on indigenous health and wellness, which may then persist for generations to come. Additionally, the resiliency by which AIAN communities have lived and thrived despite high rates of trauma and colonial practices is a testament to IP strength and abilities to adapt and survive.

Indigenous Place: "Native Americans are the Environment: The Environment is Us[2]!"

Place and Relational Orientation

For IP, the ultimate location of *place* is embedded in a profound relationship with the earth. The earth (or land) is both literally and figuratively the first and final teacher in our understanding of our world, communities, families, selves, and bodies. With such understanding it can be argued that as the land or relationship to land is impacted – physically or metaphorically – so are bodies, minds, and spirits. As La Duke (1999: 2) asserts:

> Native American teaching describe relations all around – animals, fish, trees, and rocks as our brothers, sisters, uncles, and grandpas. Our relations to each other, our prayers whispered across generations to our relatives, are what bind our cultures together. The protection, teachings, and gifts of our relatives have for generations preserved our families. These relations are honored in ceremony, song, story, and life that keep relations close-to buffalo, sturgeon, salmon, turtles, bears, wolves, and panthers. These are our older relatives, the ones who came before and taught us how to live. Their obliteration by dams, guns and bounties is an immense loss to Native families and cultures.

Indigenous worldviews recognize the interdependency between humans and nature, the physical and spiritual worlds, the ancestors and the future generations; all living things, animate or inanimate, are bound by a connection to everything else. This interconnectedness of all things is the first law of ecological thought (Cajete 1999). A *sacred* ecology acknowledges the central role of spirituality and cultural cosmology in understanding this interconnectedness; "Native American intellectual tradition still continues to express the North American landscape in intellectual and spiritual reciprocity, where the more-than-human grants qualities of mind to the human" (Sheridan and Longboat 2006). From this vantage point, human cognition or imagination is less central in the equation of defining place: ancient knowledge is so large that it has seen and known everything before. While cognitive processes are important in the articulation of ideas, it does not take a human mind to make meaning because meanings have already been set by ancestral knowledge. The meanings generated by the mind are instead seen as offerings of gratitude back to the ancestors for the wisdoms and lessons of place they have helped us discover, but which were already there. In essence, we are receptors accepting what is revealed by place. Thus, place is not a cultural product: rather, cultural products are defined by their *relationship* with and to place.

As Cajete (1999) notes, for AIAN, the relationship to place is based on an established intimate relationship with the landscape that has persisted for over 30,000 years, thus they "lack an immigrant experience within their memories" (Deloria 1995).

---

[2] Quote from Corbin Harney (Western Shoshone) as cited in Gonzales and Nelson (2001: 496).

AIAN's long-standing relationship with place leads to a "metaphysical attachment – a sacred thread – that does not bind the people so much as remind the people of the obligations and responsibilities carried forward by generations: That thread…reminds them of their past and their future, their ancestors and their offspring, their spirit and their obligations" (Watkins 2001: 42). This sacred orientation to place is a key element of an acute "ecological awareness" (Cajete 1999) that is circular, dynamic, fluid, spatial, and spherically directional. This sacred orientation is critical to understanding AIAN worldviews that bind place to relational ways of understanding the world. As Cajete (2001: 625) notes,

> Understanding orientation to place is essential in understanding what it is to be related. Many indigenous people recognize seven directions: the four cardinal directions – above, center, and below. This way of viewing [a relational] orientation creates a sphere of relationships founded on place and evolving through time and space. This is a deeply contexted and holistic reflection of relational orientation.

This sense of relationship with place is inextricably linked to indigenous traditional ways of being in relation with relatives (Cajete 1999). Metaphorical examples of the manifestations of relational place orientations are revealed in indigenous constructs of place and beings that inhabit place or space as "relatives" or "relations" as revealed in common references to "mother earth" or to rocks as "grandfathers." We converse with place as if with relatives. Place is part of our ancestral heritage, our present, and our future. It links us in immediate and visceral ways to our past, present, and future. In this sense, IP emerge from the place and have a bidirectional relationship of caring with place – place cares for us and we care for it. In a study investigating the connections between culture, health, and place in First Nations people, Wilson (2003: 88) asked First Nations (Anishinabek) individuals about their views on the influence of the land on spiritual, physical, mental, and emotional health.

> I believe that we came from the earth – just like everything is alive, potatoes, plants, anything comes alive and flourishes with flowers. The earth provides everything, wild animals, insects. The earth provides for us. The earth provides strength, that's why we call it mother. She provides life…helps us live. Without her we would not live.

In Anishinabek worldviews, the earth is seen as a feminine being and is regarded as the source of all life-sustaining things (Wilson 2003). In this interview excerpt, it is clear that this individual views the earth as a relative (mother), with whom this person shares a great deal of mutual care, respect, and honor. This relationship is experienced as core to this individual's very existence. Another description from an elder expresses similar sentiments (Wilson 2003: 88):

> Mother Earth is everything that you see. You look everywhere on earth and you see Mother Earth. The way you raise your children, the way people do things together, the way we live among our people. She is in everything we do.

As Wilson (2003: 88) notes, "the relationship Anishinabek have with the land cannot be captured by the simplified notion of being 'close to nature.' The land is not just seen as shaping or influencing identity, but being an actual part of it."

Guided by a sacred ecology and Original Instructions (OI), AIAN have an intimate knowing and being in relationship with land and place. All of nature, including plants, animals, stones, trees, mountains, rivers, insects, and other beings embodied relationships and were connected to the greater "web of life" of which each and every being has a purpose and relationship to one another that must be honored, and indeed, celebrated or renewed through ceremony and everyday living. Through making, sharing, and honoring these relationships, indigenous peoples "perceive themselves as living in a sea of relationships. In each place they lived, they learned the subtle, but all important language of relationship. It was through such a mindset, tempered by intimate relationships with various environments over thousands of years, that indigenous people accumulated ecological knowledge." (Cajete 2000: 178). This relational orientation reflects an indigenous understanding of reciprocity and the interrelatedness of all beings, all of creation over generations and has led to a deep understanding of environment and place as they are inextricably linked to behavior, practices, wholeness, and, hence, wellness. As Gonzales and Nelson (2001: 496–498) note, "we are operating from an indigenous model of wholeness, where people and place, matter and spirit, nature and culture are interrelated in a dynamic process…this reciprocal relationship goes back to creation myths [Original Instructions]…this exchange is not just one of give-and-take…giving is always the focus, not the taking." Cycles of ceremony to renew relationships and to maintain balance among all of creation are part of OI, and, through ritual, embody the immense responsibility that befalls human beings in participating in the great web of life. As Gonzales and Nelson (2001: 497) note, "to realize that, with each breath, thought, and action, we are at the threshold of creation is an enormous responsibility. IP have traditionally taken on this responsibility by following natural laws of their creation stories and by performing ceremonies to renew the earth and maintain balance between people, place, and spirits."

The recognition of the inseparability, reciprocity, and responsibility between humans and the rest of creation, particularly land and place, serves to create an ethical code of conduct in interacting and being in the world. Pierotti and Wildcat (2000) conceptualizes this orientation as traditional ecological knowledge (TEK), where TEK emphasizes that all aspects of physical space are considered part of a connected, interrelated community (humans, animals, plants, land), shifting the Western emphasis from the human to the ecological community of which humans are an integral part. According to Pierotti and Wildcat (2000), a core component of TEK is that nonhumans and nature exist on their own terms independent of human interpretation. Additionally, TEK acknowledges that IP are native to a place and live with nature – following an ethical code of conduct that exists in relation with ecosystems – in contrast to dominant Western worldviews (e.g., Manifest Destiny), which assumes humans are superior to, separated from (e.g., going "into nature"), or in opposition to – where nature needs to be tamed or conquered primarily for the benefit of humans (Pierotti and Wildcat 2000). Although many are surprised to hear of the conflicts that arise between AIAN and conservationists, the very notion of *conserving* nature reveals an underlying dominant Western orientation to the world (Pierotti and Wildcat 2000), where the assumption is that humans are or should be in control of nature, or that nature should be conserved primarily to benefit humans for economic or spiritual power. This is completely antithetical to AIAN sacred ecology where "Nature exists on its own terms," all of life has its own reasons for existence, and humans, part of the web of life, clearly play a connected and related role, but not one that assumes superiority over nature (Pierotti and Wildcat 2000). From a Native perspective, attempts to control the environment are fruitless, even harmful, and are best summarized in the sentiment, "Pity the poor Americans who cannot accept the dominion of place over them" (Watkins 2001: 42).

Finally, although we have emphasized the importance of the sacred ecology and relational worldviews of Native peoples, as Pierotti and Wildcat (2000) note, we are not subscribing to the stereotyped romanticized view of the "ecologically noble savage" (Pierotti and Wildcat 2000). In fact, sacred ecology requires Native peoples to be active participants with their environments and to engage in deep relationships with place, animals, and other beings. As Pierotti and Wildcat (2000) note, IP are not "stewards of the natural world." Rather, we are part of the natural world, the web of life, no greater than any other part, but an integral cog in the whole with responsibilities and ecological ethics that are tied to land, place, and OI (Pierotti and Wildcat 2000).

Place and Spatial Orientation

IP have unique attachments to original lands, and we carry these attachments, or sacred threads, wherever we go. These attachments are linked not only to special or sacred ritual sites but also to the whole of land and creation. In fact, the boundaries between "sacred sites" and secular sites are often difficult to define or even nonexistent as all land and locations are viewed as sacred (Zarsky 2006). AIAN belief systems and emotional intelligence descend from these attachments.

While typical mainstream conceptualizations of place often have a unidirectional and temporal order, indigenous conceptualizations do not. In her research exploring the role of healing landscapes with the Amuzgo Indians of Oaxaca, Mexico, Elizabeth Cartwright (2007: 10) cites Casey's (1993) description of place to illustrate the idea that "who we are is based on where we are":

> Place ushers us into what *already* is: namely, the environing subsoil of our embodiment, the bedrock of our being-in-the-world. If imagination projects us out *beyond* ourselves while memory takes us back *behind* ourselves, place subtends and enfolds us, lying perpetually *under* and *around* us. In imagining and remembering, we go into the ethereal and the thick respectively. By being in a place, we find ourselves in what is subsistent and enveloping.

This description illustrates a more complex comprehension of place by appreciating the past and future sensory experiences along with the enveloping and alive process of the present. It brings alive the possibility of place as not occurring at a particular instance but something that happens dynamically in all directions over time. As such, knowledge of place is deepened and broadened, allowing for alternative experience of space and time.

Additionally, while we are "in the here and now," we are simultaneously surrounded by future and past generations. Meyer (2008) notes that for IP, knowledge regarding anything is based on "sequential immortality." For example, among the aboriginal populations of Australia, dreamtime is a space and place where ancestral knowledge coexists with and interacts with contemporary indigenous experience of the physical world, and land is the core connection between these two worlds. Land is the literal and metaphorical vehicle for teaching and understanding our lessons, and as such, place cannot be referenced as a simple physical reality. Such understandings can be found in both dream and "real" time, which are never separated from one another. Traditional land-based knowledge has been passed down through generations, with each generation making its own observations, testing them, and sharing wisdom through oral, pictoral, and/or written communications regarding ecological knowledge. This ecological knowledge, although filled with intergenerational wisdom, remains flexible and adjustable to fit the current generation's historical and ecological context (Deloria 1992).

Native spatial orientation stands in stark contrast to Western Euro-American temporal orientation, "where the latter tend to look backward and forward in time to get a sense of their place in history, while native peoples look around them to get a sense of their place in history" (Pierotti and Wildcat 2000: 1334; Deloria 1992). In this traditional spatial orientation, there is no isolation from any part of nature or creation – there is no separation from biology, geography, history, land, and the cosmos (Deloria 1992). As noted by Pierotti and Wildcat (2000), spatial thinking is revealed in the seven direction orientation to offer prayers or acknowledgement by many IP – this orientation acknowledges not only respect for the space in which Native people belong but also the spiritual forces that are tied to these directions.

While this complexity of space, time, reality, and consciousness may be difficult to articulate with Western logical processes, it is the reality in indigenous spiritual cosmologies and, hence, in daily living. Thus, for IP, spirituality and ways of relating not only form the core of place understandings but also the core of everyday behavioral expressions embodied in health practices and behaviors. The oversimplification or romanticization of "being close with nature" stereotypes AIANs and trivializes the profound relationship AIANs have with place (Pierotti and Wildcat 2000). The drive to disassemble and simplify the intricate webs of indigenous relationships with space and place illustrates an epistemological stance that takes us away from the wholeness involved in indigenous cosmologies. Place is an interweaving of mind, body, soul, and spirit. Any disassembly of these essential components removes the very core of our being-in-the-world, with resulting material consequences, a process that has been played out for hundreds of years through colonization. The removal of people from the land and their land-based cosmologies and ethics through colonial processes has devastating and important implications for the health and wellness of contemporary IP.

Place, Embodiment, and Health

We are place, we are. Not those who occupy that place.
We do not exist, we are. We only are.

Comandante David and Subcomandante Marcos

Over the last several decades, there has been an emergence of the body as a key focus in the social sciences. Researchers are centralizing the body in questions of inequities in health and investigating aspects of embodiment as influenced by social, cultural, political, and economic processes (Krieger 2001; Krieger and Davey 2004). As such, it can be inferred that the body is directly impacted by place and what happens in places. In the past, bioarchaeological studies produced important information about the everyday lives of individuals and groups. From evidence of habitual motion left on bones, scientists could discern social status, race, gender, and age (Joyce 2005; Krieger 2004). Like most legacies of scientific engagement, there has historically been a split of inner and outer body as centered questions, but by looking at social epidemiological trends in health status, scientists are finding clear links between what is going on in the social world and the biological corporeal world. For example, low-birth-weight babies, a frequent problem experienced by indigenous populations, and certain bacterial infections are associated with conditions of poverty, sanitation, and access to health services (Krieger and Davey 2004). In essence, what is happening outside of the body is reflected inside and vice versa; the body is just as affected by the policies, structures, and processes that shape daily living conditions as by individual biological processes. As such, the boundaries of "the body" and the spatial context around it are now being described as "inextricably linked" (Joyce 2005: 149).

Shifting from theoretical and practical investigation of "bodies" to "embodiment" allows for deeper understanding of the complexities involved in the human experience as both biological and social creatures. While bodies are sites – records of process, animated stories of lived experience, visual/textual narratives of past and present, embodiment "is the articulation of agency and structure, causality and meaning, rationality and imagination, physical determinations and symbolic resonances" (Meskell, as cited in Joyce 2005: 151). In this way, bodies can be seen simultaneously as cultural artifacts, political entities, and representations of lived experiences (Joyce 2005; Krieger 2001, 2004).

In ecosocial theory and epidemiological research, the concept of embodiment is seen as a central component in understanding the human process of being both social and biological creatures (Krieger 2001, 2004; Krieger and Davey 2004). Emerging research and scholarship pays attention to "how actualization and suppression of people's agency, that is, their ability to act within their bodies, intimately depends on socially structured opportunities for, and threats to, their well-being" and "in the case of social inequalities and health, it likewise presumes that observed differences reflect biologic expressions of social inequality" (Krieger and Davey 2004: 95). Embodiment is an important construct that illuminates key processes for explaining the complicated ways that social worlds get lived out in bodies. According to

Krieger (2004: 1), the idea of embodiment "advances three claims: (1) bodies tell stories about – and cannot be studied divorced from – the conditions of our existence; (2) bodies tell stories that often – but not always – match people's stated accounts; and (3) bodies tell stories that people cannot or will not tell, either because they are unable, forbidden, or choose not to tell." With this framework, the high rates of chronic diseases, accidents, and suicides in indigenous communities can be viewed as bodies telling the stories of the catastrophic upheavals imposed upon them by colonial processes. This invokes the interconnectedness of all things: what happens to the land happens to our bodies, what happens to our bodies happens to our spirits, and it is happening individually, collectively, and globally. As Chief Sealth (aka Seattle), Chief of the Suquamish (1786–1866) noted:

> You must teach your children that the ground beneath their feet is the ashes of your grandfathers. So that they will respect the land, tell your children that the earth is rich with the lives of our kin. Teach your children what we have taught our children, that the earth is our mother. Whatever befalls the earth befalls the sons of the earth. If men spit upon the ground, they spit upon themselves.

Dis-placement and Dis-ease: The Impact of Historical Trauma and Land Losses on Health

> *Mother earth...we come from her, so we are part of her and she is part of us. If she is sick, I am sick, and vice versa.*
>
> Gonzales and Nelson (2001: 497)

The recognition that land, environment, and health are interconnected is an ancient understanding within many of the world's populations. For example, the Roman philosopher Seneca viewed disease (1 BCE) as "not of the body but of the place." However, for IP, disease, or literally, dis-ease (out of balance, disharmony, disequilibrium) is tied to the holistic understanding of the interconnectedness of mind, body, emotion, spirit, and land. Indigenous knowledge recognizes *place* as integral to one's sense of being which is also central to both individual and collective spiritual health and wellness. Conversely, for IP, loss of place (i.e., displacement) is akin to loss of spirit or identity. Many Native scholars have noted that place and land are directly tied to indigenous identity and health – it is the site where dynamic interactions occur among humans and all of creation (Wildcat 2001). As Deloria (1992) notes, it is through this dynamic interaction with place where a person discovers his or her identity as well as purpose. Cajete (2000: 186) refers to the dynamic relationship to the natural world as the "ensoulment of nature" or the "psychology of place" which represents the "deepest level of psychological involvement with their land and which provided a kind of map of the soul." Place literally makes us.

Moreover, connection to place not only creates healthy identities and spirit but is also protective. Watkins (2001: 42) utilizes a Navajo weaving metaphor to illustrate this health protective aspect of place:

> American Indians also share a cultural–historical relationship with the land. Their past and future is intertwined with it, as the fabric of their culture is woven of threads tied to places. The sacred locations are the foundation threads of the fabric, the warp, while the cultural connections are the weft threads. The four sacred mountains which form the boundaries of the Navajo world are the edges of the blanket, and every local landscape threads within the blanket. Thus, all individual Navajos wear a multipatterned protective blanket of their culture around them.

Nevertheless, when dis-placement occurs, social and spiritual upheaval ensues for Native people, leading to mental and physical health crises. Historically and contemporarily, dis-placement (*being* without place/spirit) of IP from their original lands and ongoing exploitation of contemporary lands have led and continue to lead to ill health and dis-ease. Specifically, Cajete (1999: 17) notes that indigenous communities have drifted or been forced from a

> …practiced and conscious relationship with place, or direct connection with their spiritual ecology. The results for many Indian communities are 'existential' problems, such as high rates of alcoholism, suicide, abuse of self and others, depression and other social and spiritual ills…Tewa people call this state… *pingeh heh* (split thinking, or doing things with only half of one's mind).

In other words, as much as connectedness to place is ensoulment, dis-placement is literally, a form of "soul loss" (Cajete 2000: 188). Thus, when historically traumatic relocations such as the *Long Walk* (forced relocation of Dine' [Navajo] to military encampment in 1864) occurred, or when dispossession from land or place forced IP to be torn from the land where the ashes of their ancestors live, this loss, which was "a symbol of their connection to spirit of life itself…led to a tremendous loss of meaning and identity… that can ultimately be healed only through re-establishing meaningful ties. Reconnecting with nature and its inherent meaning is an essential healing and transformational process for Indian people" (Cajete 2000: 188).

Historical Trauma and Health

> *When the earth is sick and polluted, human health is impossible.... To heal ourselves we must heal our planet, and to heal our planet we must heal ourselves.*
>
> Bobby McLeod, indigenous Australian (Koori)

In recent years, indigenous health has been increasingly linked to historical trauma stemming from historically traumatic events. The history of traumatic assaults experienced by IP is well documented and includes centuries of targeted attacks on indigenous people and land. Over successive generations, these attacks have included community massacres, pandemics from the introduction of new diseases, forced relocation, and the prohibition of spiritual and cultural practices, (Thornton 1987; Stannard 1992). For example, in his 1862 order to Captain Helms, commander of the Arizona Guards, governor of Arizona, John R. Baylor, called for the annihilation of all "hostile" Indians living within Arizona:

> The Congress of the Confederate states has passed a law declaring extermination to all hostile Indians. You will therefore use all means to persuade the Apaches or any tribe to come in for the purpose of making peace, and when you get them together kill all the grown Indians and take the children prisoner and sell them to defray the expense of killing the Indians. Buy whiskey…. for the Indians and I will order vouchers given to recover the amount expended. Have a sufficient number of men around to allow no Indian to escape…. I look to you for success against these cursed pests.

Historical assaults also include place-based, environmental assaults such as radioactive dumping on tribal lands, flooding of homelands, outlawing traditional hunting practices, and the introduction of diseases into communities. Some of these events, such as forced relocation and experiencing the destruction of natural habitats, are common experiences suffered historically by all IP communities. Other events such as the prohibition of whaling in Northwest coast communities are more culturally or tribally specific.

A key facet of historically traumatic assaults is that they are perpetrated with intention upon a group of people, their environment, and their sacred artifacts or burial sites for the purpose of cultural destruction, ethnocide, or genocide. Individually, each of these events is profoundly traumatic; taken together, they constitute a history of sustained cultural and ethnic disruption and destruction directed at IP (Evans-Campbell and Walters 2006). The resulting trauma is often conceptualized as collective in that it impacts a significant portion of a community, and compounding, as multiple historically traumatic events occurring over generations join in an overarching legacy of assaults. For IP, cumulative historical trauma events are coupled with high rates of contemporary acute lifetime trauma and interpersonal violence (Greenfeld and Smith 1999), as well as high rates of chronic stressors such as dealing with an ongoing barrage of microaggressions and daily discriminatory events (Chae and Walters 2009; Walters et al. 2008). Together, these historical and contemporary events undermine indigenous identity, health, and well-being (Evans-Campbell 2008) in complex and multifaceted ways. At the individual level, the impact of historical trauma on health and wellness includes impairments in family communication (Felsen 1998), symptoms of PTSD, survivor guilt, anxiety, and depressive symptomatology (Evans-Campbell 2008; Whitbeck et al. 2004). At the community level, collective responses include the disruption of traditional customs, languages, and practices (Evans-Campbell 2008; Wardi 1992) and self-reported intergenerational historical trauma (Balsam et al. 2004). Notably, despite exposure to historical and cumulative traumatic stressors, many Native people do not manifest psychopathology. Indeed, emerging research indicates that the very areas of Native culture that have been targeted for destruction (e.g., identity, spirituality, traditional practices) may, in fact, be sites of resistance.

A related field, intergenerational trauma, also recognizes collective traumatic events but is inclusive of natural disasters and other traumatic events (e.g., famine) that are man-made but not targeted with intention upon a particular group for social, cultural, ethnic, or political decimation or annihilation. Although the study of historical trauma and intergenerational trauma is still in the nascent stage of empirical examination, preliminary research indicates that the impact of these events may persist for some individuals or families over generations (Bar-on et al. 1998;

Nagata et al. 1999; Yehuda 1999), that the trauma may have a more pernicious effect on descendants of survivors if both parents experienced the event (Karr 1973), that the trauma may be differentially experienced by women compared to men (Lichtman 1984; Brave Heart 1999), and that the trauma can literally become embodied, manifesting as poor mental (e.g., depressive symptomatology) and physical health outcomes (e.g., CVD or birth outcomes) in later generations (e.g., Barocas and Barocas 1980; Jasienska 2009; Kuzawa and Sweet 2009). Research with diverse populations shows that descendants of survivors are not more likely than others to have poor mental health. Rather, they may have a higher vulnerability to stressful events, and when faced with a lifetime stressor, descendants may be more likely than others to develop PTSD or PTSD symptomatology (Solomon et al. 1988; Yehuda 1999).

Although there is strong evidence that poor health outcomes are linked to genetic, environmental, and behavioral risk factors (Olden and White 2005), the actual pathways and mechanisms, particularly biological mechanisms, for the intergenerational transmission of traumatic events are hotly contested and remain open to debate. Specifically, the relative impact of historical trauma on descendants' physical and mental health is a point of contention among Native and non-Native scholars. Some scholars have argued that the intergenerational effects of historical trauma (i.e., distal causes) would be negligible once lifetime rates of exposure to trauma (i.e., proximal causes) were accounted for, particularly physical and sexual abuse exposure (Levin 2009), while other Native scholars point to recent evidence about how extreme environmental stress in one generation can alter descendents' health risk and outcomes for generations. Specifically, these scholars point to the amassing of evidence at the cellular level that powerful stressful environmental conditions can leave an imprint or "mark" on the epigenome (cellular genetic material) that can be carried into future generations with devastating consequences (e.g., poor prenatal maternal nutrition can lead to descendant offspring CVD in adulthood; Kuzawa and Sweet 2009). Although empirical research continues to shed light on the potential pathways, mechanisms, and relative proximal and distal impact of historical and intergenerational trauma on health, IP communities simply cannot wait for the debate to be resolved – there are too many lives at stake. Native communities have developed their own community interventions to address the psychological, spiritual, and communal impact that historical (e.g., Takini Network) and contemporary traumatic events have had on physical and mental health, particularly grief and loss reactions (Evans-Campbell 2008; Walters et al. 2006; Whitbeck et al. 2004).

Historical Trauma: Removal and Relocation: Disruptions in Place

The appropriation of indigenous land by force or coercion has been a central theme in colonial interactions with IP. Land has been at the heart of colonial attempts at conquest, and historical trauma events have been the primary vehicle for land dispossession and dis-placement of indigenous people. Moreover, AIAN continue to inhabit the continent on which they have encountered historical and contemporary assaults. They live with constant reminders of historical trauma (e.g., living in areas where "massacre" sites are visited by tourists and proudly mislabeled as "battle" sites), and their subsequent trauma, resistance, and resiliency responses are markedly different from those descendent survivors who no longer occupy "place" with their perpetrators (e.g., holocaust survivors who immigrated or escaped from perpetrating countries during or post WWII). As noted by Whitbeck, there is no "safe" place to immigrate or return for AIANs. Many Native populations were forcibly relocated to lands that held (at first) little perceived monetary value or were deemed "uninhabitable or undesirable" by European-Americans. By the mid-nineteenth century, American expansionist attitudes laid the foundation for massive American Indian removal policies, particularly attitudes associated with manifest destiny and the doctrine of "discovery" – the belief that White Americans were heavenly ordained to take over indigenous lands and that American Indians would eventually "vanish" as a result. The attitudes associated with manifest destiny and the doctrine of discovery gave an exclusive justification and right to coercively dispossess indigenous rights or ties to indigenous lands. This is eloquently stated in the US Supreme Court decision (*Johnson v. McIntosh*, 21 US 543, 1823: 573, 587, 590):

> Discovery gave an exclusive right to extinguish the Indian title of occupancy, either by purchase or by conquest...the Indians were fierce savages...whose subsistence was drawn chiefly from the forest. To leave them in possession of their country, was to leave the country a wilderness.

The irony of having President Theodore Roosevelt's image sculpted into the Black Hills and desecrating a sacred landscape does not escape Native communities, particularly given the Roosevelt's attitudes and policies regarding land and American Indians. In 1894, Roosevelt noted:

> All men of sane and wholesome thought must dismiss with impatient contempt the plea that these continents should be reserved for the use of scattered savage tribes, whose life was but a few degrees less meaningless, squalid, and ferocious than that of the wild beasts with whom they held joint ownership. It is as idle to apply to savages the rules of international morality which obtain between stable and cultured communities, as it would be to judge the fifth-century English conquest of Britain by the standards of today.

Although Roosevelt is credited with the establishment of national parks, many Native communities were forcibly relocated to make room for tourists and to establish a "pristine" environment, void of human occupation.

With the passage of the Indian Removal Act of 1830, President Andrew Jackson was the first US president to implement an American Indian removal policy, thereby setting a dangerous precedent for subsequent coerced or forced removals over the next 150 years. Moreover, removal policy was set in place to acquire, by force if necessary, indigenous lands for nonindigenous consumption. This first wave of removal policy at the very least coercively, and in many cases forcibly, removed southeastern tribes living east of the Mississippi to what was then deemed as "Indian Territory" (now the State of Oklahoma), with the first wave of Choctaw removed in 1831, followed by the Seminole in 1832, the Muscogee (Creek) in 1834, the Chickasaw in 1837, and the Cherokee in 1838. Other tribes were also relocated during this period, and some tribes hid or remained in their ancient homelands (e.g., Mississippi Choctaw, the Creek in Alabama, and Eastern Band of Cherokee in North Carolina). Even before the infamous removal of Cherokee, by 1837, 46,000 American Indians from these southeastern nations had been removed from their homelands, thereby opening 25 million acres for settlement by Whites (Wikipedia 2010). Most of the waves of relocation occurred during the winter months, and many tribes were inadequately equipped or dressed with government rationing, in some cases only one blanket per family, with limited provisions to make the over 1,000 mile trek. Most suffered from exposure, disease, and starvation in the relocations, and as a result, tribes, clans, and families were decimated. For example, over 4,000 of the 15,000 Cherokee perished during relocation, giving rise to the phrase associated with this removal – *Nunna daul Isunyi* – "the Trail Where They Cried" or the *Trail of Tears*. Examples of the brutality of the relocation *process* itself cannot be underestimated. It is best captured by the Cherokee experience (as cited in the Illinois General Assembly – HJR0142 and accessed on Wikipedia 2010), where:

> In the winter of 1838 the Cherokee began the thousand mile march with scant clothing and most on foot without shoes or moccasins. The march began in Red Clay, Tennessee, the location of the last Eastern capital of the Cherokee Nation. The Cherokee were given used blankets from a hospital in Tennessee where an epidemic of small pox had broken out. Because of the diseases, the Indians were not allowed to go into any towns or villages along the way; many times this meant traveling much farther to go around them. After crossing Tennessee and Kentucky, they arrived in Southern Illinois at Golconda about the 3rd of December, 1838. Here the starving Indians were charged a dollar a head to cross the river on "Berry's Ferry" which typically charged twelve cents. They were not allowed passage until the ferry had serviced all others wishing to cross and were forced to take shelter under "Mantle Rock," a shelter bluff on the Kentucky side, until "Berry had nothing better to do". Many died huddled together at Mantle Rock waiting to cross. Several Cherokee were murdered by locals. The killers filed a lawsuit against the U.S. Government through the courthouse in Vienna, suing the government for $35 a head to bury the murdered Cherokee.

During Cherokee removal, Cherokee leaders and families prepared for the eventual return of their people to their homelands by placing Cherokee markers on trees, now known as arborglyphs, to help future generations of Cherokee find their way home and access their familial, clan, and tribal possessions. According to Forest Wade, a Cherokee descendent, the Cherokees so closely guarded the codes of the arborglyphs that they can "only be seen and deciphered by a member of the tribe or someone highly trained in this art. This knowledge, forbidden to the white race, was so secret that death was the penalty to any Cherokee who revealed it to anyone other than their own race or a blood brother." Even during the chaos and terror of removal, Cherokee elders had the importance of place for future generations of Cherokee in the forefront of their mind as they ensured there was a tie between the land, trees, and people via the arborglyphs. The trees literally bore and continue to bear witness to the historical trauma related to land dispossession suffered by the Cherokees and other tribal nations.

The Cherokee removal is but one of many historical relocations. In some removals, tribes were loaded onto trains and relocated hundreds of miles from family and tribe or forcibly moved to areas of the North American continent that were previously unknown to them (Whitbeck et al. 2004). Similar to the Dine' internment at Bosque

Redondo in 1864, in many removal and relocation cases, tribes were placed onto land that was already occupied by other IP (creating conflict among the relocates and the original inhabitants of that territory) or were forced to cohabit with "enemy" tribes on reservations. Moreover, by the 1880s, the US government was also removing children and placing them hundreds of miles from families and traditional lands into boarding schools. Torn from family, land, and ancestors, children were forbidden to practice any form of their traditional ways of life and, instead, were forced to learn Western mannerisms and speak English. Many reportedly died from "homesickness" (Evans-Campbell 2008) The punishment for speaking in a native language or attempting to practice traditional spirituality was often harsh, and children quickly learned to keep their traditional practices secret. As documented in numerous texts, physical abuse and neglect were commonplace; high numbers of children were also sexually abused. Refusing to send children to boarding schools or leaving reservations was illegal for many years and met with imprisonment, withholding of rations, or harsh physical punishment (Evans-Campbell 2008). Dis-placement during the 1800s well into the mid-1900s meant dis-placement from land, place, and with the boarding school policies as well as the Court of Indian Offense (1880s) that prohibited cultural and spiritual practices under threat of imprisonment, many tribal nations suffered greatly from disruptions from place, land, identity, family, and culture. Relocation and removal policies were and always have been fundamentally tied to material gain through land acquisition. As Hughes notes (as cited in Cajete 2000: 179), Americans of European descent:

> …saw America as wilderness, an obstacle to be overcome through settlement and the use of living and non-living resources. The land was a material object, a commodity, something from which they could gain economically. For the most part, they viewed the [indigenous] people they encountered as another resource that they would either use or abuse in accord with their agenda for material gain.

By the 1950s, the US government continued to enact historically traumatic events related to displacement of AIAN, once again to acquire indigenous land and resources. Specifically, Congress passed "termination" acts on a tribe-by-tribe basis which disbanded the tribe, extinguished their traditional rights to land, hunting, and fishing, ended any federal aid to the tribes, and eradicated tribal rights as sovereign nations. From 1953 to 1964, over 109 tribes were terminated with over 2.5 million acres of trust land removed from protected status and converted to private ownership. Over 3% of the American Indian population were terminated from tribes (over 12,000 people) during this period in US history. Public Law 280, which was passed by Congress in 1953, gave state governments the power to assume jurisdiction over Indian lands and reservations, which had previously been excluded from state jurisdiction (U.S. Department of Justice 2005). The main effect of PL 280 was to disrupt the federal trust relationship between the federal government and the tribes, leading to devastating effects on tribal sovereignty, culture, and welfare. PL 280 allowed the federal government to take over indigenous lands, particularly ones rich in mineral and water resources. Finally, concomitant with termination era policies, the federal government initiated another relocation program, the Indian Relocation Act of 1956 (aka Public Law 959) encouraging over 100,000 American Indians to leave their tribal lands with unfulfilled and underfunded promises of assistance related to job training and employment in selected US cities (e.g., major termination states and corresponding cities such as Los Angeles, Minneapolis, Phoenix, Chicago). The Bureau of Indian Affairs established Indian centers in these urban areas (e.g., Oakland's Intertribal Friendship House), and despite the economic deterioration that ensued on reservations, and unfulfilled government funding to vocational programs, urban relocation efforts unintentionally stimulated the growth of Pan-Indian social movements (e.g., American Indian Movement). Nevertheless, due in large part to PL 959, over 60% of AIAN live outside of tribal lands and communities in urban areas. Despite dis-placement from original homelands for some AIAN, AIAN continue to go "home" to tribal lands during holidays, summers, family gatherings for important events, and to fulfill ceremonial obligations, a process referred to as circular migration. Moreover, after some of the removal policies, some tribal communities remained isolated enough to have limited periods of cultural resurgence and renaissance (e.g., Oklahoma Choctaws postremoval and pre-civil war) despite the initial devastating effects of relocation and removal.

Historical Trauma and Environmental Destruction

> *In the perception of many Native cultures, their landscapes are seen as metaphoric extensions of their bodies.*
>
> Cajete (2000: 185)

Historical trauma loss also includes the systematic destruction or willful neglect of the animals, plants, flora, fauna, soil, trees, and waterways. Today, Native peoples' lands are subject to some of the most invasive, toxic, industrial, and destructive practices. Indigenous communities are targeted in part because the lands are not regulated well given the jurisdictional disputes and because Native peoples are simply easy targets given the high rates of poverty and isolation on indigenous lands and reservations. For example, according to La Duke (1999), over 317 American Indian reservations are threatened by environmental hazards, including toxic waste pollutants infiltrating land and water systems. Moreover, nuclear testing proliferates on indigenous lands (e.g., Marshall Islands) with over 1,000 atomic explosions detonated on Western Shoshone land in Nevada (La Duke 1999). Additionally, at least 16 reservations have been targeted for nuclear waste storage. Moreover, the devastating impact of environmental pollutants from corporations have left many communities with high rates of PCB contamination in their waterways or natural foods from poorly regulated industrial runoffs or in other cases high rates of radiation exposure from abandoned uranium mines leaking into soil, water, and airways (La Duke 1999). Environmental toxins not only harm the body of the People but also disrupt the communities' abilities to fulfill their lifeways and OI. For example, a Native leader noted that the mercury poisoning in their waters disrupted:

> …our way of living, the ways that our people used to live before: spirituality, culture, self-esteem, and all of that…the mercury killed everything…we lost everything… it took 30 years for them to even acknowledge what they had done to us. They compensate [other] people for natural disasters, but they don't compensate us for what they did to us. Ours wasn't an act of the Creator, it was the act of man.
>
> Frobisher as cited in La Duke (1999: 102).

Attacks on animals have also been another form of historical trauma for Native people. General Sheridan once said, "The best way to kill the Sioux is to kill the buffalo." This genocidal strategy attempts to cut off the food supply for the plains Native peoples and directly attack their relationship to the buffalo. The buffalo kills literally disrupts the people's ability to fulfill their relationship with these relatives, who are brothers, sisters, and elders to them – it is as much a direct spiritual assault as it is a material assault. In 1997, Rosalie Little Thunder was among a group of Native activists who went to pray for the buffalo that was being killed to cull the herd by the National Park service. The 1997 buffalo killing triggered a historical trauma collective memory of the Little Thunder massacre (1855) of which Rosalie is a descendant. She notes that in September of 1855 (La Duke 1999: 155):

> Then that General Harney came, the one that peak's named after [Harney's peak, known to the indigenous people as " "]. Little Thunder went out to meet him with the truce flag, and he met him, and he fed him…There was grandma there. That grandma had her ten-year-old grandson with her. She said to him, 'stay here, don't come out yet.' And she laid her shawl over him and hid him in the bushes by the tall grass. They started shooting down the people then. And when she was shot, she threw herself on top of that little boy. That way she hid him. That little boy, he was my grandfather…he remembered his grandmother's blood dripping through the shawl onto him. He stayed there until there was no sound. He and the surviving members went back to Pine Ridge on foot. Close to 70 people were killed there…this was so strange: That's what the whole scene was when they were killing the buffalo [in 1997]. That was what was coming back to me [as she witnessed the buffalo killing]. I had my ten-year-old grandson standing next to me. And they started killing the buffalo, just like that, shooting them down. I covered his face with my shawl, and told him to go [no] move…. you get the sense that nothing changes from 1855 to 1997. Actually, that time span is just a clap of thunder in our history. It's not that long.

Environmental destruction, particularly through interrupting natural waterways through redirection of water and dams, has pernicious health effects on Native peoples. Perhaps the best contemporary example of this can be seen in the rapid rise of diabetes among the Pimas and Maricopas after their water was diverted from their traditional lands for non-Native community and commercial consumption. As noted in the film, *Unnatural Causes*, "A survey conducted in 1902 found only one case of diabetes among the Pima. But within 30 years of the building of the Coolidge Dam, there were more than 500." Rod Lewis, former general counsel for the Gila River Indian Community also noted, "There is direct connection between the diversion of water in the upper Gila River and the health status and economic status of the Pimas and Maricopas…we were practically without water for almost an entire century…unable to grow crops."

Microaggressions and Place

Microaggressions are the chronic, everyday injustices that Natives endure – the interpersonal and environmental messages that are denigrating, nullifying, demeaning, or invalidating. These verbal and nonverbal encounters place the burden of addressing them on the recipient of the encounter, creating chronic stress (Sue et al. 2007; Walters et al. 2008). Microaggressive environments serve to diminish identity and render invisible indigenous presence and realities. For Native peoples, many microaggressive messages are literally carved into mountains (e.g., Mount Rushmore) or plaqued onto historical markers at sites that typically commemorate "battles," which, in many cases, were outright massacres. A prime example is the original plaque that commemorates the "Sand Creek Battle Ground" (the marker reads: "Sand Creek Battle Ground" Nov. 29 and 30, 1864). In this "battle" now known as the Sand Creek Massacre, the US military, led by Chivington, knowingly attacked a peaceful encampment and then murdered and mutilated over 200 Cheyenne and Arapaho, two-thirds of whom were women and children.

The carving up, as in the case of Mt. Rushmore, desecration, or destruction of Native places are historical traumatic events, whereas having to live with the aftermath and bear witness to place-based HT destruction in the everyday environment are environmentally based microaggressions. Other land-based microaggressions include the renaming of places with nonindigenous names. This serves two purposes in terms of microaggressions – it erases from the American imagination the indigeneity associated with that place, and it creates new protocols by which people are expected to behave. Colonial renaming is an attempt to reset protocols to place. For Native peoples, naming is a very sacred process; with a name comes relational protocols for both the named place as well as those who are in association with the named place. Naming establishes protocols and responsibilities to place, clarifies the significance of place in relation to those protocols and the people for whom it is named, and creates expectations for types of behavior to occur in relation to that place. The renaming of indigenous places quite literally supplants sacred meaning with metaphorical and symbolic colonial reminders and "conquest" messages (e.g., Mount Ranier instead of Lushootseed word Talol or Tahoma meaning "mountain of waters") of the power and privilege of colonial control. Moreover, many places, particularly sacred sites, tend to be renamed with English words that are highly offensive and insulting, such as Squawteat Peak in Central Pecos valley Texas, or Devils Tower in Wyoming (known as *Mato Tipila*, which means "Bear Lodge" in Lakota), or given nicknames such as Rum Runner Road (i.e., Snoqualmie Pass).

The seizing of land, whether justified by "Manifest Destiny," broken treaties, land allotment policy, or brute force, has exacted a spiritual, physical, and mental toll on IP. Assaults on the land are akin to assault on the body and the people; displacement from land is akin to being stripped from one's family of origin; seizing the land is akin to stealing from a relative and forbidding any Native family members their rights of access to that family member; disrespecting the land and its relatives through toxins, dumping, or mismanagement is akin to neglecting or hurting a relative. Cajete (2000: 188) notes that:

> Relationships between native peoples and their environments became so deep that separation by forced relocation in the last century constituted, literally, the loss of part of an entire generation's soul. Indian people have been joined with their lands with such intensity that many of those who were forced to live on reservations suffered from a 'soul death.' The major consequence was the loss of sense of home and the expression of profound homesickness with all its accompanying psychological and physical maladies. They withered like mountain flowers pulled from their mother soil.

Historical Land Loss: Preliminary Empirical Associations with Health Outcomes

A profound sense of loss associated with historically traumatic events tied to land and culture that happened to parents, grandparents, and ancestors continues to haunt the everyday emotional life of some tribal communities (Whitbeck et al. 2004), particularly with respect to losses associated with land. Specifically, in one study conducted with elders from two large reservation communities, Whitbeck et al. (2004) explored responses to a variety of historical and contemporary losses associated with historical trauma (e.g., loss of tribal land, forced boarding school attendance, loss of language, losses associated with broken treaties, loss of traditional spiritual ways, loss of family ties due to boarding schools). The findings indicated that although respondents were generations from historically traumatic land loss events, the trauma associated with such events was a critical factor in their emotional and cognitive life (Whitbeck et al. 2004). Specifically, when asked about how often they thought about loss of land, about one fifth of the respondents (18.2%) indicated that they thought about it several times a day or daily and over one third (33.7%) thought daily about the loss of culture (Whitbeck et al. 2004). Moreover, when asked about how often they thought about the loss of family due to government relocation [dis-placement] efforts, 10% indicated that they thought about it several times a day or daily, and nearly 16% thought about it at least weekly (Whitbeck et al. 2004). Two primary emotional themes emerged: anger and depressive symptoms. In terms of land loss, one elder noted:

> They stole our land, they stole a lot of land, and they killed a lot of people. So what do you expect us to do? Just stand here and take it?
>
> Whitbeck et al. (2004: 123)

Finally, findings from the study indicated that cognitions about historical losses were associated with emotional distress and were primarily associated with anger and anxiety or depressive symptom expression. Disentangling the effects of proximal traumatic stressors (e.g., child abuse) from the more distal stressors associated with historical trauma was not addressed in that study; however, the authors proposed that "high impact" loss individuals (i.e., those who think daily or more about historical losses) might be more susceptible to proximal stressors (e.g., microaggression distress), as they interact with historical trauma, thereby increasing emotional distress (Whitbeck et al. 2004). Evans-Campbell and Walters (2006) refer to the interaction of distal and proximal discriminatory traumatic stressors as colonial trauma response (CTR), whereby historical trauma responses may become triggered or activated by exposure to contemporary discrimination distress. Specifically, although historical trauma specifically focuses on historical collective traumatic events and responses, CTR is a complex set of both historical and current trauma responses to both collective and interpersonal events (Evans-Campbell and Walters 2006; Evans-Campbell 2008). A defining feature of CTR is its connection to colonization, whereby CTR reactions may arise as an individual experiences contemporary discriminatory event (i.e., microaggression) that serves to connect him or her to a collective and often historical sense of injustice or trauma. In their overview of CTR, Evans-Campbell and Walters (2006) presented an example of a Native woman who was called a race-based derogatory name by a stranger, and although she felt personal rage over her current experience on an individual level, she simultaneously and immediately viscerally connected to her collective sense of historical trauma and ancestral pain. Evans-Campbell (2008: 333) notes that "the connections between past and present trauma may be quite subtle, making it difficult for individuals to see the relationship between contemporary responses and a historically traumatic past. As a result, emotional responses to current microaggression may initially seem overreactive or too intense, even to those directly involved."

Empirical Findings: Historical Traumatic Place Loss and Health Among Two-Spirits

The Honor Project Study

Respondents were recruited as part of a multisite cross-sectional national health survey of Native two-spirit persons from seven metropolitan areas in the US: Seattle–Tacoma, San Francisco–Oakland, Los Angeles, Denver, Oklahoma City–Tulsa, Minneapolis–St. Paul, and New York City. Eligibility criteria included the following: (1) self-identifying as American Indian, Alaska Native, or First Nations *and* either being enrolled in their tribal nation *or* reporting at least 25% total American Indian blood; (2) self-identifying as gay, lesbian, bisexual, transgender, or two-spirit *or* having engaged in same-sex sexual behavior in the past 12 months; (3) being 18 years of age or older; (4) speaking English; and (5) residing, working, or socializing in one of the urban study sites.

Multiple sampling strategies were used to minimize selection bias including targeted, partial network, and respondent-driven sampling (RDS) techniques.

At each site, coordinators proposed six to eight diverse (by gender and age) first wave "seeds" ($n=36$) of which 33 participated. A second wave of RDS generated 58 nominees, of whom 50 participated. Volunteer respondents also were solicited through newsletters, brochures, posters, and word of mouth. We achieved a total response rate of 80.1%. There were no significant differences between RDS (seeds and nominees) and volunteer respondents for the cohort overall or by site on key sociodemographic variables (i.e., gender, education, employment, income, or housing).

Each respondent received $65.00 for completing a 3–4 hour computer-assisted self-interview. A total of 451 respondents were interviewed between July 2005 and March 2007. Of these, four respondents were later excluded due to ineligibility, leaving a total of 447 participants. The data analytic sample in the present study focused on the 354 participants who provided complete data on historical traumatic place loss.

Participants

Participants were 354 Native American adults from seven urban sites across the United States. By gender, participants were 51% male, 42% female, and 7% transgender. The mean age was 39.6 years (SD=10.7, Range=18–67), and the median monthly household income range was $501–1,000. With respect to education level, 17% had not graduated high school, 28% had graduated high school or received a GED, and 55% had some post-high school coursework but no degree. Twenty-five percent were raised in reservation or tribal lands, 36% in an urban area, 17% in a suburban area, 14% in a rural area, and 8% were raised elsewhere. Over half identified with a single Native tribe (62%) and the rest identified with two or more tribes (38%).

Measures

Historical Loss Scale: We used two items from the Historical Loss Scale (Whitbeck et al. 2004) to assess trauma associated with land loss and forcible relocation. Respondents were presented with a statement related to land loss ("*The loss of our land*") and forcible relocation ("*The loss of families from the reservation to the government relocation*") and asked to indicate the frequency with which they think about each type of loss on an eight-point scale from 0 (*never*) to 7 (*several times a day*). Higher scores reflected greater perceived loss.

Colonial Trauma Response Scale: We used two items from the Colonial Trauma Response scale (Walters 1999) to assess trauma associated with unknown burial location of one's ancestors and the consequences of land neglect. Respondents were presented with a statement related to ancestor burial ("*It is hard to grieve for my ancestors since I do not know where they are buried*") and land neglect ("People are suffering because we aren't taking care of the land") and asked to indicate their agreement on a four-point scale from 1 (*strongly disagree*) to 2 (*strongly agree*). Higher scores reflect greater perceived historical and contemporary trauma associated with ancestral place loss and land neglect.

Childhood Trauma Questionnaire: We used ten items from sexual and physical abuse subscales the Childhood Trauma Questionnaire (CTQ; Bernstein et al. 1994). The CTQ has been used previously with Native American populations (Duran et al. 2004). Furthermore, it has demonstrated convergent validity with the Childhood Trauma Interview (Fink et al. 1995). Each subscale consists of five items which were summed to create an index of childhood sexual and physical assault. Items are scored on a six-point scale ranging from 0 (*never true*) to 5 (*always true*), with higher scores indicating more abuse and the items summed to create separate a scale score ranging from 0 to 25, with higher scores reflecting greater abuse. Cronbach's alpha for the sexual and physical assault scales in the present study were 0.95 and 90, respectively.

MOS-HIV. We used the 35 question MOS-HIV health survey (Wu et al. 1997) to assess overall mental and physical health. The MOS-HIV has been shown to be internally consistent and reliable and potentially acceptable as a generic measure related to health quality of life since the instrument is not specifically anchored to HIV-related questions. The scale includes questions related to ten dimensions of health including general health perceptions, pain, physical functioning, role functioning, social functioning, mental health, energy/fatigue, cognitive functions, health distress, and general quality of life. Questions included "How often during the past 4 weeks did you feel weighed down by your health problems?" The responses were rated on a Likert scale ranging from 1 (*all of the time*) to 6 (*none of the time*). Other questions, such as "Does your health limit you from eating, dressing, bathing, or using the toilet," used a three-point Likert scale ranging from 1 (*yes, limited a lot*) to 3 (*no, not limited*). Separate indices of overall mental and physical health scores were calculated and scaled from 0 to 100 with higher scores reflecting better health. Cronbach's alpha for the overall survey was 0.95 in the present study.

Statistical Methods

We first assessed the bivariate correlations between overall mental and physical health with the four land loss variables. Correlations were evaluated for the entire sample as well as separately for males, female, and transgender participants.

Hierarchical multiple regression analyses were conducted to assess the association of land trauma with overall health. Mental and physical health was evaluated as outcomes in two parallel regression models. The primary objective of the regression analysis was to assess whether land trauma would predict variance in mental and physical health, variance not explained by other types of trauma. The secondary objective was to assess whether the associations between land trauma and overall health would differ by gender. In step 1, childhood sexual assault (predictor 1), childhood physical assault (2), and military combat exposure (3) were entered into each model to account for lifetime trauma. In step 2, trauma associated with land loss (4), forcible relocation (5), unknown burial location of ancestors (6), and land neglect (7) were entered to assess the effect of trauma connected with land. In step 3, gender [male, female, and transgender; dummy-coded as female vs. male (8) and transgender vs. male (9)] and all interactions between gender and each land trauma variable (10–17) were entered to test for moderation by gender.

Results

Overall mental health averaged 44.7 (SD=11.0, Range=13.7–66.1), and physical health scores averaged 49.5 (SD=12.0, Range=18.6–66.5). Mean childhood sexual (M=13.3, SD=7.7) and physical assault (M=11.9, SD=6.7) were in the low to moderate range of severity. Five percent of participants had lifetime military or combat experience. Self-reported thoughts regarding *land loss* (M=3.2, SD=1.6) and *forcible relocation* (M=2.8, SD=6.7) occurred in the weekly range of frequency. On average, participants disagreed that *unknown burial locations* of their ancestors made it difficult to grieve for them (M=2.3, SD=1.0), whereas on average, there was agreement (M=3.0, SD=1.0) that *land neglect* was associated with greater suffering of the people.

Bivariate correlations between the land trauma and the overall mental/physical health variables are presented in Table 10.1.

With the combined sample, all correlations were significant with the exception of the two correlations between land neglect and the mental (r=−0.02, p=n.s.) and physical (r=−0.02, p=n.s.) health variables. The magnitude and pattern of the correlations in the male sample were similar to the combined sample. However, the correlations between health and land loss were not statistically significant in the female and transgender sample. Correspondingly, the sample size of the male subgroup (n=181) was larger than the female (n=147) and transgender (n=26) subgroups.

The hierarchical regression analysis for land trauma predicting overall mental health is presented in Table 10.2.

Table 10.1 Zero-order correlations between land loss and overall mental and physical health by gender identity among two-spirit Native Americans

	All (N=354)		Male (n=181)		Female (n=147)		Transgender (n=26)	
	MH	PH	MH	PH	MH	PH	MH	PH
Loss of land	−0.22**	−0.17**	−0.24**	−0.17*	−0.14	−0.14	−0.28	−0.06
Forcible relocation	−0.15**	−0.17**	−0.17*	−0.19*	−0.12	−0.14	−0.10	−0.01
Burial of ancestors	−0.17**	−0.15**	−0.23**	−0.21**	−0.16	−0.11	0.03	−0.08
Land neglect	−0.02	−0.04	−0.02	0.03	0.05	−0.03	−0.09	−0.08

MH overall mental health, *PH* overall physical health
*p<0.05; **p<0.01

Table 10.2 Summary of hierarchical regression analysis for land trauma predicting overall mental health ($N=354$)

Variable	B	SE B	β	p
Step 1: Lifetime trauma				
Childhood sexual trauma	−0.11	0.09	−0.08	0.19
Childhood physical trauma	−0.34	0.10	−0.21	<0.01
Military combat exposure	−4.87	2.59	−0.10	0.06
Step 2: Land trauma				
Loss of land	−1.35	0.42	−0.20	<0.01
Forcible relocation	−0.02	0.41	0.00	0.96
Burial of ancestors	−1.39	0.53	−0.13	0.01
Land neglect	0.85	0.59	0.08	0.15
Step 3: Moderation of land trauma by gender				
Gender identity				
Female vs. male	−3.85	4.83	−0.17	0.43
Transgender vs. male	−0.89	9.46	−0.02	0.93
Gender identity × land trauma				
Female vs. male × loss of land	1.21	0.94	0.21	0.20
Female vs. male × forcible relocation	−0.27	0.89	−0.04	0.76
Female vs. male × burial of ancestors	0.43	1.12	0.05	0.70
Female vs. male × land neglect	−0.50	1.26	−0.08	0.69
Transgender vs. male × loss of land	−0.61	1.44	−0.06	0.67
Transgender vs. male × relocation	0.04	1.48	0.00	0.98
Transgender vs. male × burial of ancestors	3.10	2.10	0.18	0.14
Transgender vs. male × land neglect	−1.79	2.14	−0.14	0.40

Note: $R^2=0.08$, $F(3,350)=10.62$, $p<0.01$, for step 1; $\Delta R^2=0.06$, $F(4,346)=5.56$, $p<0.01$, for step 2; $\Delta R^2=0.02$, $F(10,336)=0.67$, $p=0.75$, for step 3

The lifetime trauma variables in step 1 accounted for 8% of the variance in overall mental health, $F(3,350)=10.62$, $p<0.01$. The addition of land trauma in step 2 accounted for an additional 6% of the variance in overall mental health, $F(4,346)=5.56$, $p<0.01$. Differences by gender in step 3 accounted for an additional 2% of the variance in overall mental health, a contribution that was nonsignificant, $F(10,336)=0.67$, $p=0.75$.

The hierarchical regression analysis for land trauma predicting overall physical health is presented in Table 10.3.

The lifetime trauma variables accounted for 6% of the variance in overall mental health, $F(3,350)=7.48$, $p<0.01$. The addition of land trauma accounted for an additional 4% of the variance in overall mental health, $F(4,346)=3.53$, $p<0.01$. Differences by gender accounted for another 4% of the variance in overall mental health, a contribution that was marginally significant, $F(10,336)=1.57$, $p=0.12$.

> What happens to you and what happens to the earth happens as well so we have, as I said before, common interests. We have to somehow try to convince people who are in power to change the direction they've been taking
>
> Lyons (2008: 22)

Table 10.3 Summary of hierarchical regression analysis for land trauma predicting overall physical health ($N=354$)

Variable	B	SE B	β	p
Step 1: Lifetime trauma				
Childhood sexual trauma	–0.17	0.10	–0.11	0.08
Childhood physical trauma	–0.19	0.11	–0.10	0.09
Military combat exposure	–8.01	2.87	–0.15	<0.01
Step 2: Land trauma				
Loss of land	–0.79	0.48	–0.10	0.10
Forcible relocation	–0.56	0.46	–0.07	0.23
Burial of ancestors	–1.23	0.59	–0.11	0.04
Land neglect	0.21	0.66	0.02	0.75
Step 3: Moderation of land trauma by gender				
Gender identity				
Female vs. male	–2.91	5.36	–0.12	0.59
Transgender vs. male	–4.98	10.48	–0.11	0.64
Gender identity × land trauma				
Female vs. male × loss of land	0.29	1.04	0.05	0.78
Female vs. male × forcible relocation	0.06	0.98	0.01	0.95
Female vs. male × burial of ancestors	1.00	1.24	0.11	0.42
Female vs. male × land neglect	–1.68	1.39	–0.23	0.23
Transgender vs. male × loss of land	0.54	1.60	0.05	0.74
Transgender vs. male × relocation	1.00	1.64	0.07	0.54
Transgender vs. male × burial of ancestors	1.11	2.32	0.06	0.63
Transgender vs. male × land neglect	–2.00	2.37	–0.15	0.40

Note: $R^2=0.06$, $F(3,350)=7.48$, $p<0.01$, for step 1; $\Delta R^2=0.04$, $F(4,346)=3.53$, $p<0.01$, for step 2; $\Delta R^2=0.04$, $F(10,336)=1.57$, $p=0.12$, for step 3

This chapter has provided preliminary conceptual and empirical links among land-based dis-placements and overall health and well-being among American Indians and Alaska Natives. In our empirical analyses, we found a high proportion of two-spirits who think about the impact of land-based trauma, particularly relocation from traditional homelands, land loss, and land neglect-based historical trauma on a weekly, and in some cases, daily basis. Moreover, the findings indicate that after controlling for contemporary trauma, including childhood physical and sexual abuse, as well as adult military combat exposure, historical trauma land-based events continued to have a significant effect on mental and physical health. These findings provide preliminary support that trauma related to land losses and disruptions may persist and become embodied in physical and mental health. Although we cannot conclude directionality from the cross-sectional nature of the survey data, the findings illuminate some of the place-based historical trauma factors that may lead to poor physical and mental health. Future research is needed to further discern the relationship among proximal and distal HT factors on specific health and mental health outcomes, such as PTSD and CVD, and to identify important factors that buffer against the impact of such potentially traumatic losses. Previous trauma research with Native communities indicates that trauma exposure is associated with increased risk for diabetes, asthma, and chronic obstructive pulmonary disease (Levin 2009). Moreover, although Manson (as cited in Levin 2009: 9) notes that "historical trauma, secondary traumatization and intergenerational grief need to be examined rigorously… they make only a modest contribution to risk compared to current trauma," our findings suggest that historical traumatic land-based assaults may make much more than a modest contribution to mental health risk – in fact, they may play a significant role in Native health disparities. Finally, the findings are consistent with burgeoning research indicating critical associations between environmental factors and poor health outcomes, particularly the embodiment of stress and health. As Krieger and Davey (2004: 92) note, bodies count:

> …they provide vivid evidence of how we literally embody the world in which we live, thereby producing populations patterns of health, disease, disability and death…these aspects of our being not only are predictive of future health outcomes but also tell of our conjoined social and biologic origins and trajectories.

In terms of two-spirit-specific issues, our previous studies have indicated that two-spirit AIAN are more likely than heterosexual AIAN to report high levels of historical trauma event exposure (Balsam et al. 2004). One explanation for the higher self-reported historical trauma event knowledge among two-spirits is that two-spirits might have a greater sensitivity to and awareness of discriminatory events, even historically based ones, due to their multiply oppressed status (i.e., by race and sexual orientation). However, after talking with two-spirit community members, an alternative explanation arose. Some two-spirit persons are the cultural storytellers or cultural knowledge keepers for their people, and as a result, may have historical knowledge of major events that have been passed down through generations. Two-spirits might carry this historical knowledge of trauma events as part of a two-spirit role in their respective communities. Drawing from the work of Wardi (1992), Brave Heart (1999) refers to this process as *Wakiksuyapi* where clans, family groups, or bands actually shoulder the responsibility of remembering historically traumatic events (i.e., "memorial people"). Brave Heart (1999) argues that Native communities may have a strong proclivity toward being a memorial people due to the inherent cultural emphasis on the role of ancestor spirits, collective worldview, and the spatial orientation of Native cultures.

Finally, in many Native cultures, two-spirit people held ceremonial and social roles that were tied to place. Specifically, in some tribes, they cared for the place that ancestors were buried or burned, were involved in funerary rites, which are tied to land and place, and were knowledgeable about plant medicines (Lang 1998). In these cases, place loss is not only tied directly to place, as in the case of relocation, land loss, and land neglect, but is also possibly tied to loss of place-associated ceremonial roles. Place-associated role loss potentially affects all Native community members, particularly those who hold roles associated with specific place-based responsibilities such as agricultural development, working with and taking care of plant medicines, and funerary responsibilities.

In terms of limitations of the findings, the cross-sectional nature of our data restricts our ability to infer causal direction. For example, it is possible that participants who reported poorer health and mental health were more likely to report historical trauma losses or be more cognizant of historical trauma events. Nevertheless, our findings are consistent with the extant research on the negative effects of environmental stress on health outcomes as well as research on intergenerational trauma and health impacts among descendant survivors. Moreover, our findings are concordant with our theoretical framework and Native scholarship on place and health.

Resistance and Resiliency

As noted earlier, it is important to note that not all historically traumatic events result in collective or individual mental or physical health distress. There are numerous challenges to disentangling the interrelated components of the concepts and understanding what specific mechanisms are at work (Whitbeck et al. 2004: 119). Our tribal communities, families, and individuals vary in their responses to and processing of historical trauma events. Distress based on these events is moderated to some degree by the cultural meaning attributed to the event and meaning derived from the trauma experience (Denham 2008). Thus, it is important to differentiate between the potentiating effect of a historically traumatic event and the actual or soul wound response at the tribal, familial, and individual levels. Moreover, recent research indicates that although the stress impact might actually be embodied at the epigenomic level, predisposing some to a higher propensity for poor health outcomes in descendant generations, the distress might not be expressed until certain contemporary environmental stressors act as triggers releasing the stress reaction in descendant generations. Finally, poor mental and physical health outcomes may also be buffered by important tribal, clan, familial, and individual cultural factors (Walters et al. 2002). Collective memories held by tribes, clans, and families may serve an important survival function in recovering from historical trauma events.

Collective as opposed to individual memory is integral to understanding historical trauma event knowledge transmission. Specifically, collective memory, also known as "social memory," consists of the thread of individual memories connected to a greater social fabric (Denham 2008). Additionally, individual memories, since they are from the same cloth as the collective memories, cannot exist independent of the collective. The culture and family of a tribal nation play a critical role in keeping these memories alive, and the collective aspects and, in some cases, the familial or individual memories held in common within a Native family not only keep the culture, identity, and stories alive, but they also serve, particularly in the case of familial or tribal historical trauma narratives, an important commemorative function to strengthen collective identity, to reaffirm identity and resiliency strategies employed by previous generations, and to provide important narratives of strength and hope for future generations. Denham (2008) notes that these family collective memories and the retelling of major events are "commemorative practices" and are an "embodied form of collective memory that allow one to experience and connect with ancestors and the past by working to solidify kinship bonds and experiences. Such activities have the potential to move abstract events or memories of the past into the lived present." Denham (2008) goes on to note that family members do not construct their identities and sense of "self" from a "chain of personal memories"; rather, tribal family members also "construct their sense of self from a network or chain of intergenerational memories and narratives situated within the larger sociocultural, political, and historical context. That is, narratives and memories of previous generations [over hundreds of years]...are internalized by subsequent generations" and used as a major organizing principle for tribal, familial, and individual identities. This sentiment is reflected in the Native adage, "never forget who you are or where you come from." From this perspective, historical trauma consciousness narratives of major tribal and familial events may also serve as important reminders of potential resistance, survival, and resiliency strategies employed by the ancestors that future generations can learn from and employ. Historical trauma narratives through stories, songs, and family rituals may potentially buffer family members and future generations from the deleterious effects of major historical trauma events, and provide a foundation of response strategies that can be adopted and passed on through the narrating of these major events and the telling of survival stories. For example, a Native family in the Northwest uses the metaphor of growing up with a "Rock Culture," a connection to land and place for strength and protection (Denham 2008). A family member notes:

> ...that's where we began to learn, that room where everybody was in the evening. They would pray, tell stories, they'd visit, they'd have oral history lessons, or what amounted to that, and they'd sing songs. And my brother and I learned the songs of our family, that's where we began when we were just little babies, before we could even learn to talk, they were singing to us the songs of our family. Those special songs that were maybe 1,000 years old that were handed down in this circle from those circles, those camps over there. But, these songs made there way here, to this buffer here...So that's the connection...Our father told us to never forget your Rock Culture. Practice it. One of his last breaths, he even wrote it in a letter, one of the major things he expressed is to not forget our Rock Culture.

In terms of historical trauma, family narratives tend to be strengths-based and emphasize how family members have been successful in overcoming the trauma and facing what seems to be insurmountable devastation or radical cultural changes (as in the case of relocation or other displacements) and are able to learn from these insurmountable challenges not only to survive but also to thrive (Denham 2008). Specifically, Holocaust descendant survivors utilize survival stories that emphasize overcoming the trauma as opposed to stories that focus on suffering associated with the trauma (Gottschalk 2003). This is akin to what Native communities call "transcending the trauma," which is a tribal collective, clan, familial, and individual quest to move beyond historical trauma victimization to a "warrior mind" state that transcends the trauma and allows the people to live their OI in the context of contemporary times.

Denham (2008) notes that a historical trauma response should not be required to acknowledge and validate the construct, presence, or impact of historical trauma events. Future research on historical trauma, particularly with respect to place and land loss should also consider resiliency expressions as well as the culturally protective functions of family, culture, and identity, as they may buffer the impact of historically traumatic events on wellness outcomes, particularly chronic health conditions and the embodiment of stressful events (Walters and Simoni 2002). Denham (2008: 411) notes that critical exploration of historical trauma will only strengthen it as a construct and "widen our understanding of individual and collective trauma experiences and the practical efforts to support culturally appropriate responses."

Conclusion

We are reminded that creation is an ongoing responsibility and that the sacred is as much an experience of immanence-being embodied – as it is of transcendence-being otherworldly. And, last, land is everything because without it, we simply cannot survive: survival is not just a matter of 'managing environmental resources' but of living in balance by actively participating in creation through reciprocity and world renewal ceremonies (Gonzales and Nelson 2001: 501).

The major aim of this chapter was to stimulate thinking on the relationships between indigenous place and health, specifically the embodiment of historical trauma associated with dis-placement and land loss as they are manifest in health outcomes. Theoretical and empirical findings reflect that Native health and wellness cannot be decontextualized from historical place-based processes, particularly historical traumatic event exposure and its association with physical and mental health outcomes. In terms of health and mental health practice implications, indigenous worldviews, particularly relational and spatial orientations as well as sacred ecological contexts, must be integrated into assessment and intervention design for individual, familial, and tribal or community-based interventions and prevention efforts. Moreover, these worldviews should be tailored to the contemporary context of the tribal group, family, or individual given varied histories with historical traumatic events as well as varied tribal, communal, and familial responses and negotiated resistance and resiliency strategies employed by ancestors and descendent survivors of such events. The focus on strengths-based familial and tribal survival strategies can be integrated into multilevel treatment approaches, particularly for communities and individuals who experience high rates of lifetime traumatic events (e.g., community suicides, homicides, unintentional injuries and fatalities, etc.) and high rates of corresponding population-level PTSD and depression.

Finally, on the structural level, findings indicate that place-based traumatic events, particularly historically traumatic events may have profound effects on health and wellness. Given rapid global climate change and rising ocean levels, many indigenous communities, particularly in the South Pacific and Pacific Northwest, will be hit with major land loss. Although global climate problems do not qualify as historical trauma events per se, a lack of response or indifference to the devastating land losses and relocations that will disproportionately impact Native communities can eventually become historical trauma events. Our findings support the need for early prevention efforts to minimize the physical and mental health impact of these land losses. For example, the island of Tuvalu is at the critical danger point, becoming overrun with ocean water. It is estimated that within 50 years, Tuvalu will literally be under water, thereby devastating land and place ties for the indigenous people of Tuvalu. The response to this crisis has been problematic as noted by one journalist (Woorama 2006) who stated that the:

> …unspeakable arrogance and irresponsibility for industrial nations responsible for global warming and rising sea levels to refer to Tuvalu as a "sinking island", as though its impending submersion were a fault inherent in the island and its people. It seems to make people more comfortable to talk of sinking lands, rather than rising seas, as this doesn't challenge the validity of unsustainable colonial standards of living that continue to ravage the planet.

At stake are human lives, indigenous rights and sovereignty, and ultimately, if displaced, indigenous health and well-being—all major indigenous Peoples' rights issues. As Robinson notes (2009):

> Climate change is contributing to rising prices for grains and staples that are undermining food security for millions….We know there will be more natural catastrophes in future. But they will not always involve horrific headlines and images of hurricanes and tsunamis. More commonly, they will be cumulative and unspectacular. People who are already vulnerable will be disproportionately affected. Slowly and incrementally, land will become too dry to till, crops will wither, rising sea levels will undermine coastal dwellings and spoil freshwater, species will disappear, livelihoods will vanish…Mass migration and conflicts will result. Only very gradually will these awful consequences reach those whose lifestyles and activities are most to blame. Climate change will, in short, have immense human consequences…We have collectively failed to grasp the scale and urgency of the problem…To effectively address it will require a transformation of global policy capacity.

We are at a crossroads related to Western and indigenous understanding and responsibility to indigenous place and land. It is all of our collective responsibility to address indigenous land-based injustices and to deter wherever possible, future historical trauma place-based events. All of our health and wellness depends on it. As Gonzales and Nelson (2001: 496) note, "To have a sustainable culture means having healthy land—one nurtures the other, physically and spiritually"

1. IP and individuals have the right not to be subjected to forced assimilation or destruction of their culture. States shall provide effective mechanisms for prevention of, and redress for, (a) any action that has the aim or effect of depriving them of their integrity as distinct peoples, or of their cultural values or ethnic identities, (b) any action that has the aim or effect of dispossessing them of their lands, territories, or resources (Article 8).
2. IP shall not be forcibly removed from their lands or territories. No relocation shall take place without the free, prior, and informed consent of the IP concerned and after agreement on just and fair compensation and, where possible, with the option of return (Article 10).
3. IP have the right to revitalize, use, develop, and transmit to future generations their histories, languages, oral traditions, philosophies, writing systems, and literatures, and to designate and retain their own names for communities, places, and persons (Article 13).

It is our collective responsibility to address indigenous land-based injustices and to deter, wherever possible, future historical trauma place-based events. All of our health and wellness depends on it. As Gonzales and Nelson (2001: 496) note, "To have a sustainable culture means having healthy land – one nurtures the other, physically and spiritually."

References

Anderson, P. 1995. Priorities in aboriginal health. In *Aboriginal health: Social and cultural transitions*. Darwin, NT, Australia: Northern Territory Press.

Balsam, K. F., Huang, B., Fieland, K. C., Simoni, J. M., and Walters, K. L. 2004. "Culture, trauma, and wellness: A comparison of heterosexual and lesbian, gay, bisexual, and two-spirit Native Americans." *Cultural Diversity and Ethnic Minority Psychology*, 10(3): 287–301.

Barocas, H., and Barocas, C. 1980. "Separation and individuation conflict in children of Holocaust survivors." *Journal of Contemporary Psychology*, 38: 417–452.

Bar-On, D., Eland, J., Kleber, R., Krell, R., Moore, Y., Sagi, A., et al. 1998. "Multigenerational perspectives on coping with Holocaust experience: An attachment perspective for understanding the developmental sequelae of trauma across generations." *International Journal of Behavioral Development*, 22(2): 315–338.

Bernstein, D. P., Fink, L., Handelsman, L., Foote, J., Lovejoy, M., Wenzel, K., Sapareto, E., et al. 1994. "Initial reliability and validity of a new retrospective measure of child abuse and neglect." *American Journal of Psychiatry*, 15: 1132.

Brave Heart, Maria Yellowhorse. 1999. "Oyate Ptayela: Rebuilding the Lakota Nation through addressing historical trauma among Lakota parents." *Journal of Human Behavior in the Social Environment*, 2(1–2): 109–126.

Burgess, C. P., Johnston, F. H., Bowman, D. M. J. S., and Whitehead, P. J. 2005. "Healthy country: Healthy people? Exploring the health benefits of indigenous natural resource management." *Australian and New Zealand Journal of Public Health*, 29(2): 117–121.

Burghardt, M. A., and Nagai-Jacobson, M. G. 2002. *Spirituality: Living our connectedness*. USA: Delmar.

Cajete, Gregory. 1999. "Look to the mountain": Reflections on indigenous ecology. In Gregory Cajete (Ed.), *A people's ecology: Explorations in sustainable living*. New Mexico: Clear Light Publishers. pp. 1–20.

Cajete, Gregory. 2000. *Native science: Natural laws of interdependence*. New Mexico: Clear Light Publishers.

Cajete, Gregory. 2001. "Indigenous education and ecology: Perspectives of an American Indian Educator." In John A. Grim (Ed.), *Indigenous traditions and ecology: The interbeing of cosmology and community*. Cambridge, MA: Harvard University Press.

Cartwright, E. 2007. "Bodily remembering: Memory, place, and understanding Latino folk illnesses among the Amuzgos of Oaxaca, Mexico." *Culture, Medicine, and Psychiatry*, 31(4): 527–545.

Casey, Edward S. 1993. *Getting Back into Place: Toward a Renewed Understanding of the Place-World*. Bloomington: Indiana University Press.

Chae, David H., and Walters, Karina L. 2009. " Racial discrimination and racial identity attitudes in relation to self-rated health and physical pain and impairment among two-spirit American Indians/Alaska Natives." *American Journal of Public Health*, 99(s1): s144–s151.

Deloria, V. Jr. 1992. *God is red: A native view of religion* (2nd edition). Colorado: North American Press.

Deloria, V. Jr. 1995. *Red earth, white lies*. New York: Harper and Row.

Denham, A. R. 2008. "Rethinking historical trauma: Narratives of resilience." *Journal of Transcultural Psychiatry*, 45(3): 391–414.

Duran, B., Sanders, M., Skipper, B., Waitzkin, H., Malcoe, L. H., and Paine, S. 2004. "Prevalence and correlates of mental disorders among Native American women in primary care." *American Journal of Public Health*, 94: 71–77.

Evans-Campbell, T. 2008. "Historical trauma in American Indian/Native Alaska communities: A multilevel framework for exploring impacts on individuals, families, and communities." *Journal of Interpersonal Violence*, 23(3): 316–338.

Evans-Campbell, Teresa, and Walters, Karina L. 2006. Catching our breath: A decolonization framework for healing indigenous families. In Rowena Fong, Ruth McRoy, and Carmen Ortiz Hendricks (Eds.), *Intersecting child welfare, substance abuse, and family violence: Culturally competent approaches*. Alexandria, VA: CSWE Publications. pp. 266–292.

Felsen, I. 1998. Transgenerational transmission of the effects of the Holocaust. In Y. Danieli (Ed.), *International handbook of multigenerational legacies of trauma*. New York: Plenum. pp. 43–68.

Fieland, K. C., Walters, K. L., and Simoni, J. M. 2007. Determinants of health among two-spirit American Indians and Alaska Natives. In Ilan H. Meyer and Mary E. Northridge (Eds.), *The health of sexual minorities: Public health perspectives on lesbian, gay, bisexual, and transgender populations*. New York: Springer. pp. 268–300.

Fink, L. A., Bernstein, D., Handelsman, L., Foote, J., and Lovejoy, M. 1995. "Initial reliability and validity of the childhood trauma interview: A new multidimensional measure of childhood interpersonal trauma." *American Journal of Psychiatry*, 152: 1329.

Gonzales, T. A., and Nelson, M. K. 2001. Contemporary Native American responses to environmental threats in Indian Country. In John A. Grim (Ed.), *Indigenous Traditions and Ecology: The interbeing of cosmology and community*. Cambridge, MA: Harvard University Press. pp. 495–538.

Gottschalk, S. 2003. "Reli(e)ving the Past: Emotion Work in the Holocaust's Second Generation." *Symbolic Interaction*, 26(3): 355–380.

Gracey, M., and King, M. 2009. "Indigenous health: Determinants and disease patterns." *Lancet*, 374: 65–75.

Greenfeld, L. A., and Smith, S. K. 1999. *American Indians and crime*. Washington, DC: U.S. Department of Justice.

Jasienska, G. 2009. Low birth weight of contemporary African Americans: An intergenerational effect of slavery? *American Journal of Human Biology*, 21: 16–24.

Joyce, R. A. 2005. "Archaeology of the body." *Annual Review of Anthropology*, 34: 139–158.

Karr, S. 1973. "Second-generation effects of the Nazi holocaust." *Dissertation abstracts international*, 3: 2935.

King, Malcolm. 2009. "An overall approach to health care for indigenous peoples." *Pediatric Clinics of North America*, 56: 1239–1242.

Krieger, Nancy. 2001. "Theories for social epidemiology in the 21st century: An ecosocial perspective." *International Journal of Epidemiology*, 30: 668–677.

Krieger, Nancy. 2005. "Embodiment: A conceptual glossary for epidemiology." Journal of Epidemiology and Community Health, 59(5): 350–355.

Krieger, Nancy. 2005. "Stormy weather: race, gene expression, and the science of health disparities." *American Journal of Public Health*, 95: 2155–2160.

Krieger, N., and Davey, Smith G. 2004. ""Bodies count," and body counts: social epidemiology and embodying inequality." *Epidemiologic Reviews*, 26: 92–103.

Krieger, N., Alegría, M., Almeida-Filho, N., Barbosa da Silva, J., Barreto, M. L., Beckfield, J., Berkman, L., Birn, A.-E., Duncan, B. B., Franco, S., Garcia, D. A., Gruskin, S., James, S., Laurell, A. C., Oderkirk, J., Schmidt, M. I., and Walters, K. L. 2010. "Who – and what – causes health inequities? – Reflections on emerging debates from an exploratory Latin American/ North American workshop." *Journal of Epidemiology and Community Health*, 64(9): 747–749.

Kuzawa, C. W., and Sweet, E. 2009. "Epigenetics and the embodiment of race: Developmental origins of US racial disparities in cardiovascular health." *American Journal of Human Biology*, 21: 2–15.

La Duke, W. 1999. *All Our Relations: Native Struggles for Land and Life*. Cambridge, MA: South End Press.

Lang, Sabine. 1998. *Men as women, women as men: Changing gender in Native American cultures*. Austin, Texas: University of Texas Press.

Levin, Aaron. 2009. "How much does historical trauma add to Indians' health problems?" *Psychiatric News*, 44(16): 9.

Lichtman, H. 1984. "Parental communication of Holocaust experiences and personality characteristics among second-generation survivors." *Journal of Clinical Psychology*, 40: 914–924.

Lyons, Oren. 2008. Listening to natural law. In Melissa K. Nelson (Ed.), *Original instructions: Indigenous teachings for a sustainable future*. Vermont: Bear and Company Books. pp. 22–26.

Lyons, A. C., and Chamberlain, K. 2006. *Health psychology: A critical introduction*. Cambridge: Cambridge University Press.

Mark, G. T., and Lyons, A. C. 2010. "Maori healers' views on wellbeing: The importance of mind, body, spirit, family, and land." *Social Science and Medicine*, 70(11): 1756–1764.

Meyer, M. A. 2008. Indigenous and authentic: Hawaiian epistemology and the triangulation of meaning. In N. K. Denzin, Y. S. Lincoln, and L. Tuhiwai Smith (Eds.), *Handbook of critical indigenous methodologies*. California: Sage Publications. pp. 217–232.

Nagata, D., Trierweiler, S., and Talbot, R. 1999. "Long-term effects of internment during early childhood in third generation Japanese Americans." *American Journal of Orthopsychiatry*, 69(1): 19–29.

Olden, K., and White, S. L. 2005. "Health-related disparities: Influence of environmental factors." *Medical Clinics of North America*, 89: 721–738.

Pierotti, R., and Wildcat, D. R. 2000. "Traditional ecological knowledge: The third alternative (commentary)." *Ecological Applications*, 10(5): 1333–1340.

Robinson, M. 2009. *International council on human rights: climate change and human rights – a rough guide*. As cited at http://www.ichrp.org/files/summaries/35/136_summary.pdf.

Seeman, T. E., Dubin, L. F., and Seeman, M. 2003. "Religiosity/spirituality and health: A critical review of the evidence for biological pathways." *American Psychologist*, 58(1): 53–63.

Sheridan, J., and Longboat, R. D. 2006. "The Haudenosaunee imagination and the ecology of the sacred." *Space and Culture*, 9: 365–381.

Simoni, J. M., Walters, K. L., Balsam, K. F., and Meyers, S. 2006. "Victimization, substance use, and HIV risk among gay/bisexual/two-spirit and heterosexual American Indian men in New York City." *American Journal of Public Health*, 96(12): 2240–2245.

Solomon, Z., Kother, M., and Mikulincer, M. 1988. "Combat-related PTSD among second generation Holocaust survivors: Preliminary findings." *American Journal of Psychiatry*, 145: 865–868.

Stannard, D. E. 1992. *American holocaust: The conquest of the new world.* New York: Oxford University Press.

Stephens, C., Nettleton, C., Porter, J., Willis, R., and Clark, S. 2005. "Indigenous peoples' health – why are they behind everyone, everywhere?" *Lancet*, 366(9479): 10–13.

Stidsen, Sille. (Ed.) 2006. *The indigenous world.* Copenhagen, Denmark: Eks-Skolens Trykkeri. pp. 10.

Sue, D. W., Capodilupo, C. M., Torino, G. C., Bucceri, J. M., Holder, A. M., Nadal, K. L., and Esquilin, M. 2007. "Racial microaggressions in everyday life: Implications for clinical practice." *American Psychologist*, 62(4): 271–286.

Thornton, R. 1987. *American Indian holocaust and survival: A population history since 1492.* Norman, Oklahoma: University of Oklahoma Press.

U.S. Department of Justice. 2005. *Public law 280 and law enforcement in Indian country – research priorities.* Accessed on 4/22/2010 at http://www.ojp.usdoj.gov/nij/pubs-sum/209839.htm.

Walters, Karina L. 1999. Unpublished measure, from the grant R29 AA 12010. Cited with permission of the author.

Walters, K. L., and Simoni, J. M. 2002. "Reconceptualizing Native women's health: An "indigenist" stress-coping model." *American Journal of Public Health*, 92(4): 520–524.

Walters, K. L., Simoni, J. M., Evans-Campbell, T. 2002. "Substance use among American Indians and Alaska Natives: Incorporating culture in an "indigenist" stress-coping paradigm." *Public Health Reports*, 117(s1): S104–S117.

Walters, K. L., Evans-Campbell, T., Simoni, J., Ronquillo, T., and Bhuyan, R. 2006. "My spirit in my heart: Identity experiences and challenges among American Indian two-spirit women." *Journal of Lesbian Studies*, 10(1/2): 125–149.

Walters, K. L., Chae, D. H., Perry, A. T., Stately, A., Old Person, R., and Simoni, J. M. 2008. My body and my spirit took care of me: Homelessness, violence, and resilience among American Indian two-spirit men. In S. Loue (Ed.), *Health issues confronting minority men who have sex with men.* New York: Springer Publications. pp. 125–156.

Wardi, D. 1992. *Memorial candles: Children of the holocaust.* London: Tavistock.

Watkins, J. 2001. "Place-meant." *American Indian Quarterly*, 25(1): 41–45.

Whitbeck, L. B., Adams, G. W., Hoyt, D. R., and Chen, X. 2004. "Conceptualizing and measuring historical trauma among American Indian people." *American Journal of Community Psychology*, 33(3/4): 119–130.

Wikipedia. 2010. *Trail of tears.* Accessed on 4/20/10 at http://www.en.wikipedia.org/wiki/Trail_of_Tears.

Wildcat, D. R. 2001. The question of self-determination. In Vine Deloria Jr., and Daniel R. Wildcat (Eds.), *Power and place: Indian education in America.* Golden. Co: Fulcrum Publishing. pp. 135–150.

Wilson, K. 2003. "Therapeutic landscapes and First Nations peoples: An exploration of culture, health, and place." *Health and Place*, 9: 83–93.

Woorama. 2006. *Global warming to drown Tuvalu.* Accessed on 4/22/10 at http://www.aboriginalrights.suite101.com/article.cfm/global_warming_to_drown_tuvalu.

Wu, A. W., Revicki, D. A., Jacobson, D., and Malitz, F. E. 1997. "Evidence for reliability, validity and usefulness of the Medical Outcomes Study for HIV Health Survey (MOS-HIV)." *Quality of Life Research*, 6: 481–493.

Yehuda, Rachel. 1999. *Risk factors for posttraumatic stress disorder*. Washington, DC: American Psychiatric Press.

Zarsky, L. 2006. *Is nothing sacred? Corporate responsibility for the protection of Native American sacred sites*. La Honda: CA: Sacred Land Film Project.

Part III
Justice in Places

Chapter 11
Structural Violence, Historical Trauma, and Public Health: The Environmental Justice Critique of Contemporary Risk Science and Practice

Devon G. Peña

The roots of Chicana/o environmental justice struggles run much deeper than is usually recognized (Peña 2005a:100–104). The mineworkers' strike at Cananea in 1906, led by anarcho-syndicalists affiliated with the Partido Liberal Mexicano (PLM) is one iconic example of the deep precursor roots of the modern Environmental Justice Movement (EJM). The workers at Cananea demanded an end to the company store (*tienda de raya*) that kept the workers in perpetual debt; they demanded wage equality by calling for abolition of the so-called Mexican Wage which meant the native workers were paid half as much as Anglos for the same job (Ruiz 1988:109–112). The Cananea strikers also demanded the right to unionize and to negotiate collective bargaining agreements that included clauses for greater direct worker control of production and safety conditions (González Navarro 1997).

Labor historians sometimes overlook the fact that the *huelguistas* at Cananea also demanded changes in the safety procedures at the copper mine to reduce deaths and injuries from accidents caused by hazardous working conditions and workers further demanded that management abide by previous commitments to build a hospital and parks for family recreation (Casillas 1979; La Botz 1992:115–120). The Cananea mineworkers were among the first to introduce the use of canaries in cages to warn of life-threatening gases. They recognized workplace hazards as threats to life and limb. The *huelguistas* at Cananea were among the first North American industrial workers to directly link labor rights to demands for economic and social justice, workplace democracy, and environmental protection. They were among the earliest to decry the effects of structural violence and historical trauma as sources of continued inequality and marginality degrading the health of worker and their communities.

We can fast forward to the 1960s and the first antipesticides campaign of the United Farm Workers Organizing Committee. When Dolores Huerta and Cesar Chavez began to organize farmworkers, the issues they fought over were not just the

---

D.G. Peña (✉)
Department of Anthropology, University of Washington, Seattle, WA, USA
e-mail: dpena@uw.edu

L.M. Burton et al. (eds.), *Communities, Neighborhoods, and Health*,
Social Disparities in Health and Health Care 1, DOI 10.1007/978-1-4419-7482-2_11,

rights of union recognition and a living wage. They too pioneered the struggle to end environmental racism and the unjust poisoning of working families and their communities (Pulido and Peña 1998). In a very real sense, the struggle for environmental justice has been with us as long as people of color have fought to protect themselves from risks and hazards in the places where we live, work, play, pray, and eat.

This chapter examines how places and people in these places are denied access and opportunities, resist and take action toward the inequities in their communities. I focus on the issues of environmental justice and provide a critique of contemporary efforts to include communities in the decision-making process. The use of the term, but not necessarily the concept of, "environmental justice" dates back only to the 1980s when it was first used by African American activists in the American South to describe the struggle against "environmental racism" (Bullard 2005:38–41). Environmental racism was a new and important concept because it is based on empirical studies that documented the inequalities (or better, disparate impacts) facing people of color and low-income communities who suffer disproportionate exposure to health risks from pollution in residential areas and workplace hazards. This is what we call *el racismo toxico* or "toxic racism" (Bullard 2005; Bullard et al. 2007).

While the roots of the struggles against environmental racism gave rise to a branch of activism and theory that focuses on the critique of inequalities in the distribution of environmental risks (wrongs) and amenities (rights), another branch focuses on the exclusion of people of color from participation in the planning and decision-making agencies and processes that govern environmental planning, protection, management, and regulation (see, e.g., Pellow and Brulle 2005; Peña 2005a). There is a saying among activists that expresses this concept of procedural and organizational inequity: "We are the most polluted *and the most excluded*." Indeed, one reason that communities of color are the most polluted is that they have been systematically excluded from the theory and practice of environmental protection and risk management. The two principal branches of EJ theory then are the distributive and the procedural equity schools of thought. The challenge presented for research scholars thus typically involves undertaking efforts to document distributive and/or participatory inequities and to also analyze the specific micro- and macropolitics of inequality and injustice as these play out in the application of environmental risk science in the context of decision-making practices directly affecting communities.

However, the concept of environmental justice is not just about the struggle to end the procedural, social organizational, and geographic disparities associated with environmental racism. There is another movement aphorism worth repeating: "We don't want an equal piece of the same rotten carcinogenic pie." This statement illustrates how the EJ struggle is not just about ending toxic racism or strengthening community-based participation; it is perhaps more importantly about how we define "sustainability" itself, and how communities are already organizing self-determined or autonomous pathways to a just, sustainable, and resilient society (Peña 2005b). The EJM is therefore a struggle to rethink how we work and live and how we produce and reproduce, with an awareness of the impact of our livelihoods and lifestyles on our bodies, communities, and the Earth as our shared life-support system.

The EJM seeks to redefine what is understood by the term "sustainable development" (Peña 1992; Agyeman et al. 2003). This term has been co-opted and much abused since it was first used by the Brundlandt Commission for the first Earth Summit in 1987. Corporations now use the term as if it were an exchangeable book cover and indeed the concept is usually just window dressing that masks underlying abuses and continued exploitation of workers and the Earth.

What corporations mean by sustainable development is not the same as the way the concept is used by environmental justice activists. Let me clarify. The organic agriculture sector has been taken over by the same multinational corporations that control our global food systems.[1] Cargill and ConAgra, for example, own controlling shares in five different organic food companies including such well-known product lines as "Hain Celestial" and "Hunt's Organic" and "Orville Redenbacher Organic." Do you think that farmworkers in these corporate organic farms have union recognition, collective bargaining agreements, higher wages, and better benefits? The answer I am sure you already realize is "No."

Farmworkers in the organic sector are just as oppressed and exploited as workers in conventional agribusinesses (Peña 2002). They may be slightly better off in the sense that they are not being exposed to pesticides and herbicides, but there are other remaining environmental risks in their workplaces including long hours under conditions that can induce heat strokes due to the abuse of workers by contractors and growers. The corporate takeover of organic agriculture has meant that while worker exposure to environmental risks has been significantly reduced, the social justice dimensions of farmworker struggles remain neglected.

You can be environmentally sustainable and remain unjust in your labor relations and working conditions. Indeed, many organic growers, as well as other "green" corporations, like to argue that workers in their companies do not need labor unions because this is a "New Age" of benevolent and sustainable capitalism and besides unions are just part of an old and maladaptive industrial form of organization that is no longer responsive to the needs of a globalized and information-based economy. Corporate organics is just as antiunion as the conventional agriculture sector. (Mark 2006). For the EJM this means that we cannot have an environmentally sustainable society unless we also have ecological democracy based on worker control and public participation in decision and policy-making.

Environmental Justice and Health: Structural Violence and Historical Trauma

Over the course of the past three decades that have witnessed rise to prominence of the EJM, and since the start of the movement issues related to public health have remained at the center of our struggles. Our nation faces a public health crisis that

[1] For a continuously updated and fully referenced diagram showing the growth of the corporate ownership of the organic foods sector, see: http://www.certifiedorganic.bc.ca/rcbtoa/services/corporate-ownership.html. And for the recent acquisitions of organic food companies by the top 20 largest transnational corporations, go to: http://www.certifiedorganic.bc.ca/rcbtoa/services/corporate-acquisitions.html.

is largely underpinned by the millions of workers and families that remain under or uninsured and the lack of political will on the part of Congress to pass legislation establishing a viable "public option." Everyone is hoping that the Obama Administration follows through on promises to move toward universal health coverage for all Americans. However, what about those resident workers and their families who are out-of-status immigrants? What about the millions of undocumented workers and their families who are already mistreated and misconstrued as a menace and threat to our nation's security?

There are several things we have come to understand about the public health crisis and how it is viewed within the EJM. Like any other issue related to environmental injustice, the lack of access to affordable quality health care is a significant compounding factor that makes people of color and persons from low-income communities even more vulnerable to illness and morbidity from *cumulative* exposures to toxicants and stressors. We get sick more often from toxic hazards and are also more likely than other groups to lack access to medical care for our chronic and acute health problems. By the time we get medical care, we are usually close to death in an emergency room. This mistreatment of our nation's workers must end.

In the social sciences, we have a term that is used to describe the conditions that limit access to affordable quality health care: poverty. The concept of poverty itself is very political. In our country, let's be honest, we don't like poor people and we view them as outcasts who only have themselves to blame for their presumed wretchedness; we watch with disdain while poor and homeless people rummage through dumpsters in search of their next meal and think: "See, they are just too dirty and lazy to get a job." This racist stereotype flies in the face of the fact that most of the poor in the USA are the *working* poor.

How we define and view poverty is part of the problem of how we approach the values we place on public health. Drawing from the work of my colleague Vandana Shiva (1988), a philosopher of science and ecofeminist activist from India, I want to propose that there are two kinds of poverty: The first is the poverty of a right livelihood or subsistence way of life. This is not real poverty: People who practice right livelihoods are well fed, well housed, and have access to all the resources they need to be self-reliant and healthy. Moreover, their ecological or carbon footprint is smaller than the average hyper-consuming recycler in the global North. It is only poverty because the development planners and international development agencies call it poverty since such persons and communities do not follow a western-styled high consumption lifestyle (Escobar 1996). Indeed, today the subsistence farmer is increasingly appreciated as someone who not only provides for the family but does so using traditional environmental knowledge (TEK) or ethnoecology to contribute to the protection of the earth's ecosystems. Anthropologists have a term for such people: We call them "cultures of habitat" or "ecosystem peoples" because they are able to make a living without damaging the environment (Peña 2005a:28–33). The second type of poverty is the *poverty of deprivation* and this is real poverty in the sense of a loss of independent sources of livelihoods that plunge one into a persistent state of physical, biological, cultural, and economic hardship. When you are deprived of the land, water, and other usually communal resources that sustain your livelihood, you become poor. Deprived of their homelands and their traditional ecological practices, displaced peoples move into the cities where they are becoming a "burden" to the neoliberal state that tries to manage the potential threat to corporatist order posed by displaced populations in what is rapidly becoming a "planet of slums" (Davis 2007). This represents deprivation for the Earth as well since displaced people can no longer practice livelihoods that were also critical to the resilience and protection of ecosystems and biocultural diversity. The irony is that the poverty of deprivation is almost always a result of economic development policies imposed from the outside under the spell, most recently, of the neoliberal charm of privatization and "free trade."

This brings me to another concept that has become very important ever since Paul Farmer et al. (2006) used it to describe the poverty of deprivation faced by Haitians. This is the concept of "structural violence." The term, which was first used in the 1960s and which has commonly been ascribed to Johan Galtung (1969), denotes a form of violence which corresponds with the systematic ways in which a given social structure or social institution kills people slowly by preventing them from meeting their basic needs. Institutionalized elitism, ethnocentrism, classism, racism, sexism, adultism, nationalism, heterosexism, and ageism are just some examples of structural violence. Life spans are reduced when people are socially dominated, politically oppressed, or economically exploited. Structural violence and direct violence are highly interdependent. Structural violence inevitably produces conflict and, often, direct violence including family violence, intimate partner violence, racial violence and hate crimes, terrorism, genocide, and war. Obviously, the poverty of deprivation is the most significant unacknowledged form of structural violence. Such "total" deprivation is most likely to occur in conditions that are also accompanied by political forms of violence by the state against targeted populations.

Yet, based on my own field observations, many workers in public health and environmental protection fields are largely unfamiliar with the concept of structural violence nor do they have the legal, professional, or institutional frameworks, ethics included, to address the effects of the structural violence of deprivation on the health and well-being of communities. Why should public and environmental health professionals be concerned with structural violence? Because scientific studies demonstrate that the structural violence of poverty [sic] is the single most important compounding factor associated with negative health outcomes (Farmer et al. 2006). Poverty – if I may offer a less ideologically loaded definition – is the status of living with limited resources that have been systematically and often violently denied or rendered insufficient for viable social and biological reproduction. Systemic denial and insufficiency of sustenance is a basic neoliberal tenet enforced by the state in the so-called devolution of authority for self-care to the individual and the logic of market forces. Of course, this is closely associated with lack of access to health care and medicine as the single most important compounding factor in the legacy of toxic racism and classism. We cannot address public and environmental heath disparities until we systematically address the problems associated with structural violence.

Poverty reduction, if it is understood as a reversal of the loss of independent livelihoods and the restoration of the commons, is probably our most important strategy to promote long-term health improvements in low-income and people of color communities. Professionals in public and environmental health are told that this is not within their purview or responsibility and that this is something the crumbling remnants of the welfare state are supposed to address; the elusive and ephemeral social safety net is some one else's responsibility; or not. But no one is addressing this issue and millions are falling between the cracks into what I would call a "health-care desert." The origins of the current economic and financial crisis make it clear that there is a direct link between economic exploitation, environmental degradation, and poor public health outcomes. How environmental and public health professionals link the struggle for better health care to the struggle to end the structural violence of poverty will be a pivotal turning point in this movement.

But there are other issues related to structural violence that the EJM recognizes and to some extent addresses. One of these is the problem of "historical trauma," a concept that was first developed and used by researchers studying the intergenerational health problems of Holocaust survivors and their families. More recently, Native American research scholars like my colleague Karina Walters have developed studies that focus on the intergenerational trauma experienced by native cultures and communities that have been subjected to centuries of colonial domination in the aftermath of conquest (Walters and Evans-Campbell 2004; Walters and Simoni 1999; Walters et al. 2002). This approach defines historical trauma as the "collective emotional and psychological injury both over the life span and across generations, resulting from a cataclysmic history of genocide." Moreover, the "effects of historical trauma include unsettled trauma, depression, high mortality, increase of alcohol abuse, child abuse, and domestic violence" (see http://www.historicaltrauma.com). Historical trauma is linked to structural and direct violence and is much more pervasive than acknowledged by activists in the EJM.

Indeed, a growing number of people identify themselves as part of massive postneoliberal "Mesoamerican Diaspora" – these are the indigenous Mexican immigrant workers in the USA, Canada, and Europe (Mares and Peña 2010a, b). This Diaspora indicates resilience in the face of historical trauma associated with structural violence that affects most of these displaced and itinerant populations. I have spoken with indigenous women from Oaxaca, Chiapas, Guerrero, and other parts of Mexico and Guatemala for a collaborative study of the role of Mesoamerican people in the food justice movement that involves growing participation in urban agriculture (Mares and Peña 2010a, b). Many indigenous women relate personal experiences and stories of violence at the hands of intimate partners or military personnel during village incursions. They have experienced death squads sent by rural caciques (political bosses) to displace people from ejidos or squatter communities. They have suffered from the murder or disappearance of family members who had run-ins with the hired guns and of the narco-trafficking networks. Many are enduring the face of state terrorism coupled with extensive intimate partner violence. The greatest source of historical trauma, rooted in systemic genocidal violence, may be the displacement of people from their homeland territories. The loss of one's connection to landscape, to place, has been verified as strongly associated with poor health outcomes. Place-breaking makes heart-breaking possible. Of course, try explaining this to a permit hearing officer or health inspector who is only interested in the quantifiable measures of cost/benefit analysis, a point I will return to shortly.

Environmental Justice is a Collective Action Movement

The structural violence of poverty, coupled with the cumulative effects of intergenerational historical trauma, is the principal compounding factor affecting the deteriorating health of our bodies and the degradation of our environments. I think one reason we ignore these structural factors is that we have been living and working for the past three decades under the weight of the expansion of the neoliberal ideology of privatization and deregulation. We have been limited by bureaucratic structures that resist innovation and deplore anything that makes society accountable for the collective effects of private investment and disinvestment decisions. We live in the new gilded "Age of Individual Responsibility" to go along with the so-called "Ownership Society". Both of these concepts are truly nonsensical ideologies, and every one of us has a responsibility to challenge such concepts as immoral and destructive every chance we get.

I am not against persons becoming empowered through education and economic opportunities to become independently capable of caring for themselves. There is nothing wrong with self-reliance. However, what we have in our society today is not self-reliance but the myth of the individual as a fully self-serving entity in times and under conditions that block people at every step of the way from being able to care for themselves. What I see is not self-reliance and rugged individualism but isolation and alienation from community and families. One recent study of hunger found that people, especially the working poor, are more likely to struggle on their own to find food rather than engage in a collective response to the cause of hunger, which is of course poverty (Poppendieck 1996). This is especially the case among immigrants who may have lost the connections to family and community that provide the social and cultural capital used for mutual aid and survival.

Unfortunately, as we become more "Americanized," Latina/os lose an important part of their culture: that part that has made us strong and resilient through our ties to family and community; as we assimilate, we forget how to be a "we." Richard Rodriguez recently observed, in an undated National Public Radio interview: "We only know how to be me." Thus, one of the principal barriers to environmental justice and a truly healthy community is the persistence of this banal and damaging ideology of individualism. We need to educate people, including health-care providers and environmental regulators, to recognize the healing powers of the collective and respect the fact that many people, especially those in the Mesoamerican Diaspora, do not think first of individual rights or needs but instead focus their behavior around norms related to a strong sense of communal obligations and the need for collective choices or at least personal decisions that are not detrimental to others. We need to challenge the neoliberal ideology of individual responsibility with a new community-based care ethic that values collaboration, participation, and collective action.

This loss of a sense of community and decline of a collective identity has serious implications for public health that we have not even begun to recognize let alone study. One of the intriguing implications has to do with the so-called Latino health paradox. The socioeconomic status model of health predicts that low socioeconomic status is strongly correlated with poor health outcomes. However, as the work of David Hayes-Bautista, Dolores Acevedo-Garcia, Lisa M. Bates, and other research scholars demonstrates, despite their low socioeconomic status, Latinos are healthier than many white middle-class Americans across many categories of disease and illness (Hayes-Bautista 2002; Acevedo-Garcia and Bates 2008). While Latinos tend to have higher rates of morbidity from HIV/AIDS, diabetes, and substance abuse, and gun violence, they tend to fare better across a wide range of other disease categories including those associated with certain cancers and cardiovascular illnesses. One reason for this paradox is related to the fact that our collective family and community-based assets or "social capital" provides a buffer against the negative effects of our community's low-income status.

It is precisely this form of social capital, which requires collective mobilization and community-oriented collaboration, that is most endangered by assimilation. A critical view will posit that this largely is limited to "acculturation" or better *deculturation* since we can never really become "Americans," from the distorted vantage point of reactionary forces (Aldama 2001). The environmental justice movement needs to more thoughtfully confront this intricate set of problems that link structural violence and historical trauma to declining health as a result of the compounding loss of community-based networks and social capital. Our societal institutions expect people to take care of themselves and then deny them their own culturally based and appropriate resources to do so.

Disqualifying Local Knowledge: Administrative Cultures and the Politics of "Risk Science"

I turn next to a dimension of the problem of structural violence that is too often overlooked. Earlier, I defined structural violence as a form of violence which corresponds with the systematic ways in which a given social structure or social institution kills people slowly by preventing them from meeting their basic needs. What if the way our society defines the concept of "basic needs" is itself part of the problem? We live in a society that values two things above all else: The "Individual" and "Private Property and Wealth" (or at least the money-form of wealth). Both of these are tied to the ethic that banally equates freedom with "freedom to consume." The EJM has the potential to shift our paradigm of basic needs by challenging the privilege accorded to these two concepts that are internalized to a degree and in a manner not unlike that of a religious conversion. Nothing gets most people riled up more than attacks on their notions of God or their idea that the key to happiness is for everyone to stay the hell out of the way so they can be free to pursue their private efforts at self-aggrandizement and acquisitiveness. This is the most pervasive and dangerous American myth spawned by neoliberal behavioral economics that is currently challenging our prospects for building meaningful local, place-based institutions of collective action for a just sustainability.

As long as we believe in capitalism as the "end of history" we will be plagued by this myth and its dangerous consequences for public and environmental health. The "cult of self-enrichment" and individual acquisitiveness is more than an affliction caused by a deficit of moral grounding: A popular bumper sticker reads: "He who dies with the most toys, wins." These norms imply that we must accept, as the "externality" of individual freedom, the enormous costs to other people and the environment produced by the ruthless and blind pursuit of individual wealth. Indeed, Schmitt, the Nazi Jurist, and Hayek, the Nobel Prize-winning Austrian founder of *ordo*liberalism, both agreed that the only "equality" is the "equality of inequality" (Brown 2006). This mindset is why *los chicanos*, invented the concept of *vergüenza*. The absence of shame for the harm brought to others as a result of actions designed solely for individual gain is what we call a state of *sinvergüenzas*. I learned this from my grandmother and it is a really important ethic that guides us in awareness of the virtue of *vergüenza* – a notion that invokes the existence of moral obligations to a collective, to something beyond the one self (Peña 2005a:xix).

Learning from my grandmother brings up another issue that is part of the theoretical-practical problem of environmental justice. I stated earlier that the EJM is not just against toxic racism; it is also for ecological democracy; that is, the EJM stands for the widest participation of the people in defining and settling matters of public policy and decision-making in the area of environmental protection and governance (Peña 2005a:139–146). Yet, nothing is worst than the way in which, even in an administrative culture influenced by the "Principles of Environmental Justice," most policy and decision-making practices still follow a tendency to exclude or limit the input of people in affected communities. Their disqualification is often couched in technical or technocratic concepts.

My grandmother had knowledge of the environment: She grew a polyculture home kitchen garden or *huerto familiar*; she knew wild plants and their medicinal and nutritional properties; she was an ardent seed saver and understood the importance of selecting the best and most diverse set of seeds for the next season; she warned me to stay away from Chacon Creek because it was filled with untreated sewage and she had observed other neighborhood children getting sick after playing in the tainted waters. In other words, my grandmother was an indigenous ethnoscientist. She had tremendous ethnoecological and agroecological knowledge. Indeed, most of the communities I work with have this sort of knowledge that some researchers have come to call "kitchen table science" because women gathered in the kitchen to discuss the patterns and problems of life they observe in their own neighborhoods are often the first to share this knowledge with others women in the "politically gendered" space of the kitchen (Novotny 1998). Of course, it was Lois Gibbs that received credit for this idea even if untold thousands of Chicanas and mexicanas had been doing this all along, as any liberal can see in documentaries like *Salt of the Earth.*

We have in most states, including California, an administrative culture in the fields of environmental protection and regulation that is really a "cult of experts." These experts in lab white typically do not understand or value local place-based knowledge. In fact, the current regime for environmental impact studies, risk science, and similar areas of administrative law and regulation is largely based on the single-minded pursuit of presumed neutral and objective quantitative measurement known as *cost/benefit analysis* (Peña and Gallegos 1997). This reduction of data and analysis to number-crunching exercises, that too often turn out to be based on incomplete, finagled, or tainted data, obscures many of the factors associated with perceptions of risk and risk management. The cult of expertise, and its fetish for cost/benefit analysis, dismisses or disqualifies the local knowledge of people like my grandmother who have no professional or specialized training other than that which is part of their received cultural capital and direct lived experience. Experts are privileged in their positions of authority and this often means that the process of assessment and evaluation ends up constrained by an incomplete understanding of a given situation of environmental risk (Fischer 2000; Forsyth 2002).

This disregard for local place-based knowledge is a form of epistemological violence: It is based on blatant disregard for the knowledge people develop over time by living and working in place. Over the past three decades, I have often testified as an "expert" witness in various contexts (landfill permit hearings, EIS, Title VI actions, etc.) related to environmental protection and in every single case, the experts for the corporate or governmental stakeholders demeaned and dismissed local knowledge as too "qualitative" or "emotive" and thus "unscientific." This is not just antidemocratic; it is actually more antiscientific and ill advised since too often, as I can vouch, this results in mistaken decisions based on faulty and incomplete data steered by market-oriented interests. We have to resist and transform the false participation process that leads into the cul-de-sac of the cost/benefit decision-making matrix. This leads to premeditated decisions based on the restrictive assumptions of quantitative data.

The problem in part resides in the failure for Congress to enact laws and regulations that bring the entire risk science system into sync with the actual "state of the art." There are methods and models available to develop a more holistic science of risk that (1) integrates local place-based knowledge, (2) accounts for the compounding factors of structural violence and historical trauma, and (3) provides for the analysis of *cumulative* risk factors. This should include the requirement that hearing officers, courts, commissioners, and other decision-makers accept the use of qualitative ethnographic materials as singularly appropriate to the task of presenting and evaluating data sets associated with so-called social impact assessment (SIA) or community impact analysis (CIA). We may, for example, develop and operationalize indices of "social well-being" that can "quantify" the relative weight of attributes like "sense of place" and "original instructions," since these have been shown to constitute an important part of the cognitive and emotional basis necessary for sustaining the social capital invested in community health. These are not radical ideas, but there is such a pervasive and deep-rooted quantitative bias in the risk science community that these proposals are usually waved aside as "idealistic" and "ethical" rather than scientific.

I remember attending a meeting organized by James K. Boyce for the Ford Foundation in Santa Fe back in 2001. The meeting involved EJ activist-scholars and other researchers, foundation executives, and EPA scientists and administrators. The meeting was primarily convened to discuss how to integrate the value of natural capital and related community-based assets into strategies to "democratize" environmental ownership as part of poverty reduction programs at Ford. One especially contentious issue focused on the role of federal and state regulatory agencies like the EPA, which the EJ activists viewed as limiting and manipulating the nature of risk science and environmental impact study as *deliberative* practices. The EJ activists interrogated the EPA staff members during one of the sessions because the governmental representatives insisted that we could only "meaningfully" discuss clarifying what the Clinton Administration wanted to accomplish, specifically with regard to proposals for redefining the standards for the official definition of "minimally acceptable" risk.

The EJ activist-scholars present were undeterred in deconstructing the underlying rationality of the concept of "minimally acceptable" risk. The position of the EJM on this issue was and remains clear, Richard Moore noted: EJ principles reject the concept of "minimally acceptable" risk. There is no such thing as any level of "acceptable risk" to the person affected. One death is too many. Movement activists are told this is unrealistic and impractical. For us, this is a matter of normative paradigms, and the need to challenge extant risk assessment frameworks which seem especially repugnant because industrial ecologists and environmental engineers have long been demonstrating that pollution *can be avoided*; we don't have to produce toxic wastes to produce food, shelter, and even automobiles and similar machines. *Detoxification and containment at the point of production is technologically attainable*. The neoliberal economists will object and declare that this is not profitable and therefore untenable. We would, of course, be justified in dismissing neoliberal claims in light of the world financial capitalist and credit market crises after September 2008.

Some 10 years ago, the EPA wanted us to endorse the idea that we can and should minimize risk to an acceptable level of deaths from pollution. This rather perverse philosophy is based on the notion that environmental hazards are an inevitable "externality" of our capitalist economic system. Except, of course, these are not "externalities" since toxins and other hazardous wastes are "internalized costs" to nature and people. But according to this Clintonian neoliberal view the best we can do is to "mitigate" risk through regulation and perhaps gradual incremental cleanup of the most serious air, water, and soil pollution. Everyone needs to agree to share an equal piece of the mitigated poison pie.

The EJ response to this type of "equity"-based policy is expressed most clearly in the sixth of the 17 Principles of Environmental Justice, and I mention these not as some sort of dogma but, frankly, as a rather sensible set of ideas: The sixth Principle "demand[s] an end to the production of all toxins, hazardous wastes, and radioactive materials...[and] detoxification and containment at the point of production." This approach does not mitigate pollution after it happens; it instead works to prevent the pollution in the first place. The current trend toward a "Green jobs movement" should therefore involve not just the creation of new "ecologically friendly" jobs. Perhaps more urgently, green jobs also means transforming existing production systems and practices toward systems that do not impose *avoidable risks* on the workforce or surrounding communities. This simple notion of *avoidable risk as against minimally acceptable risk* needs to become a "framing" concept we consistently place on the table as we negotiate the terms of our engagement as communities with the politics of risk science and risk management [sic].

Detoxification and containment, rather than the band-aid of "minimally acceptable" risk, remains the foremost environmental justice goal in this policy area. It is in this sense that the EJM is a struggle for democracy wedded to a campaign for environmentally safe production methods and technologies. Of course, unless we democratize the entire institutional edifice of the environmental protection and regulatory community we will never get close to realizing these demands. Discussion of these issues of democratic public access and meaningful participation in the decision- and policy-making processes is necessary. Indeed, soon enough many of the experts who make a living in these fields may find themselves replaced by a new wave of experts. Experts in toxicogenomics and mass genotyping may come to replace the standard "remote social science" purveyed by too many demographic and socioeconomic data analysts (Peña 2005a) employed by state regulators [sic] and corporations. These are the ranks of expert epidemiologists ready to ridicule and dismiss the next Native grandmother that protests black lung disease or asthma among tribal [sic] children as "storytelling." A new age of "pharmogenomics" also beckons, promising individualized medicine for the self-caring genotyped cyborg. The current experts will no longer be recognized as such by a regime based on decision-making derived from the science of genomics, bioinformatics, and their spin-offs.

Restoring the Common in the Age of the Ecology of Fear

I want to conclude by reference to a phrase I developed of restoring the "common" in the age of the "ecology of fear." This means discussing once more a concept that we too often take for granted: This is the concept of the "individual." All of our laws, and indeed much of our social identity as Americans, are based on the concept of the individual and of individual rights.

Most of the indigenous or ethnic cultures of the world do not have a word for "individual" in their Native languages. There are words like "self" and "person," and even pronouns roughly equivalent to "I" and even "me." But most of these peoples have no analog for the apparently distinctly Western concept of the "individual." Indeed, many of the Mesoamerican Diaspora people I work with along the entire length of the West Coast originate in cultures that lack a word in their native tongue for "individual." Some, like the Nahua, use the term "skin" to refer to the body,[2] emphasizing that we are human only through our connection to the social "Other," that which is, as the Lacandon Maya insist, always "my other self" (*in lak ech*). The dominant and reactionary forces in our society, which are confronted by an increasingly "shifting multicultural mosaic" nation that is indeed leading to the dissolution of borders "from the bottom-up," insist that the concept of the individual is the key to our liberal democratic rule of law, human progress, and economic prosperity. This legal regime insists that there are only individual rights. Group "rights," which native people tend to view as collective obligations to care for place, are dismissed as quaint relics, irrelevant and maladaptive norms, or worst legally impractical principles because these norms are posited as incompatible with the underlying tenets of modern Anglo American positive law (see Peña 2005b).

Obviously, I beg to differ on this characterization of place-based cultures as disappearing and irrelevant "relics." In my own family and community, I have learned that the individual has not replaced the concept of the person as a "being connected to others." Numerous Native American cultures also do not have a word for individual; they have words for "person," "being," and pronouns (like we, us), but they do not have a word for individual. What does this mean?

It means that we are in the midst of a longstanding conflict in areas of environmental protection and health and ecosystem management that, while based on recognition of collective responsibility, is still driven largely by the logic of individualized rights in a capitalist market economy. This is systematically wed to the quantification of risk and the politics of nomenclature as when technicians, bureaucrats, or permit hearing officers use concepts like "actionable" levels of exposure to risk in order to mask the underlying problems of cumulative risk and compounding factors including those associated with structural violence and intergenerational historical trauma.

Both in deference and variance to Mike Davis's use of the concept, I often use the phrase "Ecology of Fear" to describe this type of situation. Most Americans across race, class, gender, and sexuality are afraid of falling behind and not getting ahead. We are afraid to fail as individuals. We fear death from terrorism and natural catastrophes or from lack of access to health care and adequate nutrition. We are afraid of the air we breathe, the water we drink, and the food we eat. All the substances that make life now threaten to kill us. We are afraid of difference and blame the immigrant or the "Native" as a further threat and hindrance to unrealized desires in and through the "American Dream," which has clearly become a neoliberal nightmare that commodifies both risk *and* difference (Brown 2006). Women are afraid to walk alone day or night; Juarez and Tijuana have become massive killing fields filled with the victims of serial killers, rapists, and the principals and dupes of drug wars [sic]; Homes are filled with women ravaged by intimate partner violence at the hands of men that are themselves terrorized by unemployment, drugs, alcohol, and a history of abuse themselves. This is the ecology of fear. It unleashes the forces and reactions of a surveillance or Panoptican state, transforming the

[2] Tezozomoc, in personal communication to the author (April 10, 2010, Seattle, WA).

"border" – and indeed the entire territory of the "sovereign" power – into a national security/counter-terrorism/immigration control military-police action zone.

How did we get to such a condition of environmental and social deprivation and degradation where borders are both imposed and constantly transgressed? Even in the midst of all this individualized "wealth," which is ultimately extracted from our "commonwealth," the rich are also afraid of losing it all or being stripped of their acquisitions by the less fortunate. The ecology of fear, like the endemic problems of structural violence and historical trauma, is sustained by the another "cult" – of the individual rational actor. It turns out that the actor has acted rather selfishly and irrationally to the point of self-destruction, and even contemporary "Randians" complain that the Wall Street bailout was against the logic of capitalism's need for "creative destruction." In this regard, an important challenge for the EJM is the intersection of the struggles for environmental rights and community self-determination in ecological decision-making with the heightened tensions and conflicts unleashed by the insidious fascism of the "287(g) agreements" between local police forces and the Department of Homeland Security that are tearing families and communities apart. The EJ struggle has always included police–community interactions as part of our everyday lived experience in the built environment. How this connects with the ability of communities to organize for environmental and economic justice remains a central challenge today.

If environmental and food justice advocates and activists, environmental health practitioners, and environmental regulators and decision-makers are to move closer as part of a collective action movement toward a just, resilient, and sustainable future, we will have to become indignant over the conditions of a world rendered barren and distorted by this ecology of fear. To challenge that ecology of fear you will have to develop and explore more collective forms of action and mutual aid. You will have to trust in local place-based knowledge and revalue meaningful, set from the get-go, types of public participation. Indeed, we need spaces to self-mobilize around the issues brought to the forefront of policy debates by our own place-based ecological knowledge and "kitchen table science."

What I have witnessed over the past three decades is that, when Latina/os coalesce themselves into organizations for collective action, we can create our own opportunities and freedoms based on the "old-fashioned" values of self-reliance and mutual aid that our grandparents needed to survive in times not unlike ours (Peña 2005a). If we go at it alone, as individual automatons, well, sure, you may or may not get ahead for yourself by the typical measures of wealth. However, your own individual aggrandizement will do little for your community despite acts of charity. The EJM is a collective social action movement concerned with justice for all and not just "individuals" – it is about "Justice" and not "Just Us." Rebuilding our communities as places that are safe for our children requires that we reclaim the "commons" – our environmental qualities of open space, clean air and water, and homes and workplaces free of lead, PCBs, dioxins, and other toxicants. Such a movement is premised on the basic idea that the most important value of a human life is what it contributes to realizing our mutual obligations in sustaining the well-being of our families, communities, and our common life-support system, the Earth.

The politics of health and health care in this manner might be transformed from yet another free market fundamentalist trapdoor that leads to a world in which competitive desire constrains us to seek self-fulfillment based on incommensurable differences. It allows us toward resurgence as a more democratic, place-based, and collective action society that values difference without marking the entrenchment of identity politics as its ultimate referent of "self-care."

References

Acevedo-Garcia, D and L Bates 2008. Latino health paradoxes: Empirical evidence, explanations, future research, and implications. In: *Latinas/os in the United States: Changing the face of America,* eds. H Rodríguez, R Sáenz, and C Menjívar. New York: Springer, 101–113.

Agyeman, J, R Bullard, and B Evans (eds.) 2003. *Just sustainabilities: Development in an unequal world.* Cambridge: MIT Press/Earthscan.

Aldama, A 2001. *Disrupting savagism: Intersecting Chicana/o, Mexican immigrant, and Native American struggles for self-representation.* Durham: Duke University Press.

Brown, W 2006. American nightmare: Neoliberalism, neoconservatism, and de-democratization. *Political Theory* 34(6):690–714.

Bullard, R, et al. 2007. *Toxic wastes and race at twenty.* New York: United Church of Christ, Commission for Racial Justice.

Bullard, R (ed.) 2005. *The quest for environmental justice: Human rights and the politics of pollution.* San Francisco: Sierra Club Books.

Casillas, M 1979. *Mexicans, labor, and strife in Arizona, 1896-1917.* MA Thesis, University of New Mexico, Department of History.

Davis, M 2007. *Planet of slums.* New York: Verso Books.

Escobar, A 1996. *Encountering development: The making and unmaking of the third world.* Princeton: Princeton University Press.

Farmer, P, B Nizeye, S Stulac, and S Keshavjee 2006. Structural violence and clinical medicine. *PLoS [Public Library of Science] Medicine* 3(10):449.

Fischer, F 2000. *Citizens, experts, and the environment: The politics of local knowledge.* Durham: Duke University Press.

Forsyth, T 2002. *Critical political ecology: The politics of environmental science.* New York: Routledge Press.

Galtung, J 1969. Violence, peace, and peace research. *Journal of Peace Research* 6(3):167–191.

González Navarro, M 1997. Racism and mestizaje. In: *Common borders, uncommon paths: Race, culture, and national identity in U.S.-Mexican relations,* eds. Jaime E Rodríguez O and Kathryn Vincent. Berkeley: University of California Press.

Hayes-Bautista, D 2002. The Latino health research agenda for the twenty-first century. In: Latinos: Remaking America, eds. M Suárez and M Páez. Berkeley: University of California Press, 215–235.

La Botz, D 1992. *Mask of democracy: Labor suppression in Mexico today.* Boston: South End Press.

Mares, T and D Peña 2010a. Urban agriculture in the making of insurgent space in Los Angeles and Seattle. In: *Insurgent public space: Guerrilla urbanism and the remaking of the contemporary city,* ed. J Hou. New York: Rutgers University Press.

Mares, T and D Peña 2010b. Environmental and food justice: Toward local, slow, and deep food systems. In: *The food justice reader; Cultivating a just sustainability,* eds. A Alkon and J Agyeman. Cambridge: MIT Press.

Mark, J 2006. Workers on organic farms are treated as poorly as their conventional counterparts. *Grist* (2 Aug.). Accessed at URL: http://www.grist.org/article/mark/.

Novotny, P 1998. Popular epidemiology and the struggle for community health in the environmental justice movement. In: *The struggle for ecological democracy: Environmental justice movements in the United States*, ed. D Faber. New York: Guilford Press, 137–158.

Pellow, D and R Brulle (eds.) 2005. *Power, justice, and the environment: A critical appraisal of the environmental justice movement.* Cambridge: MIT Press.

Peña, D 1992. The brown and the green: Chicanos and environmental politics in the American Southwest. *Capitalism, Nature, Socialism* 3(1):79–103.

Peña, D 2002. *Environmental justice and sustainable agriculture: Linking social and ecological sides of sustainability*. Occasional Paper Series, Second National People of Color Environmental Leadership Summit, Washington, D.C. 23–27 October. URL: http://www.ejrc.cau.edu/summit2/SustainableAg.pdf.

Peña, D 2005a. *Mexican Americans and the environment: tierra y vida.* Tucson: University of Arizona Press.

Peña, D 2005b. Autonomy, equity, and environmental justice. In: *Power, justice, and the environment: A critical appraisal of the environmental justice movement,* eds. D Pellow and R Bruxex. Cambridge: MIT Press, 131–152.

Peña, D and J Gallegos 1997. Local knowledge and collaborative environmental action research. In: *Building community: Social science in action*, eds. P Nyden, A Figert, M Shibley, and D Burrows. Thousand Oaks, CA: Pine Forge Press.

Poppendieck, J 1996. Hunger in America: Typification and response. In: *Eating agendas: Food and nutrition as social problems*, eds. D Maurer and J Sobal. Hawthorne: Aldine DeGruyter.

Pulido, L and D Peña 1998. Environmentalism and positionality: The early pesticide campaign of the United Farm Workers' Organizing Committee, 1966-71. *Race, Gender, and Class* 6(1):33–50.

Ruiz, R E 1988. *The people of Sonora and Yankee capitalists*. Tucson: University of Arizona Press.

Shiva, V 1988. *Staying alive: Women, ecology, and development*. London: Zed Books.

Walters, K and T Evans-Campbell 2004. *Measuring historical trauma among urban American Indians*. Paper presented at the University of New Mexico, School of Medicine, Albuquerque, NM (February).

Walters, K and J Simoni 1999. Trauma, substance use, and HIV risk among urban American Indian women. *Cultural Diversity and Ethnic Minority Psychology* 5:236–248.

Walters, K, J Simoni, and T Evans-Campbell 2002. Substance use among American Indians and Alaska natives: Incorporating culture in an "indigenist" stress-coping paradigm. *Public Health Report* 117(Suppl. 1): S104–S117.

Chapter 12
Environmental Justice and the Well-being of Poor Children of Color

Michael S. Spencer, Amanda Garratt, Elaine Hockman, Bunyan Bryant and Laura Kohn-Wood

Researchers and activists in the environmental justice movement have long argued that socioeconomically disadvantaged communities of color are disproportionately exposed to various forms of environmental hazards and risks (Boer et al. 1997; Mohai and Bryant 1992; Pulido 1996; Sadd et al. 1999). Children living in these communities are among the most vulnerable members of our population (Bearer 1995). The disparity in exposure to environmental hazards that poor children of color endure has serious implications for their health and well-being and for the health of future generations. One mechanism to help resolve this problem is for communities to devise strategies that address issues of environmental injustice. This chapter describes a community-based, participatory research (CBPR) study that aims to increase awareness of the impact of environmental hazards among parents of children enrolled in Head Start programs in the City of Detroit. We describe how features of places can be used to enact meaningful social change in a community. The study was intended to build the capacity of parents to develop strategies for protecting their children and the children within their community from the harmful impact of environmental hazards. Specifically, the study uses Photovoice (Wang 1999), a participatory action methodology that blends photography and social action, as a tool for increasing awareness and promoting grassroots response to address the problem in Detroit Head Start communities.

Race, Socioeconomic Status, and Children's Well-being

Numerous studies have documented the effects of poverty and environmental risk factors on children's well-being, such as long-term deficits in physical health, motor coordination, problem solving, attention, and academic achievement

M.S. Spencer (✉)
School of Social Work, University of Michigan, Ann Arbor, MI, USA
e-mail: spencerm@umich.edu

L.M. Burton et al. (eds.), *Communities, Neighborhoods, and Health*,
Social Disparities in Health and Health Care 1, DOI 10.1007/978-1-4419-7482-2_12,

(Brooks-Gunn and Duncan 1997; Capaldi and Patterson 1994; Dryfoos 1990; Hammen and Rudolph 1996; Huston et al. 1994; Pollitt and Gorman 1994; Werner and Smith 1992). The effects of poverty on the well-being of children appear to be mediated through a number of factors including exposure to environmental toxins (McLoyd 1998). Evidence for the inverse association between low socioeconomic status and environmental hazards, such as hazardous wastes and other toxins, ambient and indoor air pollutants, water quality, and ambient noise, exacerbate the deleterious effects of poverty on the health and well-being of poor communities (Evans and Kantrowitz 2002).

Numerous studies have found that poverty alone does not fully explain the disproportionate distribution of environmental hazards in the USA and that race is a more potent predictor of this disparity. For example, in the landmark study of race, toxins, and hazardous waste landfills, commissioned by the United Church of Christ (1987), researchers found that race was the most significant variable tested in association with the location of commercial hazardous waste facilities. Furthermore, although socioeconomic status appeared to play an important role in the location of commercial hazardous waste facilities, race still proved to be the most significant factor.

Since the United Church of Christ report, subsequent studies have repeatedly demonstrated how racial and ethnic minority and low-income populations are disproportionately burdened by environmental hazards and how race is a greater explanatory variable to the distribution of environmental hazards than income (Burke 1993; Faber and Krieg 2002; Gelobter 1987, 1992; Goldman 1994; Hockman and Morris 1998; Lopez 2002; Mohai and Bryant 1992; Morris and Hockman 1997; West et al. 1992). While some researchers have argued that there are insignificant racial differences on a national scale after controlling for income and other covariates that account for the location of environmental hazards (Anderton et al. 1994a, b), other studies indicated that environmental disparities by race do exist at the national level (Been 1994, 1995; Been and Gupta 1997).

Environmental Hazards and Children's Well-being

It is well recognized that children, because of their physiologic characteristics, are particularly susceptible to the toxic effects of environmental hazards and pollutants (see Bearer 1995 for review). Children's exposure to lead is a salient example. Lead-based house paint is the primary source of lead for young children, whether by eating paint chips or breathing the lead dust from deteriorating paint. Using data from the NHANES III, Brooks-Gunn and Duncan (1997) found that children living in poverty (families with income less than 130% of the poverty threshold) were 3.5 times more likely to have lead poisoning (blood lead levels 10 μg/dL or greater). Also, the study reports that overall blood levels were highest among 1–5-year olds from low-income African-American families in large central cities and that the mean levels were almost three times greater than for all 1–5-year olds.

Furthermore, a study by the Agency for Toxic Substances and Disease Registry found that even when controlling for family income, African-American children under the age of 5 were nearly twice as likely to have elevated blood lead levels than white children, providing further evidence of the significance of race above and beyond poverty. Young children may also be at risk through exposure to carbon monoxide, radon, mercury, polycyclic aromatic hydrocarbons such as those found in cigarette smoke, and arsenic and creosote through some treated woods used in playground equipment. Due to their higher metabolic rate, children consume more oxygen relative to their size than do adults and have breathing zones closer to the floor, where heavier chemicals and large breathable particulates settle out, thereby making them more vulnerable to exposure (Bearer 1995). Furthermore, children's vulnerability arises from their inability to protect themselves from these toxins and pollutants.

Place-Based Response

The problems and concerns around race, socioeconomic status, and children's well-being often require the education of parents and policymakers who have the ability to take action. Parental involvement in the well-being of their children through the schools provide one possible avenue for fostering a new generation of local people concerned about environmental injustices and involved in environmental justice activities. CBPR provides a methodology through which this can be achieved. The methodology emphasizes participation in the process of creating knowledge, embodied in constructivist and critical theory paradigms that highlight the socially created nature of scientific knowledge (Israel et al. 1998). When the locus of control of the research partnership is shared with the community, we make the assumption that people are wise and capable of solving their own problems. In many instances, community or nonprofessional people have shown their capability of participating constructively in research, problem solving, and planning activities (e.g., Brown 1991; Brown and Tandon 1993; Carr and Kemmis 1986; DiPerna 1985; Gaventa 1998).

In the environmental justice arena, community people have been successfully involved in a number of community-based research activities. People in Rocky Flats, Colorado, conducted health surveys that played a role in leading to a campaign against nuclear poisoning. In Love Canal, Buffalo, New York, the results of such surveys led to the cleanup of toxic dumpsites (Gaventa 1998). In Woburn, Massachusetts, Harvard-trained community people collected information to substantiate the hypothesis of a housewife that childhood leukemia was associated with drinking water from a local well (Brown 1991; DiPerna 1985). In Appalachia, people collected information from county tax rolls to identify undertaxed properties of absentee landlords, which put pressure on landlords to pay their fair share to support needed social services and fire and police protection.

In summary, poor communities of color have reason to address environmental injustice issues, particularly with their children's well-being at stake. The following is a description of a study that promotes capacity and empowerment of parents of children in Detroit Head Start programs around addressing environmental justice in their communities. We describe the use of Photovoice process, the mechanism through which we identify community perspectives on the problem, involve and educate parents, and promote social action.

The Project

The study was conceived from an interdisciplinary collaboration between Detroit Head Start staff, the Family Development Project at the University of Michigan, School of Social Work and the Environmental Justice Initiative located in the School of Natural Resources and Environment. We utilize a community-based participatory research methodology where we involve community members in all aspects of the research process including problem definition, data collection, analysis, and dissemination.

The setting. The City of Detroit is a large urban center in Wayne County with a very diverse population close to one million people. Until recently, it experienced a sustained period of economic decline. Detroit is one of the most diverse cities in the USA and at the same time one of its most racially segregated. Within its boundaries are Latinos, European Americans, Asians, and American Indians, but African Americans constitute nearly 82% of the city's population (U.S. Census 2000). Eight delegates of the Detroit Head Start program lie within the city boundaries. Our CBPR study was conducted in Detroit's largest delegate agency that incorporates 26 Detroit ZIP codes. In Table 12.1, we present data from the U-M Environmental Justice database, which includes the most current environmental hazards information from publicly available sources, including the 2000 US Census, Michigan Department of Environmental Quality, Environmental Protection Agency (EPA), and the Centers for Disease Control and Prevention (CDC). We include demographic characteristics and various indices of environmental toxin exposure, including the asthma index for children over an 8-year period, number of incinerator records, children's lead levels, number of leaky underground storage tanks (LUST) sites, toxic release inventory (TRI) citations, and a pollution density index, representing the number of pollution sources (TRI, Act 307, LUSTs, landfills, hazardous waste facilities, and incinerations) per square mile. The data illustrate exposure to environmental hazards in the ZIP codes where Head Start children live compared to the 28 other ZIP codes in Detroit/Wayne County. We found significant differences between the ZIP codes for all variables except the number of LUST and TRI. Figure 12.1 presents a map of Detroit with pollution density in standard deviation units by ZIP code. The labeled ZIP codes are those where Detroit Head Start children live. The map displays higher levels of pollution density in ZIP codes where Head Start children live, with many ZIP codes where pollution density was two standard deviation units or more. Analysis of variance (ANOVA) for comparing

Table 12.1 Environmental hazard exposure for ZIP codes where Head Start children ($n=26$) live compared to other Detroit/Wayne County ZIP codes ($n=28$)

Variable			
African American (%)	Detroit Head Start	88.71	$p<0.05$
	Other Wayne Co.	13.72	
Household income (Median)	Detroit Head Start	$27,653.38	$p<0.05$
	Other Wayne Co.	$55,563.18	
Adults with high school education (%)	Detroit Head Start	67.11	$p<0.05$
	Other Wayne Co.	83.59	
Low birth weight (%)	Detroit Head Start	12.23	$p<0.05$
	Other Wayne Co.	4.70	
Asthma index for youth over 8-year period	Detroit Head Start	2.32	$p<0.05$
	Other Wayne Co.	0.88	
Number of incinerator records	Detroit Head Start	41.92	$p<0.05$
	Other Wayne Co.	17.36	
Lead	Detroit Head Start	0.086	$p<0.05$
	Other Wayne Co.	0.001	
Number of leaky underground storage tank (LUST) sites	Detroit Head Start	13.65	
	Other Wayne Co.	15.00	
Toxic release inventory (TRI) citations	Detroit Head Start	10.73	
	Other Wayne Co.	9.61	
Pollution density per square mile	Detroit Head Start	15.56	$p<0.05$
	Other Wayne Co.	4.92	

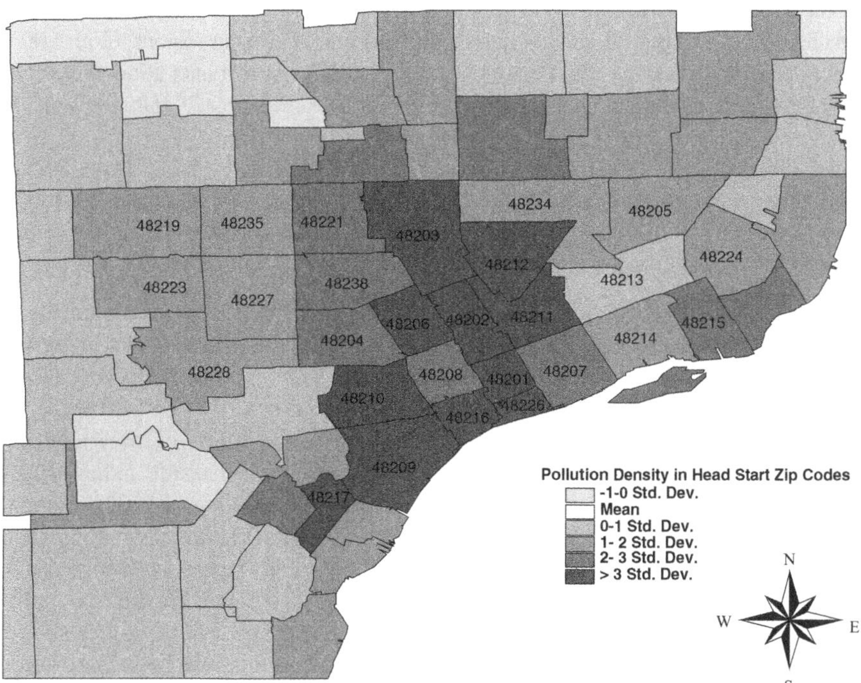

Fig. 12.1 Pollution density in Detroit Head Start ZIP codes in standard deviation units

mean pollution density by Head Start, other Wayne County, and 835 other Michigan ZIP codes found statistically significant differences between the three groups ($F=179.62$, df=870, $p<0.001$).

The sample. A total of 20 parents were recruited to participate in the Photovoice project in 2004–2006. All the participants were of African-American descent. The parents were recruited from the Media subcommittee of the Parent Policy Council. This group was selected by Head Start staff because the group met regularly and represented parents who have a history of involvement in Head Start and its governance. The demographics of the Head Start delegate agency from which our sample was taken include 90% African Americans, 5.5% Hispanic, 2.4% White, 0.5% Asian, and 0.1% Native American, 50.5% Female, and a mean age of 4.8 years of age. The mean household size was 3.5; about 69% of the households were headed by a single parent, and 62% received public assistance at enrollment into Head Start.

Photovoice is a participatory action research methodology that provides people with cameras so they can record and represent their everyday realities. The method is based on the understanding that people are experts on their own lives (see http://www.photovoice.com). Photovoice has three main goals: (1) to enable people to record and reflect their community's strengths and concerns, (2) to promote critical dialogue and knowledge about important issues through large and small group discussion of photographs, and (3) to reach policymakers (Wang and Burris 1997). Photovoice has been applied to a number of local and international settings, including village women in the Yunnan Province, China (Wang et al. 1996, 1998), the homeless in Michigan (Wang 1999; Wang et al. 2000), and youth in Flint, Michigan (Strack et al. 2003; Wang et al. 2004). Using the Photovoice methodology, participants allow their photographs to raise the questions, "Why does this situation exist?" "Do we want to change it, and if so, how?" Also, Photovoice has been adapted for use in clinical nursing practice and research (LeClerc et al. 2002; Riley and Manias 2004), among African-American breast cancer survivors in rural North Carolina (Lopez et al. 2005), Black gay men and lesbians in South Africa (Graziano 2004), and African-American Early Head Start parents on the topic of school readiness (McAllister et al. 2005).

Procedure. The researchers worked with a local environmental justice organization, Detroiter's working for Environmental Justice, to conduct two trainings for interested parents of Head Start children in Detroit. The participants learned the history of the environmental justice movement, important terms related to environmental justice, national and global facts on environmental injustices, the effects of environmental hazards on child development, an overview of environmental hazards and injustices in Detroit, and information on how to identify environmental injustice. The training included a slideshow presentation, a short video, discussion of current environmental policies and statistics, and dialogue among the participants regarding their personal experiences with environmental injustice. At the conclusion of the training, we introduced the Photovoice project and provided a brief training on this method.

In the Photovoice training, the Head Start mothers learned how Photovoice could be used as a community assessment and social action tool. Participants also learned about photography tips and the mechanics of taking good pictures.

Following the training, all consenting participants received one disposable camera. All but one individual participated in our Photovoice project. For 3 weeks, the mothers spent time in their homes and neighborhoods, observing their environments and looking to identify both the elements that contributed to the healthy well-being of their children and the elements that had a damaging effect on the well-being and development of their children. The participants selected six photos to share with the group at the follow-up meeting 3 weeks later.

Focus groups and planning meetings. At the completion of the photo-taking stage, the mothers got together along with the researchers to view and discuss the photos by the parents. Across three meetings, the participants shared and learned from one another as they identified common themes that arose in their discussion. The participants each chose their two favorite "positive" or "healthy" and two favorite "negative" or "unhealthy" photos and wrote captions for each of them, describing the content and their reasons for selecting the particular image.

Throughout the photo analysis process, the participants discussed what they could do to address issues of injustice in their neighborhoods. The focus groups were followed by a series of meetings with the specific objective of drawing out the ideas the parents had for stimulating positive change around environmental justice, as well as for identifying the resources directly available to the group. The group reviewed the outcomes and common themes of the photo analysis and brainstormed possible avenues for action.

At the end of this process, it was decided that the group would organize and host a community forum on environmental justice where the Head Start parents would display and present their Photovoice results to policymakers, the media, the Detroit community, and the general public. The group designed the forum to allow for discussion and contributions from policymakers and the general public. The forum, named by the mothers, was entitled: "Hidden Dangers in our Own Backyard: Does Detroit Deserve Clean Air?" There were more than 80 attendees at the forum, which included community members, policymakers, and media. The half-day event met the following objectives: (a) to give the mothers participating in the Photovoice project a space and time for their voice to be heard and their expertise to be shared, (b) to allow the participants and other members of the community to speak frankly with public officials and policymakers about the environmental issues in their communities, (c) to include academic experts and members of the public to learn and share with one another the realities of environmental justice in Detroit and across the country, and (d) to raise greater public awareness through the incorporation of media coverage.

Community Findings

The Photovoice process revealed that parents tend to see the place effects on children's health through the physical environment. For the purposes of this chapter, we focus on two positive (supportive institutions for their children, e.g., churches and schools, and new housing development) and two negative (abandoned buildings, illegal dumping) perceptions that parents had about their physical environment.

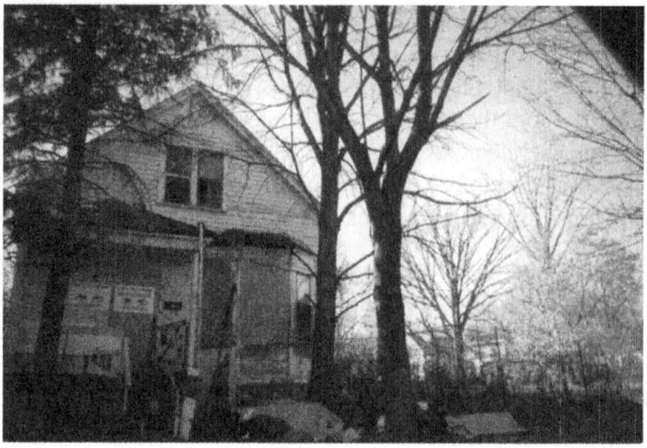

Fig. 12.2 Abandoned home that acts as a physical and psychological hazard for children's well-being

Abandoned homes and buildings. Dramatic photos of abandoned homes and buildings were represented in many of the photos with windows broken, warning signs posted, roofs caved in, and signs of fire prevalent (see Fig. 12.2). Several parents commented on how beautiful the homes and buildings used to be. These brick homes and apartments were well built with many featuring different kinds of stained glass, which has now been destroyed.

Although this abandonment was clearly viewed as an eyesore, parents were more concerned about what their children might find in these homes and what may lurk behind the doors of such abandoned homes. For example, parents feared that their children may wander inside the abandoned structures and possibly encounter drugs or drug paraphernalia, dangerous individuals, or simply have these structures collapse on their children. The location of these abandoned homes and buildings was also a factor. Parents commented on how close these structures were to school zones, playgrounds, and places where children play. For example, one parent stated:

> "This is really scary. This is a house. It has a tarp over it, I have no reason to know why, but it's in the middle of the block and the school is two blocks from this house. There's children playing up and down the street and there's people that live on each side of this house."

Other parents talked about how these homes and buildings have been this way for a while. They wondered why the city allows these buildings to remain. There was a sense of bewilderment; "just unbelievable" it was to see the once well-kept buildings and streets "all broke up." One parent described her photo of an abandoned home in the following way:

> "It's a house that at one time was very nice, but there's just a lot of debris. I believe a tree has fallen (onto the house) and it's right around the corner from the school. If I could find this, how come the city can't find this as a danger zone for children?"

One parent described what a nuisance and danger these types of abandoned and destroyed homes pose to their community and their children. "This house has been there for quite awhile, it is available to squatters, crack heads, homeless folks, and drug dealers. It is an eyesore to parents who don't like seeing it walking their children to school everyday and our kids could be subject to rape or abuse (by those using that building)."

Another parent described the negative image of a destroyed and rotting bus terminal in her community and the lack of action by the city to provide proper maintenance and upkeep of a once thriving bus terminal. "Where is the effort? The windows are busted, there is garbage everywhere for rodents to play in. This is a depleted building who knows what is stored in there? What can they use these buildings for but drugs or dead bodies."

This parent noted the importance of community effort in changing the look and image that this building places on their community. The parents not only explained the lack of the city's effort, but they also validated the importance of the community's voice. "I feel really bad, wow look at all that mess. It's the Mayor's responsibility to make people want to stay in our communities, but people didn't enforce (them to work) in our neighborhood so the city didn't take care of it. If the community demanded that the city do something better, it would happen."

Illegal dumping. Abandoned lots located in close proximity to Head Start children's homes are consumed with debris. Residents are often baffled why the city does not play a major role in the maintenance of abandoned property. Some parents are concerned that the location of the illegal dumping is alongside elementary and middle school routes, essentially exposing youth to opportunities to play, touch, and smell hazardous material. For example, one parent stated:

> "It's like someone used this area for a dumping ground. It smelled so bad, it's like trash and everything around there and it's near the school."

Other parents talked about how the streets are not clean enough for children to play. "The alley is just not clean and it does promote a hazard to the children playing around that area, a biohazard because their waste is not properly stored."

The parents also described the lack of effort by the city and other politicians to remove negative images like these from their community. "No one cares about the poverty level, especially when there are cuts in funding. We (the community) needs to find help, resources, get on the phone or send letters to congressmen telling them about these eye sores and nuisances."

More than the physical dangers of these properties, parents worried about the psychological damage that these buildings and properties had on their children. The parents talked about the sense of hopelessness that could arise from children who have to walk past these places every day. They were further worried that without this sense of hope for their children's future, the children would lose their sense of will to do well in school and to become successful and productive members of society.

Schools, churches, and new development. The parents noted the positive features of places that include schools, churches, and new housing developments in the city.

Schools are particularly important because they represent education. They described the positive impact that schools have on their community and their families. "This is in the middle of the neighborhood and this neighborhood doesn't really have anything else positive in it but the school. Education is important, the school gives the positive image of a positive outlook."

The parents described the quality that education in their community brings to their family, and how for them it is one of their only hopes for their children's future. They explained that as parents, they did not attend college, but education is the focus for their family and their children. "I'm for it 100% to keep my kids going to school everyday."

A positive thing about the community is the development of new playgrounds on school grounds. The addition of new playgrounds created a positive atmosphere in which community members and youth could feel more comfortable and healthy within their environment.

The church also was a dominant positive theme of the photographs. One parent described the church as a place of empowerment for her family and community. The parents noted that the church is a place of refuge for many community members and provides more than just spiritual services. "I see the church as a place for our children and youth to receive instructions and values that will help to change our community and our city in a positive way. This is a place for our children to get off the streets, away from drugs and other vices and to captivate their time not just on Sundays but through after school programs, day care, Head Start, and through other programs. The church helps you from the cradle to the grave."

Another parent described the ways in which the church helps to bring the community together, more than just on Sundays. "The church is the foundation and the backbone of many African American families. It helps individuals and families come together to worship, socialize, and establish relationships in order to help fellow man."

Finally, new housing development was a major theme among the positive photos that the parents took. The City of Detroit is currently going through a process of redevelopment that has converted old buildings into loft apartments and abandoned lots into gentrified housing. The parents saw these developments in a positive light, despite the fact that these homes are likely to be economically out of reach. Nonetheless, they represented a sense of hope, for their city and children. Even if they are never able to afford these places, new development represents a new future for a struggling city. It is something that they and their children could aspire to. It also represents safety, both physical and psychological.

The decision of the researchers to take not only negative pictures but also positive ones was intentional and had a helpful impact on the study as a whole. Many parents were empowered by this process stating: "taking pictures provided me with an experience of going out in the neighborhood I live and to see both the good and the bad, with hope of them improving this. It's a gradual process, but there's a lot of things that they could do that would be less detrimental or dangerous to residents."

Discussion

This study describes the process and findings of a Photovoice project conducted with parents of Head Start children in Detroit, Michigan to understand the impact of environmental hazards on children's well-being and to promote action around environmental justice advocacy. The parents identified both positive and negative themes related to their environment. Themes from the photos identified by the parents were primarily physical structures, such as houses, buildings, schools, and churches. This is not entirely unusual given the urban landscape in which these families live. In particular, the parents talked about how these structures impact the lives of their children: the "eyesores" of abandoned homes and buildings that pose safety concerns and make children question the hopefulness of their future, and the schools and churches that provide education and support for families. These findings are consistent to those obtained from researchers and activists in the environmental justice movement who posit that socioeconomically disadvantaged communities of color are disproportionately exposed to various forms of environmental hazards and risks and that these pose both physical and psychological risks for families (Boer et al. 1997; Mohai and Bryant 1992; Pulido 1996; Sadd et al. 1999).

Although the intent as well as a major goal of the Photovoice project was to engage parents in social action around environmental justice, the researchers were not entirely sure what to expect or how successful the project would be. The resulting action to date from the Photovoice process certainly met the expectation of the researchers. Although the group was small in size, its impact is far reaching and is sustained through its ongoing activities. The first of these action-oriented activities was a presentation of their photo display at a citywide Town Hall Meeting to address the closing of a large incinerator. The meeting was attended by community members, environmental justice advocates, media, city officials, and politicians. Several of the parents brought their children, which prompted a number of those giving testimony at the meeting on the impact of the incinerator on children and the future of Detroit.

Second, all the participants as well as other parents within the Head Start community were invited to attend an environmental justice training session. A professional in the environmental justice field, who was also a member of a prominent social services organization in the community, led this training. The training session included information on environmental hazards as well as ways to protect one's children from the negative effects of these hazards. The training session also introduced participants to the work of community advocacy groups and ways in which they could become involved to implement policy changes concerning environmental injustices in their community.

After the environmental justice training session, numerous parents from the project were anxious to begin an advocacy campaign of their own and formed the Environmental Justice Advocacy Committee (EJAC). This committee of about five to seven parents developed a mini-training session and script on environmental justice advocacy similar to the professional training session that they had gone through themselves. With minimal researcher assistance, the parents devised a 15 and 30 min script that they then presented to the entire Detroit Head Start Parent Policy Committee a few months later. The mini-training participants were provided with materials, such as the script and environmentally friendly goody bags (that had magnets on lead poisoning, seeds to plant ground cover, dust cloths for mold removal in homes, and various other items) to then take back to over 50 Head Start sites. The Policy Committee members then presented the script to their schools so that in the end over 400 parents were exposed to the EJAC's session.

Additionally, two parents from the EJAC also joined the City of Detroit's Healthy Homes/Healthy Start Program as representatives from their community. This program helps to decrease the effects of environmental hazards such as lead poisoning throughout the City of Detroit. Furthermore, the Head Start Parent Involvement Coordinator that collaborated with us on this project was asked to sit in on a meeting with the Governor of Michigan's Environmental Policy Board.

The project has presented its research at two national conferences to date. The first of the two presentations was the National Head Start Association Annual Training Conference, where researchers, Head Start staff, and parent representatives of the EJAC trained attendees in environmental justice issues presented the findings of the Photovoice project. The second presentation was the Administration for Children and Families (ACF) Head Start National Research Conference in Washington DC, where we presented our process and the resulting accomplishments.

In addition to the intended effects, the Photovoice project also yielded unanticipated results. For example, the parents clearly focused on physical structures not typically associated with environmental hazards. The researchers anticipated that parents would take pictures of more traditional icons of environmental injustice, such as incinerators, exhaust from cars, or peeling paint chips filled with lead. Rather, the community-based, participatory approach, which allows participants to identify the problem, directed the parents toward other structures that may impact children more directly. It also provides evidence for the importance of the physical environment in the lives of community residents and its priority in the hierarchy of social problems they encounter. While lead poisoning and air pollution may be serious problems, it is what you "see" that becomes important, but from there, other issues that arise from these problems can be addressed. It is from this place that social action can occur. Environmental hazards in disenfranchised communities have immediate implications for the health and well-being of urban youth and also suggest direction for action and further inquiry. The study also demonstrates how community-based participatory approaches can be used to help poor communities of color gain an understanding of the risks that their children are exposed to while constructing strategies for addressing environmental injustice through action – one cannot occur without the other. As Beverly Tatum (1994) stated, raising awareness without also raising awareness of the possibilities for change is a prescription for despair. It is unethical to do one without the other.

References

Anderton, D.L., A.B. Anderson, J.M. Oakes, and M.R. Fraser. 1994a. "Environmental equity: The demographics of dumping." *Demography*, 31: 229–248.

Anderton, D.L., A.B. Anderson, P.H. Rossi, J.M. Oakes, M.R. Fraser, E.W. Weber, and E.J. Calabrese. 1994b. "Hazardous waste facilities: 'Environmental equity' issues in metropolitan areas." *Evaluation Review*, 18(2): 123–140.

Bearer, C. 1995. "Environmental health hazards: How children are different from adults." *Critical Issues for Children and Youths*, 5(2): 11–26.

Been, V. 1994. "Locally undesirable land use in minority neighborhoods: Disproportionate sitting or market dynamics." *The Yale Law Journal*, 103(6): 1383–1422.

Been, V. 1995. "Analyzing evidence of environmental justice." *Journal of Land Use and Environmental Law*, 11: 1–37.

Been, V. and F. Gupta. 1997. "Coming to the nuisance or going to the barrios? A longitudinal analysis of environmental justice claims." *Ecology Law Review*, 24: 1–56.

Boer, J.T., M. Pastor, Jr., J.L. Sadd, and L.D. Snyder. 1997. "Is there environmental racism? The demographics of hazardous waste in Los Angeles County." *Social Science Quarterly*, 78: 793–810.

Brooks-Gunn, J. and G.J. Duncan. 1997. "The effects of poverty on children. The future of children." *Children and Poverty*, 7(2): 55–71.

Brown, L.D. 1991. "Bridging organizations and sustainable development." *Human Relations*, 44: 807–831.

Brown, L.D. and R. Tandon. 1993. *Multiparty collaboration for development in Asia*. New York, NY: United Nations Development Programme.

Burke, L.M. 1993. "Race and environmental equity: A geographic analysis in Los Angeles, CA." *Journal of Geographical Information Systems*, 3(9): 44–50.

Capaldi, D.M. and G.R. Patterson. 1994. "Interrelated influences of contextual factors on antisocial behavior in childhood and adolescence for males." pp: 165–198. In *Progress in experimental personality and psychopathology research*. Edited by D.C. Fowles, P. Sutker, and S.H. Goodman. New York, NY: Springer.

Carr, W. and S. Kemmis. 1986. *Becoming critical. Education, knowledge and action research*. Lewes: Falmer.

DiPerna, P. 1985. *Cluster mystery: Epidemic and the children of Woburn, Mass*. St. Louis, MO: Mosby.

Dryfoos, J.G. 1990. *Adolescents at risk: Prevalence and prevention*. New York: Oxford University Press.

Evans, G.W. and E. Kantrowitz. 2002. "Socioeconomic status and health: The potential risk of environmental risk exposure." *Annual Review of Public Health*, 23: 303–331.

Faber, D.R. and E.J. Krieg. 2002. "Unequal exposure to ecological hazards: Environmental injustices in the commonwealth of Massachusetts." *Environmental Health Perspectives*, 110(2): 277–289.

Gaventa, John. 1998. "Participatory research in North America." *Convergence*, 24(2–3): 19–28.

Gelobter, M. 1987. *The distribution of outdoor air pollution by income and race, 1970–1984*. Master's Thesis, Energy and Resource Group. Berkeley, CA: University of California.

Gelobter, M. 1992. "Toward a model of environmental discrimination." pp: 64–81. In *Race and the incidence of environmental hazards: A time for discourse*. Edited by B. Bryant and P. Mohai. Boulder, CO: Westview.

Goldman, B. 1994. *Not just prosperity: Achieving sustainability with environmental justice*. Commissioned for the National Wildlife Federation Corporate Conservation Council Synergy '94 Conference.

Graziano, K. 2004. "Oppression and resiliency in a post-apartheid South Africa: Unheard voices of black gay men and lesbians." *Cultural Diversity and Ethnic Minority Psychology*, 10(3): 302–316.

Hammen, C. and K.D. Rudolph. 1996. "Childhood depression." In *Treatment of childhood disorders*. Edited by E.J. Mash and R.A. Barkley. New York, NY: Guilford Press.

Hockman, E. and C. Morris. 1998. "Progress towards environmental justice: A five-year perspective of toxicity, race and poverty in Michigan, 1990–1995." *Journal of Environmental Planning and Management*, 41: 157–176.

Huston, A.C., V.C. McLoyd, and C. Garcia-Coll. 1994. "Children and poverty: Issues in contemporary research." *Child Development*, 65: 275–282.

Israel, B., A. Schultz, E. Parker, and A. Becker. 1998. "Review of community-based research: Assessing partnership approaches to improve public health." *Annual Review of Public Health*, 19: 173–202.

LeClerc, C., D. Wells, D. Craig, and J. Wilson. 2002. "Falling short of the mark. Tales of life after hospital discharge." *Clinical Nursing Research*, 11(3): 242–263.

Lopez, R. 2002. "Segregation and black/white differences in exposure to air toxics in 1990." *Environmental Health Perspectives*, 110(2): 289–297.

Lopez, E., E. Eng, R. Randall-David, and N. Robinson. 2005. "Quality-of-life concerns of African American breast cancer survivors within rural North Carolina: Blending the techniques of photovoice and grounded theory." *Qualitative Health Research*, 15(1): 99–115.

McAllister, C., P. Wilson, G.B. Patrick, and J. Baldwin. 2005. "Come and take a walk: Listening to early head start parents on school-readiness as a matter of child, family and community health." *American Journal of Public Health*, 95(4): 617–625.

McLoyd, V.C. 1998. "Socioeconomic disadvantage and child development." *American Psychologist*, 53(2): 185–204.

Mohai, P. and B. Bryant. 1992. "Environmental racism: Reviewing the evidence." pp: 163–246. In *Race and the incidence of environmental hazards: A time for discourse*. Edited by B. Bryant and P. Mohai. Boulder, CO: Westview.

Morris, C.M. and E.M. Hockman. 1997. *A multivariate analysis of the relationship among pollution, ethnicity, poverty, and public health in Michigan, 1990–1996*. ACSP 1997 Annual Conference. Fort Lauderdale, FL. November 6–9.

Pollitt, E. and K. Gorman. 1994. "Nutritional deficiencies as developmental risk factors." In *Threats to optimal development: Integrating biological, psychological, and social risk factors. The Minnesota Symposium on child psychology*. Volume 27. Edited by C.A. Nelson. Hillsdale, NJ: Lawrence Erlbaum Associates.

Pulido, L. 1996. *Environmental and economic justice: Two Chicano struggles in the southwest*. Tucson, AZ: University of Arizona Press.

Riley, R. and E. Manias. 2004. "The uses of photography in clinical nursing practice and research: A literature review." *Journal of Advanced Nursing*, 48(4): 397–405.

Sadd, J.L., M. Pastor, Jr., J.T. Boer, and L.D. Snyder. 1999. "Every breath you take… The demographics of toxic air releases in southern California." *Economic Development Quarterly*, 13(2): 107–123.

Strack, R.W., C. Magill, and K. McDonagh. 2003. "Engaging youth through photovoice." *Health Promotion Practice*, 5(1): 49–58.

Tatum, B. 1994. "Teaching white students about racism: The search for white allies and the restoration of hope." *Teachers College Record*, 95: 462–476.

United Church of Christ Commission for Racial Justice. 1987. *Toxic waste and race in the United States: A national report on the racial and socio-economic characteristics of communities with hazardous waste sites*. New York: Public Data Access, Inc.

U.S. Census. 2000. *Demographic profiles*. Washington, DC: U.S. Census Bureau.

Wang, C.C. 1999. "Photovoice: A participatory action research strategy applied to women's health." *Journal of Women's Health*, 8(2): 185–192.

Wang, C.C. and M. Burris. 1997. "Photovoice: Concept, methodology, and use for participatory needs assessment." *Health Education and Behavior*, 24(3): 369–387.

Wang, C., M. Burris, and Y.P. Xiang. 1996. "Chinese village women as visual anthro-pologists: A participatory approach to reaching policymakers." *Social Science and Medicine*, 42: 1391–1400.

Wang, C.C, K.Y. Wu, W.T. Zhan, and K. Carovano. 1998. "Photovoice as a participatory health promotion strategy." *Health Promotion International*, 13(1): 75–86.

Wang, C.C., J. Cash, and L.S. Powers. 2000. "Who knows the streets as well as the homeless?: Promoting personal and community action through photovoice." *Health Promotion Practice*, 1(1): 81–89.

Wang, C.C., S. Morrel-Samuels, P. Hutchison, L. Bell, and R.M. Pestronk. 2004. "Flint photovoice: Community-building among youth, adults, and policy makers." *American Journal of Public Health*, 94(6): 911–913.

Werner, E.E. and R.S. Smith. 1992. *Overcoming the odds: High risk children from birth to adulthood*. Ithaca, NY: Cornell University Press.

West, P.C., L. Fly, and R. Marans. 1992. "Minority anglers and toxic fish consumption: Evidence from a State Wide Survey of Michigan." In *race and the incidence of environmental hazards: A time for discourse*. Edited by B. Bryant and P. Mohai. Boulder, CO: Westview Press.

Part IV
Epilogue

Chapter 13
Attachment and Dislocation: African-American Journeys in the USA

Carol B. Stack

Introduction

I went to rural Mississippi in the summer of 1968 when I was pregnant with my son, Kevin. I took the Illinois Central south from Chicago to Holmes County on June 4th. A couple of hours after midnight on June 5th, the passengers were awakened by tears and people crying out. Bobby Kennedy had been assassinated. It was devastating. Those of us riding the train together stayed up the rest of the night. Friends and strangers slumped into one another's arms. I got off the train in Holmes County with some folks with whom I had shared the night.

I had traveled to Mississippi to help out in a head start program that was launched by the local parents and civil rights workers in the County. During that summer, I learned and eventually recorded many family stories about the Great Migration. My very first publication, "The Kindred of Viola Jackson" (Stack 1970) told a story of family migrations from rural Mississippi to St. Louis, Chicago, and Benton Harbor.

What astonishes me now, as I review my own writing from the perspective of the present, is that in *All Our Kin* (Stack 1974), I did not write anything, not one word, about that journey north, about the process of displacement, or the strong emotions that often accompany a mass exodus to urban places. The families in *All Our Kin* appear in the city in a neighborhood called The Flats, as if they were ancestors of the city, living in a timeless space, so to speak. In a sense, you might say, these urban families were "mis-placed" in my own writing.

Way back in 1974, I did place these families within the specific economic and policy context of the times. I documented the impact of social inequities – racism, low wages, unemployment, and AFDC – on their lives, but I totally ignored the larger picture – that is, what forces propelled their exodus to the North. I did not pay attention to the social or psychological impact of dislocation, to the knots that bind

C.B. Stack (✉)
Professor Emeritus, Graduate School of Education, University of California,
Berkeley & Visiting Professor, Duke University, 1818 Martin Luther King Blvd., Suite 116,
Chapel Hill, N.C. 27514
e-mail: stack@berkeley.edu

L.M. Burton et al. (eds.), *Communities, Neighborhoods, and Health*,
Social Disparities in Health and Health Care 1, DOI 10.1007/978-1-4419-7482-2_13,

urban kin to family ties back home, nor to the complexities of obligations to kin who remained in the South.

We were trained back then in anthropology to think of urban and rural as separate and distinct. I remember the famous anthropologist Max Gluckman who reminded young scholars that a tribesman is a tribesman, and an urban dweller is an urban dweller. At the time, rural and urban were seen as separate and distinct. We were also taught that "the urban" symbolized progress – and that people did not look back.

At several moments during the research for *All Our Kin*, I noticed that children were missing. Donald, who was 11, had disappeared, and Brenda, who was 12, was gone. I asked where the children were and people told me "they went back south," but no one made anything of it. I jotted a few words in my field notes that I set aside and disregarded. Conventional wisdom held that most migrants to northern cities would never go home. The Great Migration, I assumed, was a one-way trek (Stack 1970).

In the early 1970s, I missed clues before my eyes that foretold the subject of my new book, *Call to Home* (Stack 1996). Hundreds of thousands of children had participated in cyclical migrations between the North and South. They are the children of the Great Migration. Children and young adults dominate migration streams at all geographic scales – local, national, and international. People below the age of 24 make up the vast majority of migration streams to Third World cities. And, close to one third of all interregional movers in the USA are children below the age of 15 (Cromartie and Stack 1989).

In the research for *Call to Home*, I could not possibly overlook the children, 70,000 in the Carolinas alone, who had moved back and forth between families in the North and South. I dug up my old field notes from *All Our Kin* that had been packed away for years. The missing children were accounted for. Brenda had been sent to care for her younger sister and Donald to help an aging aunt and uncle.

Returning south for my research for *Call to Home*, I found that isolated, rural communities were teeming with children in very poor and working poor families. Already back home for the second or third time from schools in Harlem, in Brooklyn, in Philadelphia, and Washington, D.C., many of these children were awaiting the return of their own parents, grandparents, aunts and uncles, siblings and cousins. This is another omission that is difficult to admit. These oversights were embedded in my earlier work, *All Our Kin.*

In the course of doing ethnography on return migration, I learned about many community and personal dramas embedded in the return movement. For one, the Great Migration out of the South lasted a long time, longer than living memory, more than long enough to accumulate terrible strains on poor people whose large families were stretched thin across America. In reverse, the Great Return Migration within the USA has been evolving as individuals and families respond to the destruction of American urban lives. This return movement represents a dramatic reversal of a 50-year-long migration trend.

By 1990, the South had *regained* from the cities of the North the half-million black citizens it had lost to northward migration during the 1960s. The Census Bureau predicted that the southward trend would continue well into the next century, and it has. For 8 years, mostly in the 1980s, I talked to people who had left the South and then moved back home again: professionals, unemployed, land-owning folks who had lost their land, and Vietnam vets, to name a few. Most of those who returned had been young adults when they first left home, though many had spent summer and school years with families up north. As this generation came of age in the 1960s and 1970s, and graduated from high schools in the South, they went north in their parents' footsteps. They too found what jobs they could and started families and sent their own children home to Carolina to be raised (Stack 1996).

Per family tradition, these migrants moved far from home, but many did not really ever leave their parents: when they arrived in Newark or Philly, they often moved right down the block from their parents and cousins and uncles and nieces, if not into the same apartment. They played old roles in old family tales, but for this particular generation, the old stories would have surprising new endings. At each step, along the route that they thought they knew, these young people felt the ground spin out from under them in the cities. When the boys of this generation set out to go north and go to work, as their fathers before them had done, they found themselves drafted and shipped off to Vietnam. If they made it back to the USA, back to the city, they found themselves in a society in which the image of young black men had taken a sordid and malignant turn – and jobs were scarce. Black Vietnam veterans were no longer viewed, as their fathers had been, as potential ditchdiggers; they were reflexively regarded, with a shudder, as a probable heroin addict, Black Power troublemakers, or worthless, unemployable and unwelcome. Even if they made their peace with all that disparaging talk, even if they somehow found some kind of job and set about developing ordinary family routines, whenever they looked around them, they saw more squalor and sorry streets.

Their parents had found steady work up north, often in factories, or in civil service. The next generation came to realize that thousands of those jobs were flat-out gone, engineered or budget-cut out of existence, or packed off around the globe, or had moved close to southern cities, a hundred miles or more from their home places; the Sunbelt patina had not brightened the outlook for rural regions of the black South. The jobs these men and women could find up north were not steady, and the conditions were sometimes at the sweatshop level.

The North, the *Promised Land*, the land of freedom and opportunity, had become the Rust Belt. Industrial decline was the overwhelming fact of life in big cities across the Northeast and Midwest; ongoing decline was the heart and soul of the regional economic outlook. Even people fortunate enough to find more or less full-time work saw their wages fall far behind the cost of living. They may or may not have been active in the political turmoil that characterized their years of exile, the civil rights movement, or community-organizing efforts. They may or may not have been in the streets when demonstrations raged or cities burned. But, they got a political education; however, they came by it.

When they quit big cities and returned to rural home places in eastern North and South Carolina, many were still men and women in the prime of life – in their thirties and early forties. Folks told me that not a whole lot had changed in Carolina while they were away. But, they had changed. The people they had become found the move back home jolting, exhausting, and sometimes paralyzing. But, the process of readjustment was also exhilarating. As one person said "When you have to fight old demons to make a place for yourself in your own home, you learn a lot about who you are and who you want to be."

Many people in the place where I did my research returned to small, all-black, hamlets – rural home places like Boney's Bend, Chowan Springs, New Jericho, and Rosedale – in the Carolinas. They arrived with a sense of history and destiny that drove them homeward. And, back home again, they could not settle for what earlier generations had taken or left. They were men and women with a mission. Many who returned had some work experience, or business experience, or education, or organizing experience – in housing projects, or in Vietnam. Donald Hardy, who graduated from college and eventually became a city planner, said that he did not prepare mentally for his return, while Doris Coleman spoke of feeling profoundly different. Earl Henry Hydrick, who appears in a chapter of my book called "Soul Searching," owned a small business after he returned from Vietnam. Earl proposed a metaphor that seems to capture many of the complexities of return: "when you return to your homeplace", he told me, "you go back to your proving ground, the place where you had that first cry and gave that first punch you had to throw in order to survive."

In the prime of their lives, people might return to a proving ground to assess their progress, thinking to themselves: "If I can succeed away from home, I can do it here." Returning becomes "a test – a test and a half." People are indeed tested, in many different ways, when they move back home. They have to find a way to make a living, a way to relate to their families, and often a new way of entering the larger community. They have to change themselves, make compromises, take risks – and sometimes they also have to try to change the society around them. These challenges and transformations generate complexities in their lives. A return movement influences not only the course of individual lives but also the unfolding of entire communities.

Eula Grant told me one afternoon on her porch in Burdy's Bend, "You can definitely go home again. You can go back. But you don't start from where you left – to fit in, you have to create another place in that place you left behind." These men and women were not the first people to return to rural home places and talk about the terms on which it might be possible for exiles like them to come home again. They share with thousands upon thousands of other return migrants a certain restlessness about the way things are going back home, and an ongoing quest for self-respect and self-knowledge, for a working space and honest understanding in the community.

Part I: Methodological Challenges

Over the course of studying return migration, I found myself facing four methodological uncertainties: the *historian's question* and the *demographer's question,* which were inspired by two colleagues; the *superintendent's dilemma* and *Clydes's dilemma* which emerged out of my long-term ethnographic engagement. Tangling with these questions over several years of the study allowed me to render the complexities of the return movement and place ethnographic and demographic data side by side in the conversation across generations of these migrants' lives.

The Historian's Question

First let us turn to the joys and hazards of working across four generations. A colleague at Duke University, Sydney Nathans, a historian, and I talked endlessly about my study. He had followed the beginnings of my research for *Call to Home* and knew what I was doing then. But, one day he asked me a very simple question. *Who are you studying?* I was caught short. He knew that I was then traveling to northeast North Carolina, studying individuals and families who had left several northern cities and were returning to rural home places. What did his question mean? My colleague proceeded to put a simple timeline on a piece of paper suggesting I locate the returnees along the timeline to show how different generations of individuals and families passed through time, and how time moved through their lives.

The vast majority of southern-born African-American families born before the 1920s did not migrate north. However, as grandparents and great grandparents caring for children, they were active participants in the Great Migration. For convenience, I refer to them as the first generation in the Great Migration. World War I marked the beginning of a mass northbound movement among African Americans. The second generation, born between 1920 and 1940, joined the migration to northern cities but often sent their school-aged children home to reside with grandparents. There is considerable evidence of back-and-forth movement in this generation, and the seasonal shifts between factory and farm. Many members of this generation, now in their late forties to sixties, say that they plan to go home to retire. Members of third generation, born between 1940 and 1960, were primarily southern born but generally split their childhood between the North and the South. By age 20, many members of this generation had moved north to join their parents and other relatives. They were part of the exodus that peaked between 1940 and 1970.

This third generation currently makes up the majority of return migrants. Older than typical migrants, they are now returning to southern home places ahead of their own parents. They are joining households of grandparents, and quite often, they are joining their own children who were already sent home whom I refer to as the fourth generation. The fourth generation, born between 1960 and 1980, were often sent south at a young age to live with kin. Unlike their parents, more members of this generation are northern born. However, like their own parents, these school-aged children have lived in both the North and the South, and spent large parts of their childhood in the South. These young children – the fourth generation – have moved back and forth as dependents; then, as adolescents and teenagers, they were sent back home to care for younger children or older relatives – they were also sent away to escape inner city schools and ghetto life.

The Demographer's Question

By the mid-1970s, their parents – the third generation – began to follow their own children back home. There is something special about the third generation. It is the largest age group to return to rural home places in the Carolinas between the 1970s and 1990s. This generation has played a special role in the context of return migration, but they are missing or obscured in census materials. One of the first challenges that I faced when I turned to the US Census and PUMS data was how to make sense of who counts as a returnee. Geographer and colleague, John Cromartie, posed a question: why was I not interested in so-called new migrants to these southern counties. I knew on the basis of 5 years of ethnographic research that few outsiders moved into the rural, isolated, impoverished communities in the Carolinas: few newcomers had moved back to the eight counties where I did my study in northeast North Carolina. It is safe to say that return migration is at heart, a closed system. The people who are arriving are linked to local members of these communities by kinship, land, and memories.

People moving back to these rural home places made up 88% of the population gain between 1975 and 1980. This includes people born in the South, along with their children, and those acting on familial place ties, including spouses.[1] However, between 1975 and 1980, the US Census identified only 29% of the children under 18 moving to the eight county region of my study as returnees. The rest were classified as newcomers – that is nonreturn migrants. This was a surprise to me. When I began to look deeply at the life histories, I collected, of young people who returned, it was clear that many of the children had lived their lives in both the North and South. They spent their early childhood back south: 1st through 4th grade in the North, 5th and 6th grade in the South, 7th through 9th grade in the North, and by 10th, 11th, or 12th grade they were in the South again.

When these children were born in the North, the US Census and the PUMS data – the Census Bureau's Public Use Microdata Sample – classified them as newcomers. It became obvious that we needed a new method of identifying return and nonreturn migration that reflected the importance of intergenerational ties to destinations, intergeneration migration strategies, and the household context of migration. These young people – and their parents (some of whom were also born in the North) – did not start from scratch in selecting destinations. Children who were born in the North were sent home as soon as they could be of help to grandparents down south; they are also summoned north by their parents to care for newborn babies. A few years later they traveled south with those younger siblings and attended southern schools once again. Demographer John Cromartie and I looked at the PUMS data. The PUMS files provide a detailed portrait of the familial and household situations

[1]The assumption a "closed system" of migration (in which all migrants, both to and from the area, were linked to their original cohorts) is based upon Stack and Cromartie's comparison between county-based census data and ethnographic research among extended families in these same counties.

of individual migrants. The status of migrants in the data is determined by place of birth. Classifying children who were born in the North as newcomers obscures the momentum of the return migration movement and the character of intergenerational strategies. Together, we reinterpreted THE PUMS DATA in a publication in the following way: Any mover into the region who resides in a household that includes a native of the state (whether the native is a returnee or a stayer) is reclassified as a return or what we call a homeplace *mover*. This reclassification changed the demographic portrait of children under 18 in these rural counties. After reclassification, 75% instead of 29% were deemed homeplace movers[2] (Cromartie and Stack 1989). The children I came to know so well during my ethnographic study were no longer missing. The Census data did not reveal the magnitude of the return because family dynamics regarding childhood and migration were invisible.

The Superintendent's Dilemma

Social theorists, demographers, economists, anthropologists, and the media had been caught by surprise by this return movement. Let us turn to the communities themselves and take a look at local knowledge on the return movement. My field notes show that officials and school administrators at the local level in these rural communities had also been caught by surprise by the return. A White school Superintendent I spoke with asked me: "Where did all these kids come from?" He said, "We keep closing down our local schools because folks are moving north, but our classrooms are getting very crowded." Conventional wisdom held by administrators in these counties that people would never return obscured the facts, or the children, before this administrator's eyes.

In 1985, I spent several weeks speaking with school superintendents and teachers searching for records on the comings and goings of children in the school district. What I was looking for was in the realm of an anthropologists' dream. I asked if schools kept records on the migration of children and was assured that nothing existed, nothing, absolutely nothing. Returning one day to an overcrowded front office, I noticed Mr. Parks in his office through the open door and waved. "Come on in," he urged me, "I was just thinking about you. You might be interested in our "tuition drawers." These mysterious long file drawers were packed tightly with 3 × 5 cards kept since the late 1940s. Each card was a record of every "new" student who entered or reentered the school district, whose parents lived outside the county or state. Each card had the handwritten name of the new student as well as the name and location of the child's parents (usually in the northeast),

[2]Fifty-seven percent of in-migrants were returning to their home state, and an additional 31% were nonnative homeplace movers; together, they made up 88% of all in-migrants. Even this may be an underestimation, since many of the remaining 12% nonnative in-migrants who established their own household may also be acting on familial place ties.

the name and relationship of the local "responsible" relative, and the location of the last school the child attended. These records were used to collect tuition payments.

The tuition drawers opened up a wealth of labor-intensive records on household and migration patterns; the cards provided a picture of distinctive migration patterns between origin and destination for the county and refined the patterns found in detailed Census data in two ways. First, they provide vivid evidence of cyclical migration from the 1950s through the 1970s. One year, a child's name would appear in the tuition drawer, and then 2, 3, or 4 years later, the same name would reappear, showing the leaving and returning of each child moving between north and south, with the location of parents in the North. Second, the cards made it possible to track parents' movements from one urban destination to another. Parents might be living in New Jersey, for example for one school term, but 2 or 3 years later, when the child returns south, the entry may record her mother as now living in Philadelphia.

County by county, the cluster of destinations coalesced into a predictable pipeline, with each rural county effectively supplying migrants to a slightly different array of urban locations. The cards showed relatives from one rural southern county moving, for example, between the Philadelphia–New Jersey "connection," with kin residing in both places, others moved between Brooklyn and Harlem. Census data provides snapshot information on the last location before a move rather than the sequence of moves

By the late seventies, the tuition drawers grew slim as parents joined their children back home, or as children and parents returned south together. The tuition drawers quietly foretold the return migration. As the tuition drawers dwindled, the number of children in the rural school systems increased. Understanding this phenomenon was a challenge to the school district and to the superintendent I mentioned earlier.

Clyde's Dilemma

Responding to a family crisis may jeopardize all the dreams of a lifetime, and even mature and loving individuals may come forward only reluctantly. When timing is a problem, when substantial sacrifice is required, when a family is too poor to buy services that might mitigate the burden, and when no individual seems well suited to a particular task, family ingenuity as well as commitment can be tested. The families returning to Burdy's Bend, New Jericho, Chowan Springs, and Rosedale – along with the families receiving them there – were devising new patterns of assigning kin-work and writing new scripts for old family values. The men and women in New York and other cities who are keeping an eye on goings-on in places like Rosedale and Burdy's Bend often find that one particular turn of events back home stands out as painfully salient: the grandparents and other relatives who raised them are aging, ailing, and dying. No one is ready when parents or grandparents can no longer take care of themselves, even if preparations have been laid. Not everyone responds by quitting work and moving right back home. But, poverty limits choices, and cultural values fashion expectations. Returning to take care of an aging relative may seem like the only thing to do. Many people regard a call for such help as their most immediate call to home. Once they are resettled back home, people often decide to stay.

Clyde's "letter" is a research construct designed to elicit discussion of tensions between personal agendas and family pressures. The vast majority of people who spoke with me about Clyde's dilemma were able to recount their own personal experience caring for older family members. In some families, a summons to provide such care was directly linked to an individual's decision to move back home, and in other families, it was part of the background of expectations that molded a whole series of moves and decisions. In order to learn about the pushes and pulls that family members faced, I worked with people living in Burdy's Bend to construct the following dilemma regarding aging parents in bad health and in need of care back home. I then interviewed people who had returned using the locally constructed dilemma below. Here is Clyde's dilemma:

> Dear Abby,
>
> I am an unmarried man who lives in Washington, D.C. I work part-time as a security guard. My parents live back home in Rosedale, which is a small town out in the country, about 250 miles south of D.C. My mother has been bedridden for a couple of years, and my father has sugar and recently lost a leg, so he can't take care of her any more. My two sisters have both had a turn taking care of them. They live in New Jersey and hope to move back home eventually, but right now the older one has a good job and the younger one just got married. Both of my sisters think I am the one who should go back home and take care of my parents. What do you think I should do?
>
> Clyde

Below is one of many responses to this dilemma that make up my field notes and are included in *Call to Home*. Collectively, these responses fine-tuned my understanding of how people negotiated what they felt they owed themselves and what they owed others, and how the force and pull of family ties plucked at their heart and changed the course of their lives.

Clayton, age 42:

C: By me being a man, I got no business even bathing a daughter no more after 3 years old. And I don't think the mama would want her son bathing her.

I: Why do you think that?

C: Is she confined to a bed? That mean she has got to be bathed and everything. They are some sorry daughters if the son have to do it. And how those daughters going to feel if their mama don't live. In a family with three or more children, out of those offspring you usually have one who wants to come back and oversee the home and the finances. Since Clyde's the only male in the family, and his sisters decide to stay in D.C., Clyde is next in line in terms of manly responsibilities.

C: In my opinion, if Clyde really love his mama and she wants him to come home, I say, yeah, don't let her end up in a rest home somewhere. You know, a lot of people love a dollar, and they tend to love a dollar better than they love human beings. It's up to the individual.

I: What about if it were you?

C: If it were me instead of Clyde? Oh, lord. I guess I would come home and take care of her. Somebody has to do it. You wouldn't want to put them in a nursing home. I think families should take care of families. Getting old is no disgrace. It's a cycle. They had to feed us and wipe our butt. We just do the same for them. That's the way I feel about it.

For every rhetorical flourish on the theme of rugged individualism, there are ten celebrations of the long list of old-fashioned family virtues: respect for elders, sacrifice for others, long-term commitment, self-restraint, discipline for children, and so on. Family life is a resource, sometimes the only readily available resource, that poor people can turn to in times of trouble. Turning to your family is no small matter, however, for most of us we feel a certain shame and a fear of indebtedness. It is often a course of last resort, and even then, it does not always solve problems. For example, spreading scarce resources thinly throughout a large, poor family is no solution to the problem of poverty. It may help people get through tough times, but it does not lift them into economic security. And, while the most sentimental among us might argue otherwise, if the cupboard is just flat-out bare, there is no dosage of family values that will put bread on the table. Families can be battered into oblivion. But, it is so very hard to say no. And, responding to a call for help provides, all too often, the only lifeline available.

Part II: Writing Strategies and Storytelling

As ethnographers, we experience our fieldwork in many different ways and through the eyes and voices of many different actors and institutions in the communities we study. In *Call to Home*, I spent time with individuals and clusters of kin across generations: at work places, at schools, in day-care centers, and the like. Of the many voices in the text, I wish to bring attention to a special subset of voices that speak out and make arguments that theorize, and interpret, right before the ethnographer's ears and eyes. Strong voices shape the text in ethnographies. You might even say that some voices come to have more *say so* in books, as they attract the researcher's attention. Sometimes these strong voices emerge out of a cacophony that forms a new collage of voices. Let me explain.

In the beginning stages of my study of return migration, I had stimulating conversations with many people who were return migrants. As my research networks emerged, I noticed that I tended to interview clusters of people who led me to others in their network. Eventually this snowballed into multiple overlapping networks, but in the early stages of research, in small communities, there was always overlap. Within these small networks, the word got out that I was interested in those who came back from the northeast. This stirred lively conversations among the people I had met. In those conversations among people who had returned, they listened to one another and recreated their migration stories. That is, people began to make small changes in their stories: they remade their stories in response to one another. New stories with slightly different edges were constructed out of on-going conversations, debates, or situations. People appropriated material from one another. The stories began to sound the same. As I listened, day by day, I realized that I was following the orbit of self-rendering that was shaped and reshaped collectively by my presence and focus, and in spite of it.

People in these rural communities were having conversations about the meaning of their return and making and creating individual and family stories, and political interpretations of these rural communities. In my presence and with one another, they talked. My challenge as a researcher was to disentangle the bits of collage and remaking of stories from the particular, from one person's particular experience across large extended family networks. In this process, as researchers, we uncover many perspectives that are particularly illuminating, especially since individuals themselves argued with and against the newly assembled collective stories. I was lucky to be a part of these many forms of conversation with individual people and, of course, in groups. Over the course of several years, the people I met were changing, and local communities were indeed transformed by the people who had returned home. Conditions in northern cities changed, and sites of oppression became sites of resistance. Returnees learned that they were able to use the social capital they brought home if they took the time to relearn local culture and social structure. They learned to listen to local voices across generations, to have conversations, to try out their theories of social change on their friends and kin, to listen to people whose views rendered the complications of local life, and to hypothesize on politics and social change.

Moving among those who returned and narrated their own stories, many angles of vision emerged. People who returned were in the process of constructing their own narratives: they listened to many voices, some highly contradictory, creating their own ethnographic narrative and course of action. Their practices and mine coalesced. Such is the nature of collaboration.

References

Cromartie, John and Carol B. Stack. 1989. "Reinterpretation of Black Return and Nonreturn Migration to the South, 1975-1980." *Geographic Review*. 79(3): 297–310.

Stack, Carol. 1974. *All Our Kin: Strategies for Survival in a Black Community*. New York: Harper & Row.

Stack, Carol. 1970 "The Kindred of Viola Jackson: Residence and Family Organization of an Urban Black American Family," Pp. 303–312, in *Afro-American Anthropology: Contemporary Perspectives*, edited by N. E. Whitten and John F, Szwed. New York: The Free Press.

Stack, Carol. 1996. *Call to Home: African Americans Reclaim the Rural South*. New York: Basic Books.

Index

L.M. Burton et al. (eds.), *Communities, Neighborhoods, and Health*, Social Disparities in Health and Health Care 1, DOI 10.1007/978-1-4419-7482-2,

Lightning Source UK Ltd.
Milton Keynes UK
UKOW06n2156301015

261770UK00001B/40/P